William Stokes

Lectures on Fever

Delivered in the Theatre of the Meath Hospital and County of Dublin Infirmary

William Stokes

Lectures on Fever
Delivered in the Theatre of the Meath Hospital and County of Dublin Infirmary

ISBN/EAN: 9783743395817

Manufactured in Europe, USA, Canada, Australia, Japa

Cover: Foto ©Thomas Meinert / pixelio.de

Manufactured and distributed by brebook publishing software (www.brebook.com)

William Stokes

Lectures on Fever

DELIVERED IN THE THEATRE OF THE MEATH HOSPITAL
AND COUNTY OF DUBLIN INFIRMARY.

BY

WILLIAM STOKES, M.D., D.C.L. Oxon., F.R.S.,

REGIUS PROFESSOR OF PHYSIC IN THE UNIVERSITY OF DUBLIN,
PHYSICIAN TO THE QUEEN IN IRELAND.

EDITED BY

JOHN WILLIAM MOORE, M.D., F.K.Q.C.P.,

ASSISTANT PHYSICIAN TO THE CORK STREET FEVER HOSPITAL,
EX-SCHOLAR AND DIPLOMATE IN STATE MEDICINE
OF TRINITY COLLEGE, DUBLIN.

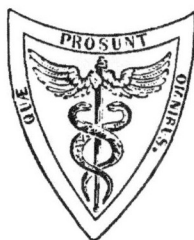

PHILADELPHIA:
HENRY C. LEA.
1876.

THE FOLLOWING PAGES

Are Dedicated to

HENRY WENTWORTH ACLAND, M.D., LL.D., F.R.S.,

REGIUS PROFESSOR OF MEDICINE IN THE UNIVERSITY OF OXFORD;

HONORARY PHYSICIAN TO H.R.H. THE PRINCE OF WALES.

WHOSE ENLIGHTENED EFFORTS TO SHOW THE RELATIONS OF CURATIVE AND

PREVENTIVE MEDICINE TO THE HIGHEST INTERESTS OF

MAN HAVE EARNED FOR HIM THE GRATITUDE

OF ALL HIS FELLOW-WORKERS.

PREFACE.

It seems fitting I should mention that the following Lectures, the delivery of which has been spread over a considerable period of time, were not given in any regular sequence, so as to form a continued or systematic course. On the contrary, most of them were delivered at irregular intervals, and all as extemporary discourses. In one remarkable instance, this has led to the repetition of a very peculiar case of internal abscess in convalescence from Fever with icterus. As stated in the text, I was at first inclined to regard the liver as the primary seat of the abscess; but at page 149 I have given reasons for concluding that the lesion was originally in the spleen. Several years intervened between the delivery of the first, and that of the second, lecture in which the case is mentioned.

The place in which I spoke should be remembered—namely, the theatre of a General Hospital, containing, indeed, separate fever wards, but also wards for the treatment of cases other than those of essential disease. And so, with the view of publication, it became necessary to employ a good deal of selection as to the subject-matter of each lecture. Some of them, so far back as the year 1854, were edited by my friend and former pupil Dr. Lyons, and appeared in the *Medical Times and Gazette* under the head of "Clinical Lectures on Fever."

Since that time, I need not say, the study and the teaching of Fever have been continued in the Meath Hospital, with at least one important result—namely, the valuable and original work of my trusted friend and late colleague Dr. Hudson, a work worthy to follow that of Dr. Graves for its learning, judgment, and practical worth.

It appeared to me that lectures addressed to successive classes of clinical students, and grounded on constantly renewed observations in the sick ward throughout many years, would have a value different in kind from, if not superior to, any exhaustive history of fever, especially as regards the various theories of the disease or the observations made by others.

I have ever believed that the great object of a clinical instructor is twofold—first, that he should teach rather by example than by precept; and, secondly, that he should act more as a fellow-student than as a master.   In this way the members of his class, associated with him in investigation, will learn as much or more by his example as they would by his precepts.   They will taste the pleasure of original work and the value of self-instruction, and perceive that their great object is less to be taught by another than, in following his steps, to learn to teach themselves.   This shows the superiority of clinical over systematic teaching in medicine.   The former admits of immediate demonstration; and, from the ever-varying combinations and characters of essential disease, no one lecture can, as it were, repeat another.

But while his discourses must vary from time to time, according as they may deal with the infinitely varied complications of local secondary disease, or in relation to the "epidemic character" of the essential or general malady, the duty of the teacher should ever be to imbue the minds of his hearers with the state of his own convictions on the subject in general.   Thus he will furnish them with a knowledge less of particulars or of theories than of those broad principles which in after-life will guide them in dealing with disease.

In the following Lectures I have considered in some measure the question of the separate identity of typhus and typhoid fevers, but I have not entered into it as fully as the labours of other observers in various countries might have encouraged me to do.   I have preferred to dwell on the great subject of the relation of the secondary affections of fever to the essential malady, and in the light of that relation to discuss the question of treatment.

No one can deny that a normal case of typhus will show striking differences from a normal example of typhoid; yet that these differences belong rather to species than to genera, and that the principles of treatment of the two affections are the same, must, as it appears to me, be admitted.   In fact, the study of the points of agreement between the two forms of Continued Fever under discussion will be more valuable than that of their differences.

They are both essential affections, in which the local anatomical changes are secondary to, or resulting from, the fever.

They are both subject, although in varying degrees and at different times, to the Law of Periodicity.

The characters of the constitutional and local symptoms in both vary as to intensity, amount, seat, combination, period of appearance and of cessation, and effect upon the primary disease.

In both, the local symptoms may be only functional, or more or less connected with anatomical change.

In both, local change may interfere with the law of periodicity, or even be attended by cessation of the constitutional symptoms. This has been observed more frequently in typhus than in typhoid.

In both, the action of the law of periodicity applies not only to the general condition, but also to the secondary affections.

In both, the local or secondary malady may take on a consequent condition of reactive irritation, thus adding a symptomatic to the primary fever.

The essential and local characters of both vary with the "epidemic constitution" of the time being.

The symptoms of local disturbance, which are reliable as a guide to diagnosis where essential disease does not exist, in a great measure lose their significance in the presence of both forms of Continued Fever.

In both, any or all of the functions may be disturbed singly, collectively, or successively, with or without corresponding anatomical change.

In both, deposits of tubercular matter may occur as a secondary local affection.

Similar exciting causes seem occasionally capable of giving rise to either form of fever.

In "relapse cases"—I do not mean cases of Relapsing Fever—the character of the second attack may differ widely from that of the first. Thus typhus may give place to typhoid, or *vice versâ.*

The petechial or the measly eruption of typhus may coexist with the rose-spots of typhoid.

Both forms are contagious, although in different degrees.

As I have said, the principles of treatment in both are the same.

These Lectures do not pretend to give even a sketch of all that is known or believed to be known respecting Fever. Nothing will be found in them relating to histological research, the chemico-vital states of the fluids or organs, or the analysis of the laws of crisis. The wide questions of the correlation or convertibility of essential disease are barely touched upon. Some of the facts connected with the change of type of disease, especially as regards the local affections of essential maladies, are mentioned. I have also spoken of the short-comings of the numerical system in medicine, of which Professor Trousseau, in the introduction to his immortal work,[1] writes as follows:—

"Si la statistique appliquée à la médecine n'élevait pas trop haut ses prétentions, si elle se considérait non comme la clef de voûte de toute science, mais comme un procédé un peu moins imparfait que la plupart de ceux que l'on suivait jusqu'ici,, je ne songerais qu'à la louer, qu'à la présenter à votre choix, parce que réellement je la crois utile ; mais elle fait tant de bruit pour de si pauvres résultats, qu'on ne peut, en conscience, l'aider à tromper la jeunesse par une sorte de charlatanisme d'exactitude et de vérité."

The difficulties attending the application of the numerical system are nowhere greater than in the study of essential fever, because of the ever-changing nature of the epidemic type of the disease and of its secondary local affections.

I cannot close this Preface without expressing my deep sense of obligation to my distinguished colleague Dr. Arthur Wynne Foot for a valuable record of temperatures in Fever, collected for the most part under his personal supervision in the wards of the Meath Hospital during the last three years.

[1] Clinique médicale de l'Hôtel-Dieu de Paris, deuxième édition, tome 1er, Introduction, p. xliv.

CONTENTS.

PART I.

ESSENTIAL FEVER AND ITS SECONDARY AFFECTIONS.

LECTURE I.

PAGE

INTRODUCTORY—Injurious influence on the student and practitioner of having studied surgical cases exclusively—Influence of timidity from want of intimacy with bed-side treatment of fever—Erroneous views in relation to the frequency of inflammatory disease—Inflammation not the primary cause of many local though acute affections—Errors of Broussais—Abuse of the antiphlogistic treatment. 1

LECTURE II.

CHANGE OF PRACTICE as regards the treatment of fever—Change of type in disease from sthenic to asthenic—Views of Alison—Sir Robert Christison—The author's views—Evidence (1) from symptoms, (2) from appearances of blood drawn by venesection, (3) from pathological appearances of internal viscera, and of serous membranes, (4) from isolated sthenic cases, and (5) from influence of treatment—Signs of a return to sthenic forms of disease—*Vital* character of disease   10

LECTURE III.

FEVER DESCRIBED, but not defined, as "a condition of existence without any known or necessary local anatomical change and subject to new laws, different from those of health"—Error committed by the school of Broussais—The "Law of Periodicity"—Danger to the fever patient due to the primary disease or to its secondary complications—Secondary affections of continued fevers more inconstant than those of the exanthemata—Classification of diseases: (1) Diseases having *an anatomical character;* (2) *neuroses,* having no known anatomical character; (3) *fevers,* subject to the law of periodicity, causing secondary affections, transmissible by contagion 20

LECTURE IV.

CONTAGION—Exclusive doctrines are to be deprecated—Endemic disease arises independently of contact—The numerical system of Louis fails in practical medicine—Evidence in favour of contagion from the *Doctrine of Chances*—Investigations of Dr. Whitley Stokes and the Bishop of Cloyne; with Dr. Paget's remarks thereon—Variation in the degree of contagiousness of acute essential diseases 27

LECTURE V.

CAUSES OF FEVER—Preventive and Curative Medicine contrasted—Risk of error in limiting the number of the causes of disease—The *correlation* and the *convertibility* of disease two important questions, the answers to which are not as yet fully or satisfactorily determined 34

APPENDIX A 40

LECTURE VI.

PAGE

VARIETIES OF FEVER as observed (1) in different epidemics, (2) in the same epidemic, and (3) in members of the same family, living under the same conditions —This last-named fact is corroborative of the doctrine of the essentialism of fever—Definition of the term *epidemic character* of fever—Outbreaks of 1818-19, 1826-27, and 1847 contrasted—*Typhus* and *typhoid* or *enteric* fever appear to be but species of the same genus— Contagiousness of typhoid fever—Dr. Flint's memoir—Principles of treatment of fever of any type must be based on an acquaintance with the *law of periodicity*, to which the disease is subject . . 42

LECTURE VII.

POINTS OF RESEMBLANCE in the various forms of fever a more practical subject for investigation than their distinctions—As regards the principles of prognosis, diagnosis, and management, the various forms of fever lose their separate and individual significance—Points of resemblance between typhus and typhoid— The famine fever in 1847—Recapitulation 49

LECTURE VIII.

DIVISION OF FEVERS INTO ESSENTIAL AND SYMPTOMATIC—No anatomical expression for the disease—Secondary affections of fever—These may, and do, frequently produce organic changes—The presence of essential disease invalidates the ordinary rules of diagnosis—Illustrations of the truth of this statement—Local symptoms of fever are (1) *functional* or *nervous*; (2) *anatomical*, i. e., depending on special anatomical changes: (3) *secondarily inflammatory*, i. e., arising from reactive inflammation, itself due to the typhous infiltration of some part or organ of the body—Similar symptoms may arise from essentially opposite conditions in disease—Illustrations of the proposition that *fever is capable of producing local symptoms without organic change* 55

LECTURE IX.

LOCAL CHANGES IN FEVER are symptomatic, subject to *law of periodicity*, and probably depend on the presence of a specific typhous deposit—This deposit possesses a *vital*, specific character—Illustrations of this statement—The principal pathological conditions in fever are (1) *functional*, (2) *intercurrent* and *secondary irritations* of (*a*) mucous membranes, (*b*) parenchymatous structures, (*c*) serous membranes, (3) *secondary irritations associated with typhous deposits*, (4) *independent typhous deposits*, (5) *reactive inflammations* due to these deposits, (6) *softening of organs*—Effect of *locality* in determining the seat of secondary affections of fever—Effect of *social rank* in the same direction—Prognosis unfavorable and treatment by stimulation so far contra-indicated in cases where nervous symptoms preponderate 64

LECTURE X.

SECONDARY BRONCHIAL AFFECTION OF FEVER—*Pneumo-typhus* of Rokitansky— Views of this author as to the *anatomical expression* of typhus and typhoid respectively—Description of the bronchial affection of fever; frequent absence of symptoms therein—Râles sonorous, mucous, or crepitating; no increased sonoriety—This affection is not ordinary "bronchitis"; it comes on silently and subsides spontaneously—Argument from the effects of treatment by stimulation—Modes of termination of the affection 72

LECTURE XI.

BRONCHIAL AFFECTION OF FEVER, *continued*—Alternating secondary affections—Imperfect convalescence due to reactive bronchitis—Cases resembling phthisis— Three forms of tubercular disease, as a sequela of fever, (1) *coexisting tubercle*, (2) *acute consequent tubercle*, (3) *consequent softened tubercle*—Diagnosis based on *the want of accordance between physical signs and symptoms* in suspected phthisis after fever—Expectoration of small calculi some months after bronchial typhus —*Tubercular fever* in the typhus epidemic of 1826-1827—This fever may be contagious 78

LECTURE XII.

PAGE

SECONDARY PNEUMONIC COMPLICATIONS OF FEVER—Secondary *congestion* or *consolidation* of lung—The term "typhoid pneumonia" is incorrect—"Acute asthenic pulmonary disease," or "typhoid pneumonia," appears under *seven* forms—" *Aborted* typhus" in connection with the occurrence of lung consolidation—Local disease may assume a *sthenic* type even in the presence of a general *asthenic* condition—Description of the secondary pulmonary affection of fever under its *three* principal forms—Differential diagnosis between this disease and *acute primary pneumonia*, based on both pathological and anatomical grounds 89

LECTURE XIII.

PNEUMONIC COMPLICATIONS OF FEVER, *continued*—"Typhoid pneumonia," so called, is not dependent on a coexistent gastritis—Correct view is that both pulmonary and intestinal lesions spring from the one parent condition, that of fever—Physical signs of ordinary pneumonia are often found, but in an irregular succession, in the secondary pneumonic affection—Sign of *tympanitic resonance* in latter, first described by Dr. Hudson—Probable causes of the production of this percussion sound—The author's views—Dr. Lyons' views—Three explanations of the production of the sign—Frequent absence of *crepitus redux* in resolution of secondary typhous disease—When inflammatory affections do occur in fever, they are reactive or tertiary in their nature—Typhous affection of the larynx—Rokitansky's "laryngo-typhus" 98

LECTURE XIV.

THE HEART IN FEVER—The state of the pulse, especially in typhus, not always a reliable guide—Weakening of the heart may coexist with a full, bounding pulse—*Slow* pulse in convalescence is consequent on a typhous weakening of the heart—*Rapid* pulse in convalescence is of unfavourable import, pointing to (1) *tuberculosis,* or (2) secondary *reactive inflammation of the mucous glands of the intestine,* or (3) *phlegmasia dolens*—In such cases the local malady assumes the prominence hitherto presented by the essential disease—Illustrative case of hepatic (?) abscess in convalescence from the yellow fever in 1826–1827—Intermittent fever at close of epidemic in 1827—Frequency of phlegmasia dolens—Bleeding in cold stage, after Dr. Mackintosh—Failure of quinine in cases of simulative ague, arising from (1) phlegmasia dolens, (2) urinary disease, and (3) the puerperal state 106

LECTURE XV.

THE HEART IN FEVER, *continued*—Louis' conclusions, based on *post-mortem* observations—Typhous softening of the heart *during life* first studied at the Meath Hospital in epidemic of 1837–39—As regards state of the heart, fever cases fall into *three* categories: those accompanied by (1) *no alteration in heart's action,* except of rate; (2) *weakness after a few days,* consequent on depressed vital power; (3) *cardiac excitement*—Neither a depressed nor an excited state of the heart in fever necessarily implies organic change—*Dynamic* condition of the heart a more important indication for treatment than presence or absence of any structural change—True carditis very rare in fever—Typhous weakening predominates in left side of the heart—State of involuntary muscular fibre in acute essential disease is of great importance—Laennec's theory as to typhous softening of heart erroneous, for there is no correspondence between the softening of voluntary and involuntary muscular structures—Illustrations from yellow fever of 1826–27—Exemption of heart from typhous affection is a ground for a favourable prognosis—Continued excitement of heart equally a ground for a bad prognosis—Excited heart with compressible pulse most unfavourable—Transfusion of blood under these circumstances—Absence of red blood after death, the only noteworthy pathological appearance in this case—Blood-waste in fever to be met by administration of nourishment . . 114

LECTURE XVI.

PAGE

THE HEART IN FEVER, *continued*—Depression of the heart, more marked in typhus than in typhoid—Signs of the change connected with (*A*) the impulse, (*B*) the sounds—The phenomena attending depression are variable—Description of their development, generally from the *fourth* day.
A. IMPULSE:—Possible sources of error in diagnosis: (1) constitutionally feeble impulse, (2) emphysema of lungs—Necessity for comparison of condition of heart from day to day—Peculiar modification of impulse in certain cases—Vermicular action—Effect of *position* on impulse of heart—Loss of impulse generally progressive, sometimes rapid—" Where differential diagnosis is difficult or impossible it is often unnecessary as a guide to immediate practice"—Retrocession of the local malady is gradual.
B. SOUNDS :—*First phase of lesion:* second sound becomes relatively, but not positively, augmented. *Second phase;* disappearance of first sound. *Third phase:* disappearance of both sounds (a condition of most unhopeful augury)—Fœtal character of the sounds in some cases—Speculations as to failure of *second* sound—Loss of impulse and failure of sounds generally advance *pari passu*, but not invariably so—As failure of sounds begins at the left side, so in recovery the phenomena follow the inverse course 121

LECTURE XVII.

THE HEART IN FEVER, *continued—Post-mortem* appearances in extreme typhous softening—This affection not followed by chronic disease of the heart—Periods of invasion and of retrocession—Diagnosis of actual softening depends on (1) the character of the fever, and (2) the presistence of physical signs of failure of the heart—Simultaneous lessening of both sounds (fœtal heart)—Its bearing on the treatment by stimulants—SLOWNESS of pulse in convalescence from typhous softening—Analogy to fatty degeneration of heart with slow pulse—In latter case the phenomenon, however, is constant—Occasional reversal of the order in which the signs of typhous softening show themselves—*Prognosis* more favourable with depressed than with excited heart—Former condition is more amenable to treatment—Report on an epidemic of typhus at Stockholm in 1841, by Professor Huss—CARDIAC MURMURS in fever, especially in advanced stages of typhoid and relapsing fever are generally *basic* and *systolic* functional in character, and occasionally accompanied by venous murmurs in the neck—Difficulty of distinguishing the first and second sounds of the heart in certain cases of disease: (1) *chronic bronchitis*, with weak and irregular heart and congested liver: (2) late stages of some forms of fever—Example of the latter—*Diagnosis drawn from a want of accordance in the symptoms* . . . 117

LECTURE XVIII.

SECONDARY INTESTINAL COMPLICATIONS OF FEVER—General and introductory remarks—A generic resemblance between the various forms of fever—Secondary abdominal complications are more frequently observed in typhoid fever, but do not exist as its necessary anatomical character—Dothinenteritis was largely prevalent in the typhus epidemic of 1826-28—Fever must be observed independently in each epidemic and in every country—Typhoid fever almost without characteristics symptoms—Illustrative case ; extensive intestinal ulcerations found after death—Vital symptoms of intestinal complication: (1) thirst, (2) swelling of belly, (3) diarrhœa, (4) ileo-cæcal tenderness, (5) increased action of abdominal aorta, (6) rigidity of adbominal muscles—Three forms of abdominal swelling: (1) early and moderate tympany, (2) doughy condition, (3) slight ascites—Increased action of abdominal aorta—Case of, in perforation of the stomach—Analogous local arterial excitement in (1) whitlow, (2) rheumatism—Diagnosis from aneurism—Intestinal complications seem to interfere largely with action of the law of periodicity—Early elevation of local irritation checks deposit, and so prevents future mischief—Hence relief of symptoms by early depletion as practised by Broussais, who misinterpreted the matter, and was led to look upon the general fever as but symptomatic of a local lesion 135

LECTURE XIX.

PAGE

INTESTINAL COMPLICATIONS OF FEVER, *continued*—They resemble all the other secondary affections of fever in their general characteristics and relations to the primary essential malady—More frequent in typhoid, but occurring in typhus also, as, for example, in the epidemic of 1826–27—Pathological appearances observed in the intestinal tract in fever—Yet these appearances were not necessarily found after death even where severe abdominal symptoms existed in life —Eruption of rose spots in fever 142

LECTURE XX.

INTESTINAL COMPLICATIONS OF FEVER, *continued*—Division into *three* categories, with reference to the vital symptoms: I. These symptoms are absent, although the *silent* disease may be great in amount; II. Local symptoms are evident; III. Symptoms and pathological changes are both well marked—Further description of the epidemic of 1826–27—Sudden access of intense abdominal pain, followed by icterus and gangrene—Fatality of this complication—Splenic(?) abscess occurring in the first case of recovery, and discharging through the lung—Resemblance of this form of fever to the yellow fever of the tropics—Dr. Lawrence's observations—Dr. Graves' observations 146

LECTURE XXI.

INTESTINAL COMPLICATIONS OF FEVER, *continued*—Organic changes—Perforation of intestine—Of common occurrence in 1826–29: (1) Generally rapidly followed by symptoms of peritonitis; (2) but may be unattended by local symptoms in progressive cases, or again may induce only limited peritonitis (adhesions); (3) Symptoms of perforation may be veiled by the coexistence of intense irritation in another cavity of the body—Illustrative case—Time of occurrence of perforation as observed in *six* cases—Diagnosis of internal solutions of continuity is based on sudden development, without apparent exciting cause, of new, local, violent, and often rapidly fatal symptoms—Cases to which this rule of diagnosis is applicable—In effusion into a serous sac the degree of resulting inflammation is determined chiefly by the quality of the effused fluid—Examples—Influence of an irruption of pus in producing serous inflammation contrasted with that of an irruption of blood—Physiological difference between pus corpuscle and white-blood cell—The formation of conservative adhesions seems to be rarer in peritonitis than in pleuritis—Case of hepatic abscess in which adhesious occurred and recovery followed (diagnosis from abdominal aneurism) . 151

LECTURE XXII.

SECONDARY NERVOUS OR CEREBRO-SPINAL COMPLICATIONS OF FEVER—When they predominate, prognosis is unfavourable—Of all secondary typhous affections they are least connected with organic change—Probable reason; mucous membranes and skin undergo anatomical change more readily than serous membranes—Cerebral inflammation rarely observed in fever—Purpuric fever of 1867 an exception—Absence of organic change in typhous cerebral derangement does not lessen its importance as regards prognosis and treatment—Inadmissibility of routine treatment, either antiphlogistic or by stimulation, in fever—Results obtained by Louis as to relation between head symptoms and pathological change in fever—Actual cerebritis, when it does occur in fever, is a *tertiary* phenomenon—Dr. Hudson's cases—Study of analogies is of importance in essential diseases; thus relief of headache in early stage of smallpox by leeching is analogous to good results of moderate depletion in early stages of some cases of fever—Further examples of the effect of lessening vascular supply in controlling development of smallpox eruption—Analogy in case of secondary affections of fever—Nervous symptoms arise from *three* conditions: (1) influence of fever-poison, (2) uræmia, (3) specific secondary inflammation, probably erysipelatous in character 159

LECTURE XXIII.

PAGE

NERVOUS COMPLICATIONS OF FEVER, *continued*—*Cerebro-spinal fever*—Phenomena of fever inconstant and variable, except, perhaps, the phenomenon of increased temperature—*Type* of fever also varies in different epidemics—Two examples: (1) *yellow fever* of 1826-27, (2) *malignant purpuric*, or *cerebro-spinal fever* of 1867—Dr. E. W. Collins' report on latter—There exists a "constitutional element" in the disease, so that the cerebro-spinal arachnitis can hardly be held to be a primary, idiopathic affection—Evidences of essentiality from presence of other phenomena in connection with the skin, etc.—Reports to the *Medical Society of the King and Queen's College of Physicians in Ireland* on the epidemic of 1867—Inconstancy and variability of the symptoms in the outbreak—Dr. H. Kennedy's views—Symptoms of the disease—Petechiæ—Early setting in of putrefaction—*Retraction of head*; sometimes persistent after disappearance of other local and general symptoms, and sometimes persistent after death—Recapitulation: Points to be considered in connection with epidemic of 1867: (1) yellow fever of 1826-27, (2) cerebro-spinal arachnitis of 1846 (Dr. Mayne), (3) coincidence of cases of malignant measles in 1867, and (4) hemorrhagic and purpuric smallpox in epidemic of 1871-72 165

LECTURE XXIV.

NERVOUS COMPLICATIONS OF FEVER, *continued*—*Hysteria*—Occurrence of hysteria, especially at an early stage, of unfavourable import—View that hysteria is always symptomatic of uterine excitement is quite erroneous—Nymphomania only a local and accidental manifestation—Hysteria is observed in males as well as in females in fever—Case of erotic symptoms in typhoid fever occurring in a young girl, reported by Dr. A. W. Foot—In early stage of fever hysteria generally is the precursor of severe nervous symptoms—Its appearance may lead to serious complications later in the disease—Illustrative cases—Hysterical symptoms are sometimes connected with actual or organic disease, *especially in acute affections*—Dr. Cheyne's observation: *Hysteria a ground for a good prognosis in every disease, fever alone excepted*—Outbreak of hysteria, affecting the abdomen, in female fever ward of Meath Hospital—Anomalous symptoms in advanced stages of fever often due to hysterical state—Case of typhous hysteria in the male followed by cerebritis 173

PART II.

TREATMENT OF FEVER.

LECTURE XXV.

INTRODUCTORY REMARKS—Principles on which the treatment of fever is to be based—True meaning of the word *empiric*. Historical retrospect—The Symptomological, the Anatomical, the Rational or Eclectic Schools—*Essence* of fever cannot be determined by pathological anatomy—*Etiology* of fever is indefinite . . 177

LECTURE XXVI.

No specific line of treatment—Respect to be had (1) to the essential disease, (2) to its local and secondary effects—Failure of specifics in early stage of fevers—Want of success in the endeavour to found a science of therapeutics on experimental physiology or pathology—Effects of the action of the law of periodicity wrongly attributed to the adoption of therapeutical measures—Sustenance by *food* and *stimulants*—Two sources of danger to the fever patient: (1) primary effects of the fever poison in causing depression, (2) supervention of secondary local disease—Views of Dr. Graves on the subject of giving food in fever . 185

LECTURE XXVII.

PAGE

STIMULANTS IN FEVER—Views as to the nutrient properties of stimulants are to be received with caution—*Anticipative* use of stimulants—Meaning of the term—Considerations to be taken into account in resolving upon this method of treatment: (1) prevailing epidemic character of the disease, (2) previous condition of the patient—"Sinking of vital power"—Illustrative case—Stimulation often unsuccessful in the intemperate, and in those whose brains are over-worked, (3) development of symptoms of severe typhus, (4) development of *fever odour*—Contrast between typhus and typhoid as regards period at which stimulation is called for—*Condition of the heart, a guide*—Physical signs of cardiac weakening 193

LECTURE XXVIII.

STIMULANTS IN FEVER, *continued*—Signs in connection with the heart of the agreement of stimulants: (1) return of impulse, (2) return of first sound, (3) gradual fall in the rate of the pulse—In cases of "fœtal heart" great boldness in stimulation is needed—No certain rules as to quantity of wine and whiskey or brandy required—Examples of free use of stimulants in malignant typhus—Case of Hardcastle (typhoid fever)—Eruption of vesicles as a secondary complication—Bed-sores 201

LECTURE XXIX.

STIMULANTS IN FEVER, *continued*—Case of Hardcastle, continued—Treatment by food and stimulants in extreme cases—Presence of cerebral symptoms to a great extent unfavourable to the exhibition of stimulants—Necessity for daily observation to the effects of the treatment in each case—Signs of disagreement of stimulants—*Routine* practice is in every instance to be deprecated—Fallacies of the numerical system in therapeutics—History of *routinism*—Its results—Description of routinism in the treatment of fever 212

LECTURE XXX.

TREATMENT OF THE LOCAL SECONDARY AFFECTIONS IN FEVER—Relative importance of these affections as regards *prognosis*—BRONCHIAL AFFECTION—Necessity for administration of stimulants and nourishment—Danger of exhibition of tartar emetic—Failure of emetics—Turpentine-punch—Dry-cupping, poulticing, blistering—*Internal remedies:* bark, ammonia, spirit of chloroform, turpentine—ACUTE CONSOLIDATION OF THE LUNG—Its *three forms*—Treatment of the first form by dry-cupping, blisters, quinine, turpentine, and wine—Of the second form by local depletion simultaneously with the administration of wine—Of the third form, *externally* by iodine and blisters, *internally* by tonics and iodide of potassium 222

LECTURE XXXI.

TREATMENT OF INTESTINAL SECONDARY AFFECTIONS—Two chief indications: (1) alleviation of symptoms, (2) modification of typhous deposition—Poulticing—Local depletion in early stage—Analogy in variolous eruption—Danger of alterative or purgative treatment at the outset of Continued Fever—Necessity for caution—*Constipation—Diarrhœa*—Poultices, demulcents, sedative astringents, injections of flax-seed tea—*Tympany*—Turpentine injection—*Diet* in diarrhœa—*Perforative peritonitis*—Opium our sheet-anchor—Danger of the antiphlogistic method—Dr. Murchison on the treatment of this accident—Bran poultices and warm fomentations—*Hemorrhage* from the intestine in fever—Not to be interfered with unless continued and excessive—Treatment by astringents, opium—Illustrative case 227

LECTURE XXXII.

PAGE

TREATMENT OF THE NERVOUS SECONDARY SYMPTOMS OF FEVER—HEADACHE—Cold
lotions, warm fomentations, moderate leeching, shaving the head, cold affusion,
ice—DELIRIUM—Treatment depends on (1) period of case, (2) presence of hyper-
æmin of the brain, or otherwise—Ice, leeches, shaving the head, cold affusion
in *active* delirium—Nourishment and wine in *passive* or anæmic delirium—
SLEEPLESSNESS—Moderate leeching, cold affusion, ice—Turpentine in constipation and tympany—Catheterism in distended bladder—Sedatives—Opium,
tartar emetic and opium, hyoscyamus, bromide of potassium, chloral, wine—
CONVULSIONS—Most formidable in fever—Uræmic, due to (1) *retention* of urine:
catheterism; (2) *suppression* of urine: dry cupping and poulticing over kidneys,
diluents, diuretics, aperient enemata, promotion of action of the skin   .   . 287

LECTURE XXXIII.

PHLEGMASIA ALBA DOLENS—The swelling is not always painful, or white in appearance—Symmetry of the affected limb not lost—Professor Trousseau's views as
to the etiology of the affection—Phlegmasia (1) of puerperal women, (2) in
scrofulous and (3) cancerous cachexiæ—Pulmonary *embolism* caused by phlegmasia—Case of phlegmasia after typhus fever—TREATMENT of the affection—
GENERAL CONCLUSION   .   .   .   .- . 245

     APPENDIX B   253

INDEX 257

LECTURES ON FEVER.

PART I.

ESSENTIAL FEVER AND ITS SECONDARY AFFECTIONS.

LECTURE I.

INTRODUCTORY—Injurious influence on the student and practitioner of having studied surgical cases exclusively—Influence of timidity from want of intimacy with bedside treatment of fever—Erroneous views in relation to the frequency of inflammatory disease—Inflammation not the primary cause of many local though acute affections—Errors of Broussais—Abuse of the antiphlogistic treatment.

SEVERAL of the hospitals in Dublin, considered as schools for clinical study, have the advantage of being essentially medico-chirurgical hospitals—that is to say, that in them the student, in connection with his surgical pursuits, may see and study most forms of the so-called medical diseases, which include not only the acute and chronic local diseases, but the various forms of essential affections, including continued fevers.

I am anxious to draw the attention of the surgical student to the all-important subject of fever; for when we consider the enormous extent to which this fell disease, or group of diseases, prevails over the world, and also that it is in itself a special study, we cannot help believing that the student who has not dealt with fever, no matter how ably he may have been educated in surgery and in the history of visceral diseases, has but half learned his business.

The importance of a practical knowledge of fever, as distinguished from that obtained from books or lectures, is not yet sufficiently impressed on the surgical student. If such a one possesses a reflecting mind, he will have abundant and bitter causes of regret at having neglected his hospital opportunities, whereby alone he can obtain that intimacy with the subject which will be his guide and safeguard in after-life. It is in the fever-wards alone that he can learn the priceless lesson that there is a large class of diseases, whose nature and property it is to get well of themselves, which require little or no

1

medication or daily interference. This lesson is not to be learned from purely surgical studies, one effect of which leads in medicine to the *nimia diligentia*, so common a fault in practice, so clear a sign that the medical mind has not been formed. He will see that what the patient requires is in many cases only time, and to be kept from sinking by proper support. He will come to learn how this great fact of the spontaneous cessation of disease bears on all therapeutical research in fever by showing him that he is not to confound the *post hoc* with the *propter hoc*. He will learn that there are few questions more difficult of determination than the effect of any special remedy, or even general mode of treatment in diseases which are under the law of periodicity; and thus he will be taught caution in drawing conclusions as to his own practice, while he will be charitable in reflecting upon that of others. Take for example the case of rheumatic fevers. How long have physicians been seeking for a specific treatment? Venesection, blistering, mercury, opium, bark, alkalies, acids, have all had their advocates, whose statements are supported by genuine cases, and yet the question remains unsolved; would not the disease have subsided of itself as well, and as quickly, as under any specific treatment? And in case of recovery, may not this even have occurred *notwithstanding* the treatment?

I heard with great pleasure the report by my distinguished friend Dr. Sibson, read at the meeting of the British Association at Newcastle-upon-Tyne, in which a long series of cases of rheumatic fever was detailed as having been successfully treated without any medicine beyond small doses of peppermint water—given, I presume, to satisfy the minds of the patients that something was being done for them beyond keeping them warm in bed till the disease subsided.

It is not to be understood that Dr. Sibson does not recognize the frequency of local inflammation in rheumatic fever, and the necessity of meeting it in many cases. But his researches are directed to show the comparative uselessness of a specific treatment.

I well remember the time when surgeons, who had been otherwise well educated, but had never in their student days seen or attended a case of typhus fever, objected to deal with such a case, and were of course, from apprehension of contagion, more or less ineffective when brought to perform any operation such as catheterism, and so on.

All students who are looking to the public service, whether in the civil, military, or naval department, should be taught by those who assume their direction or instruction that they cannot tell when they may have to deal with fever even on a great scale, and that, as the principle of treatment of all fevers is the same, the study of the disease at home will fit them to meet the yellow fever, the bilious remittent, the camp fever, the plague of the Levant, and the cholera of India.[1]

How few of our surgical students are aware of the fact shown by Sir Gilbert Blane that in the Peninsular War more men died of fever than from all other causes, including the sword.

But, further, the student who confines himself to merely a surgical ward often enters on his profession unfitted by timidity to meet his foe. I have known several instances where surgeons in civil practice, though willing to do their duty, were always nervous on entering a fever ward. I do not say that such men were cowards in the ordinary sense of the word, or that the feeling of danger would make them shrink from discharging their duty; but there is a condition which may be described as physical fear, distinct from moral fear; a condition of susceptibility to contagion, which is doubtless lessened by intimacy with disease. I know of a gentleman who was called to inspect the body of the first victim of cholera in the earliest and great epidemic of 1832. The case occurred some miles from Dublin. During his return he had many of the symptoms which threaten an attack of cholera. He had the abdominal pains, the feeling of imminent death—"the cold meditation of death" of the old authors—cramps, and other symptoms. For two days these recurred. The epidemic shortly afterwards burst out with violence in the city, when, feeling that if this condition persisted he would be unable to do his duty, he entered a crowded temporary cholera hospital, where he remained for thirty-six hours in close attendance on the sick. During the first eighteen hours seven patients died, it may be said, in his arms. I need not say that all the yielding of the system he had shown rapidly disappeared. I know of another case, where a gentleman, now an eminent member of the profession, was cured of repeated attacks of cholerine by undertaking the office of house surgeon to a large cholera hospital, where, under the direction of the late Dr. Mackintosh, he had to conduct the treatment by venous injection in many cases. To mention a third instance, the case of Mr. West and his party is quoted by my father, Dr. Whitley Stokes, in his pamphlet on Contagion.[2] During the expedition to Egypt under Sir Ralph Abercrombie Mr. West was ordered to take charge of a pest hospital at Rosetta in the beginning of May, 1801. In this house he was shut up for four months. His staff consisted of an assistant surgeon, an Italian; an English soldier; and of Arab servants. "No one of the party took

---

[1] See Swan's Edition of Sydenham, page 75.
[2] Observations on Contagion, 2d edit.. Dublin, 1818.

the disease, although Mr. West operated and dressed the buboes himself, and treated sores from anthraces so extensive that half a pound of flesh sometimes came off by sloughing; and although the servants washed the sheets, bedding, and bandages, rubbed the patients with mercurial ointment extensively, supported the faint, tied the delirious, and buried the dead. In short, they were exposed as fully as possible to contagion. At this time the plague was so severe at a village twenty-five miles from Rosetta that one-fourth part of a population of 400 died within a month. I have said that none of the party took the disease. Great attention was paid to cleanliness, and the house was a roomy building, situated on an elevated bank over the Nile and exposed to the northwest sea breeze.

On this singular result Dr. Stokes remarks, "Mr. West's deep interest in the discharge of his duty and in the improvement of his profession must have contributed to turn his mind from the selfish melancholy contemplation of his personal risk, a risk which one of our best officers fairly compared to that of a hundred battles. Such has been the triumph of good sense, temperance, firmness, and industry; and Mr. West has earned a civic crown which some men will venture to compare with the laurels of the greatest conquerors."

The surgical student who has not studied fever in the living subject, and himself felt the responsibility of its management, is in this position: the doctrine of the universality—or of the extraordinary frequency, whichever you will—of inflammation has been impressed on his mind in every possible way, for the ordinary practice at the commencement of a course of surgery used to be to occupy the student for many weeks with the history of inflammation. Inflammation is thus placed in the foremost rank. It is the great thing to which his earliest attention is directed, and naturally it appears to him to be the key to all medical and surgical knowledge. It is still more impressed upon him by the kind of experience he gets during a considerable part of his studies. That experience is obtained in a surgical ward, and it is hence very natural that he should have exaggerated notions of the importance and frequency of one morbid process. Too often at the end of his course he finds that he has been taught only inflammation, he has seen little else than inflammation, and he *believes* in little else than inflammation. A great many students are educated in this way, and they go forth to the world ignorant of two facts in practical medicine and surgery, the importance of which cannot be overrated. The first is the existence of an enormous number of acute and dangerous diseases which are not inflammatory—of diseases, as I said before, which are acute, which are dangerous, and still further, which are febrile. The idea has never been impressed on their minds that there may be a local, acute, febrile, and most dangerous disease which is not only, to use the words of a recent author, not inflammation, but something the very opposite of inflammation. When we consider that it is in the various forms of fever that these conditions are met with, and when we recollect the extent to which fever prevails over the world, we are justified in declaring that when we compare diseases in which inflammation is the primary condition with those in which it is not, the former fall immeasurably short of the latter in number and importance.

The other great fact is that the student has not learned the error of exclusive antiphlogistic treatment in the management of ordinary primary inflammation. From not having had to deal with local diseases, which require not the lancet, not starvation, but rather tonics and wine, he has never become accustomed to, or familiar with, the latter remedies. He is timid in the use of these measures, and even in the ordinary primary diseases he follows too long the common rule of antiphlogistic treatment instead of changing in time to one of a tonic and stimulating nature. The erroneous application of the antiphlogistic method arose subsequent to a change of doctrine from humoralism to solidism.

In order to get a clearer notion of this matter, let us go a little back. Before pathological anatomy became a science it was held that a large number of diseases depended on the alterations of the fluids. But when anatomy was directed to the investigation of disease medical opinion underwent a change, and solidism succeeded to humoralism. Disease was then an alteration of the solids, the living tissues of the body. Now, I wish to impress upon you that solidism, as was then understood, soon came to mean more than its original name would imply; and solidism *plus* the doctrine of inflammation became the ruling dogma of the day.

For the same mode of investigation, which established the frequency and variety of alterations of the solids, showed that in many cases there was a common character recognized as the result of inflammation. This paved the way for the introduction of the so-called physiological doctrine, which referred all diseases to alterations of vitality in the solids—not generally as affecting the whole system, but local—not differing from one another by any special characters, but in degree only. A disease was, then, either a *plus* or a *minus* vitality in the affected organ, and its symptoms were explained by the sympathies of that organ. But as so many diseases were attended with vascularity, deposition, and increased sensibility, it was inferred

that most local affections, and the more important diseases, were examples of augmented vitality in the part, producing not only the
local symptoms but those also which arose from the sympathetic
irritation.   This doctrine spread rapidly, and there were many reasons why it should do so.   It was specious, simple, and had for its
founder a man of extraordinary energy and eloquence.   In this world
any doctrine which is novel and has an energetic and eloquent apostle
will not want for converts, and Broussais was a man of great talent,
experience, and practical knowledge.   He was, however, deficient in
reasoning power, and, in my opinion, an imperfect pathological anato-
mist.   The doctrine became popular on the Continent from the facility
which it promised in the treatment of disease, for as the great majority
of diseases was symptomatic of the *plus* vitality of some organ, we
had only to discover the part in which this excess of life was seated,
and to modify it, of course, by antiphlogistic treatment.

When the investigations of Broussais and his followers were directed to the examination of fever cases, it was found, on the Continent
more especially, that local disease frequently existed in the gastro-
intestinal tube.   At once, then, the doctrine followed, that fever
formed no exception to the rule—that it was symptomatic of a *plus*
vitality of the gastro-intestinal tube; and we were led to believe that
fever could be at once cured by leeching, by starvation, by poultices
to the belly, and by such means.

It is curious that there are some circumstances connected with fever
which greatly tended to prop up this doctrine.   We shall see by-and-
by, that an essential condition of fever is periodicity; that it is a
disease which has a tendency to spontaneous termination at a given
time.   It is like a paroxysm of ague, only prolonged as it were.   This
will give the best idea of fever.   This mysterious law of periodicity
implies that the system has the power of curing itself—that is to say,
that the diseased action will spontaneously subside either suddenly or
gradually.   Now, it is found that there are a variety of circumstances
which interfere with the operation of this extraordinary law of spontaneous cure.   One of these is the existence of a local irritation in
any part of the system.

We see this remarkably exemplified in cases of ague.   We shall
very often find that in cases of intermitting fever the treatment by
bark will not succeed; and when we come to inquire the cause of this,
we find that there is some local inflammation present.   If we can
remove that local inflammation, then the treatment by bark succeeds.
Broussais appealed strongly to the following fact: that in cases of
fever, after free depletion of the abdomen, the patients speedily re-

covered. So they did ; but the nature of the fact was misinterpreted. Those patients had a local secondary disease in the intestine, which interfered with, or prevented, the operation of the law of periodicity. When that local disease was modified or removed, the law of periodicity came again into action, and the patient recovered. The fever did not subside because it was symptomatic of a disease of the intestine; but it subsided because, the disease of the intestine being removed or modified, it was reduced to its normal state, as it were to its state of simplicity, and then the law of periodicity was enabled to act.

The doctrine of the purely symptomatic nature of fever was received extensively on the Continent, in America, and in England and Ireland, but not so extensively in the schools of the two latter countries. There was a much greater reluctance to the reception of the physiological doctrine in this country and in England than on the Continent, or in America, and this is highly creditable to the British and Irish medical mind. Many reasons might be adduced to explain why this was so, but we shall not enter at length into them. I may, however, observe that English medicine had received a great degree of excellence from the writings of the old masters in England—from the writings of Sydenham, Haygarth, Fothergill, and other men of that order. These great medical observers had, unknowingly, taught the true medical philosophy. They had taught a rational eclecticism, and hence they implanted in the minds of the British medical investigators great reserve and extreme caution in the reception of new doctrines.

Still, however, upon the younger members of the profession the doctrine had a wonderful influence. A large number of the junior members of the medical and surgical profession in this country, during the last quarter of a century, or perhaps the last half century, were strongly imbued with this doctrine, and went forth to practise over the world, influenced by the theory of inflammation being the sole cause of diseases, and believing that the whole practice of medicine was reduced to the removal of local inflammation.

Another cause, however, I cannot help noticing here. About this time, owing to the unhappy and calamitous division of the profession into medicine and surgery, arose those corporate distinctions that have done so much to retard the progress of science in these countries; exclusive schools of surgery sprang up, and consequently, as I observed at the commencement, a large and increasing number of young men were educated without having ever seen a case of fever. They were educated in surgery ; they were educated in a surgical ward, and were sent forth naturally advocates of inflammation, because they had

seen nothing else; and thus, ill prepared, they went forth to combat
fever—that disease which numbers more victims than any other—
over the wide dominions of the British crown, in America, in the
West Indies, in Asia, in Africa. These men in hundreds—I may
say thousands—went out ignorant of the fearful enemy they had to
encounter, and trusting in the teachings which compared the ordinary
phenomena of ophthalmia, or those of the healing of an incised wound,
or those of the cicatrization of an ulcer, with the symptoms of that
terrible group of diseases which embraces the plague, the yellow fever,
the bilious remittent, the malignant ague, and the typhus fever.

There is nothing more difficult, gentlemen, than for a man who
has been educated in a particular doctrine to free himself from it,
even though he has found it to be wrong. There is something in
a human mind which renders the reception of a doctrine, if it be a
bad one, a most dangerous circumstance. It is like the imbibition
of a particular poison or miasma. We find that some men who have
been once exposed to the miasmata which induce intermitting fever
will, for nearly the whole course of their lives, be incapable of getting
rid of that influence which has been once received. And thus it is
not only with physical but with moral or intellectual impressions.

I have said that it is difficult to unlearn. This fastening of false
doctrine in the mind is one cause; but there are other causes too.
The indolence of many men prevents them taking the trouble to
unlearn. The pride of many men has the same effect; and, above all
things, there is this, that a very large number of students, not only
of surgery, but of medicine, although they were taught the technicali-
ties of the profession—the alphabet of their profession, as it were—
were not taught what is infinitely more important, namely, how to
teach themselves. Now, this ought to be the grand object of every
teacher of medicine, and, indeed, of any science of observation. I
believe that no man can be fully and entirely taught anything. He
must teach himself. And what the teacher has to do, and what I have
ever set before myself as my highest duty, is to endeavour to teach
you how to teach yourselves.

We can easily anticipate what the result of all this must have been;
and I believe I am not saying too much when I declare that a large
proportion of the fearful mortality to which our gallant army has been
subjected in the colonial service has been owing to the circumstances
to which I now draw your attention—the fact of the medical officers
going out with erroneous doctrine fastened in their minds.

This name of inflammation is an unfortunate one, and it is to be
regretted that it was given to the process in question. It gives the

idea of a fire which must be quenched by its opposite, water; of a heat which must be quenched by its opposite, cold; of vascularity—fulness of the bloodvessels—which must be met by measures which will empty those vessels. It gives the idea of a fever, an excitement which is only to be met by abstinence, by starvation, or, as the French term it, *diète absolue*, which means no diet at all. The fact is, gentlemen, that the formula of *contraria contrariis* has as little title to respect in legitimate medicine as that of *similia similibus* in quackery. Both are false; and I really believe that any exclusive application of either formula is both ignorant and mischievous in the highest degree.

The next great error was, that although the surgical student had plenty of opportunities of seeing symptomatic fever, he had no opportunity of seeing the essential fever, and he naturally confounded the two together. And hence, in this country and abroad, for many years the abuse of the antiphlogistic treatment was carried to an extent which it is frightful to contemplate. Conditions of the system which required wine, bark, stimulants, careful nutrition, were met by the lancet, by leeches, and by starvation. I remember when I was a student of the old Meath Hospital, there was hardly a morning that some twenty or thirty sufferers from acute local disease were not phlebotomized. The floor was running with blood; it was dangerous to cross the prescribing hall for fear of slipping; and these scenes continued to be witnessed for many years. The cerebral symptoms of typhus fever were met by opening the temporal artery, or by a large application of leeches to the head; and it sometimes happened that the patient died while the leeches were upon his temple—died surely, and almost suddenly. An eminent apothecary in this city assured me that when he was serving his apprenticeship there was hardly a week that he was not summoned to take off a large number of leeches from the dead body. I mention these circumstances to show to what extent, even in our own country, the abuse of this doctrine had been carried. It is not so now. Those who have been in the habit of attending fever hospitals in this country will bear me out when I say that the lancet is an instrument now very seldom indeed employed in our wards. But while all this is true, it must be understood that I am far from going the length of some modern physicians in their wholesale condemnation of the antiphlogistic treatment in various forms in the management even of essential fever. To this subject I purpose to return in my next lecture.

LECTURE II.

CHANGE OF PRACTICE as regards the treatment of fever—Change of type in disease from sthenic to asthenic—Views of Alison—Sir Robert Christison—The author's views —Evidence (1) from symptoms, (2) from appearances of blood drawn by venesection, (3) from pathological appearances of internal viscera, and of serous membranes, (4) from isolated sthenic cases, and (5) from influence of treatment—Signs of a return to sthenic forms of disease—*Vital* character of disease.

BASED on the doctrine that local inflammation or irritation was the exciting cause of febrile disease, we observe the wide-spread adoption of an antiphlogistic treatment in fever. The doctrine of essentiality of disease was ridiculed. Venesection in fever was common, and its traditional employment was supported by modern theory; the use of wine and other stimulants was forbidden, and many a life was sacrificed to this unphilosophical method of looking at disease.

But for nearly half a century we observe a change in practice in the opposite direction. General blood-letting is rarely practised; local bleeding in a very modified way ; while stimulants have been, by one school, clearly employed in an unjustifiable manner.

So complete was the change in practice, that venesection, from being a routine treatment, the performance of which was entrusted to junior students, became the rarest of surgical operations. Within the last twenty years I have known several surgeons who had never performed or even witnessed the operation. I remember having to instruct a hospital surgeon of remarkable ability in the operation. For a period of nearly twenty years the use of the lancet was unknown in our wards, and in latter times, when venesection was occasionally practised here, it was instructive as well as amusing to see how the class crowded round to witness for the first time a proceeding so unusual.

We can hardly conceive a revolution in practice more complete. In place of the loss of blood we have the exhibition of stimulants. In place of a system of almost starvation we have the careful use of nutriment.

This change in practice, depending on change in the vital character of disease, was followed by the charge against many of our predecessors and teachers that they were mistaken practitioners, ignorant of true pathology, and little better than blind followers of traditional error. Not only have their powers of observation been questioned, but even their morality and honour have been assailed; and it has been suggested that the whole doctrine of change of type in disease was an invention to cloak former errors.

It is interesting to note that this is not the first time that charges of a similar kind have been brought against the profession. Thus Broussais arraigned the existing and former practitioners for not treating fevers and acute diseases by local bleeding and starvation. Can there be stronger evidence than this that our modern practice is not a novelty? All his predecessors were in error, because they practised as we do now. I say that this charge was remakable, inasmuch as the author's views largely influenced European practice for many years.

But the thinking man finds it hard to believe that the fathers of British medicine were always in error, or that they were bad observers and mistaken practitioners. They, indeed, have rested from their labours, but their works remain; and he who reads the writings of Sydenham, of Haygarth and of Fothergill, of Heberden and Fordyce, of Gregory, Cullen, Alison, Cheyne, or Graves, must have a very inapprehensive mind, if he fail to discover that there were giants in those days, and that the advocacy of such ideas only indicates a state of mind not consonant with the modesty of science.

The declaration that it has been or can be proved by a more advanced pathology that bleeding never was the proper remedy for fevers and inflammations has as yet no scientific ground. It is not yet given to us, notwithstanding all our advance in normal and in morbid anatomy, in the physiology of health or of disease, to be able to say, from the most minute examination of the dead organ or structure, what were *all* the conditions which attended it during life, under the influence of disease; what were its local vital phenomena; what was the accompanying constitutional state, whether sthenic or asthenic.

But, let us ask, which is the more probable of these two suppositions? First, that our predecessors were bad observers, incapable of divining the truth, and blind adopters of an antiquated and mischievous method—or, secondly, that the type of disease has changed, and that almost in our own time. It fortunately happens that we can examine a living witness of great authority in this matter, and can refer to the works of two more who have left us their written testimony. Sir Robert Christison is still among us, in health and intellectual vigour—long may he be so—Dr. Alison and Dr. Graves have been but lately removed.

Now, all these testify that the character of disease has changed from a sthenic to an asthenic type; that is to say, from a condition in which inflammatory action was the prominent feature to another where that state was absent, or, if present, only ephemeral—a condition observable in essential and local diseases, in which the antiphlogistic treatment agreed well, and was productive of great relief, to one in which a tonic, stimulant, and supporting *régime* was found the best method of guiding the system to a happy termination of the disease.

It is very important to note that these views were not formed from any historical study of the recorded labours of others, but come before us as the actual observations of the great men whose names I have stated. They tell us that which they know—that which they themselves have seen. If we refuse this collective though separate and independent evidence—if we hold, with Professor Bennett and with Dr. Markham, that the doctrine of change of type is untenable—we must believe one of two things : either that these distinguished men were deceived or were themselves deceivers. From this alternative there is no escape.

Let us hear Dr. Alison : " When we reflect on these facts, we cannot think it unlikely that the result of the inquiry which I have stated as so important may be to show either that all causes capable of exciting diseased action in the animal economy, or, more probably, that the liability to diseased actions in the different departments of the animal economy itself, are subject to variations, which are made known to us only by the variation of such phenomena themselves; occurring merely in the natural course of *time*—an element affecting all vital phenomena quite differently from its agency on inanimate nature ; and the effects of which, on living beings, we must take as ultimate facts, to be carefully observed, arranged, and classified, but which we are not to expect to be resolved into any others, which the study of this department of the works of Providence presents."

When I read these words of Alison, the best man I ever knew, it is with a feeling of wonder how it has happened that men should forget what reverence is due to his memory, whether we look on him personally as a man of science and a teacher ; or at his life as an exemplar of that of a soldier of Christ.

Sir Robert Christison[1] shows that the change of treatment in acute diseases is to be considered with reference to fever as well as to local affections. He bears witness that the abandonment of bleeding in idiopathic fevers preceded by a good many years its abandonment in acute inflammation ; and that this change in practice took place gradually in all acute inflammations, not alone in pneumonia, because of the improved diagnosis of the disease, but in all others, in many of which

---

[1] Memoir on the Changes which have taken place in the Constitution of Fevers and Acute Inflammation in Edinburgh during the last Forty-six Years. 1856.

no sensible progress in diagnosis had been made. Looking at the fever epidemics of Edinburgh from the beginning of the present century, he shows conclusively that in 1817–20, and in 1826–29, their characters were those of Cullen's synocha and synochus—inflammatory, relapsing, critical.

Speaking of the epidemics of 1817–20, he dwells on the hard, incompressible pulse, the ardent heat of the skin, the florid hue of the venous blood and the impetus with which it escaped almost *per saltum* from the vein, the vivid glow of the surface, and the distracting pain and pulsation of the heart and chest.

Similar phenomena occurred in the epidemic of 1826–29, and in both bleeding was largely practised with the happiest effects; so that in the former epidemic the mortality, which was at first one in twenty-two, fell to one in thirty—a result which disposes of the charge of malpraxis against the profession.

But in 1834 Sir Robert found that probably for two years previously a change had been going on; synocha had disappeared; synochus had lost the vehement reaction of its early stages; typical typhus was much more common; and what did not come up to Cullen's mark of fully formed typhus was what physicians would now commonly call mild typhus, with more of introductory reaction than we observe at present, but with less than in the two epidemics of 1817–20 and 1826–29.

"In epidemic fevers," says this distinguished physician, "a change may take place in the constitutional part of the fever; and this change has been exemplified in Edinburgh during the last forty years, by a transition from the sthenic or phlogistic character in the first twelve years to the asthenic or adynamic character in the twelve years which have just elapsed."

And he adds these most remarkable words:—

"If this change be admitted to have been proved, there is an end to all difficulty in accounting for the abandonment of blood-letting in the treatment of our fevers. In point of fact, I am able to state very positively that the abandonment of bleeding in fever was suggested by the observation of a change in the constitution of fever, and in the effects of the remedy on it, and not by any other circumstance, whether extraneous or intrinsic. It is impossible to ascribe such change of practice, as Dr. Bennett has done in the instance of pneumonia, to an improved knowledge of disease. We have improved our knowledge of fever so far as to have been for some time well acquainted with the form of enteric typhus (dothinenteritis), which was unknown, or not recognized, at the commencement of our epidemics. But this is a rare form of fever in Edinburgh, scarcely belonging to its epidemics at all. And as to our only undoubted epidemic fevers, typhus and synocha with their intermediates, we cannot be truthfully said to be the better acquainted with them in 1857 than we were in 1830.

"I have given, I hope, a sounder explanation, less flattering perhaps to the rising generation of physicians, but surely more honourable to physic itself, more creditable to medical observation and experience, more consonant with the advanced state of medical philosophy. My own convictions on the subject are so strong that I regard nothing as more likely than that in the course of time some now present will see the day when a reflux in the constitution of fever will present it again in its sthenic dress, and again make the lancet its remedy. And in that event it is not impossible that, while we are now charged with giving up blood-letting, because it was discovered to have never been the proper method of cure, we shall hereafter be assailed by some new enthusiast in blood-letting, who, in imitation of Dr. Welsh, and regardless of the fate of his doctrines, will accuse us, with equal justice, of having our late fevers asthenic and typhous by blindly withholding their fittest remedy."

Since the delivery of my address on "Change of Type in Disease" before the British Medical Association at Leamington, in the year 1865, I have received numerous letters on the subject from many leading physicians in England and Ireland. The testimony of these gentlemen has been of the strongest character in favour of the occurrence of an asthenic type of local inflammatory disease within the last forty years.

That the type of both local and essential disease varies within certain limits of time we must believe. That a more asthenic form of disease has for nearly half a century prevailed in these countries is, I hold, an incontrovertible truth, and a time may come when those whose experience is of a later date will speak of the practice of their predecessors with greater modesty and more reverence.

I may now add the results of my own experience in this matter. I remember the period when the change of type took place in Ireland, and am under the impression that it was observed earlier in this country than in Scotland, or at least in England. The great epidemic of fever in 1827 was a remarkable one from its compound nature, and seemed to be made up of synocha, synochus, and enteric typhus. But nothing was more remarkable than the vehemence of the inflammatory reaction in many cases; and it is a curious fact that this was sometimes seen at its highest pitch in the relapses, when it was often far more violent and dangerous than in the first attack. Local bleed-ing was largely employed. In many cases venesection or arteriotomy had excellent results ; so that, although there were abundance of cases with prostration, and others marked by the typhoid condition, the old sthenic character had not disappeared. The amount of wine used at that time in hospitals was quite insignificant as compared with its consumption in more recent times.

Between 1822 and 1828 the sthenic character of essential and local disease existed, and the lancet was freely used—often, as I believe and have elsewhere stated, with too great freedom. But I well remember observing the frequent occurrence of the phenomena mentioned by Sir Robert Christison—the vehement action of the heart, the incom-pressibility of the pulse, the vivid redness of the venous blood, and the force with which it spouted, almost *per saltum*, from the orifice in the vein. I have myself taken as much as sixty ounces in a case of active cerebral congestion, with hemiplegia, before any impression was made on the arterial excitement ; in this case complete success followed. In rheumatic fever, too, we found the use of the lancet in the early stage of the disease to be productive of great relief. Vene-section was seldom employed more than once, but its effect was to shorten the duration of the disease, to lower the fever, to lessen the liability to the so-called metastases, and to render the whole case much more amenable to treatment.

But I have not bled in rheumatic fever for the last thirty years, for the whole character of the disease has changed. We have not had for many years the bounding pulse, the exaggerated heat and sweating, or the same liability to acute inflammations of the internal parts. The action of the heart is often feeble, and the tonic and supporting plan seems called for from an early period. Another point worthy of remark is, that cardiac and aortic murmurs of the anæmic kind have for many years been much more frequently observed, both during the attack and in the convalescence, and these demand the use of iron for their removal.

In judging of this question the evidence of those who have been intimate with acute diseases in this country during the period of 1820 to 1830 or 1835 must be attended to on this point. As already stated, I have received a vast number of communications from experienced and practical men, who had no theory to support, all telling the same tale, all testifying to the fact that a change in the vital character of acute disease was observed. This was particularly seen in rheumatic fever, which gradually lost its quality of high reaction, as shown by the great heat of the skin, the bounding and resisting pulse, the vigour of the heart's action; the frequency and severity of metastasis, not only as regards external but internal structures whose functions were violently disturbed. Cases, too, of visceral inflammation, independent of rheumatic complication, and marked by high reaction, pain, and great functional disturbance, were common. This was well seen in the cases of pleuropneumonia, in pericarditis, and in peritonitis, in all of which violence of symptoms, high reaction, and great pain and rapidity of morbid processes were the rule. Now, since the asthenic character of acute disease has set in, all this has changed. The violent acute and commonly suppurative pneumonia is rarely met with. We frequently meet cases of pericarditis in which, but for the physical signs, the disease could not be recognized, or its being overlooked would be excusable—you have seen many cases with little or no oppressive distress or throbbing of the heart. And as to acute peritonitis, formerly so well known, there has rarely been seen in any of our wards a case of it that did not result from the perforation of the intestine in enteric fevers.

It is needless to add examples; let us rather turn to another kind of evidence. Hitherto the change of type has been recognized and determined less by anatomical observation than by the observation of symptoms, and still more by the application of therapeutical tests. Remedial measures of a certain kind were found to fail and to be hurtful, where they were formerly safe and successful; and, conversely, the use of a supporting system of tonics, and the free employment of stimulants, were found necessary and safe where formerly they did mischief.

That morbid anatomy adds its testimony to the truth of the doctrine of the change of type in disease will, I believe, appear from considerations based on observed facts. Thus, after or about the time when an asthenic tendency was first noticed in Ireland, a change was detected in the condition of the blood drawn by venesection. The buffed and cupped character became very rare, and I well remember expressing my surprise at the absence of the fibrinous coat in cases in which we had fully expected its presence. In place of the small, dense, almost spherical crassamentum, we had a soft clot, with little if any separation of serum; while, instead of the buffy coat with inverted edges, we had a thin sizy pellicle. This circumstance was one of those which led us to be more and more cautious in the use of the lancet.

Again, the specimens of acute disease have had for many years a character very different from that commonly met with in Dublin between 1820 and 1830. As a general rule, these specimens all showed appearances indicative of a less degree of pathological energy. In pneumonia, for example, the redness, firmness, compactness, and defined boundary of the solidified lung was seldom seen; and that state of dryness and vivid scarlet injection, to which I ventured to give the name of the first stage of pneumonia, became very rare.   In place of these sthenic characters, we have had a condition more approaching to splenization—the affected parts purple, not bright red; friable, not firm; moist, not dry; and the whole looking more like the result of diffuse than of energetic and concentrated inflammation.

Let us now turn to the serous membranes, and the same story is repeated.   The high arterial injection, the dryness of the surface, the free production, close adhesion, and firm structure of the false membranes in acute affections of the arachnoid, pericardium, pleura, and peritoneum, which had been so familiar, ceased in a great measure to make their appearance.   The exudations began to assume a more or less hemorrhagic phase, serous or sero-fibrinous effusions tinged with colouring matter replacing the old results of sthenic inflammations. The effused lymph lay like a pasty covering, rather than a close and firm investment as before; it was thin, ill-defined, and transparent in varying degree.   All this tallied exactly with the change in the vital character of the disease.

It has happened to me—and I mention this in evidence that we were not mistaken with reference to cases of the sthenic character—that a few instances of disease in its old phase of high inflammatory reaction have appeared in isolated examples and at irregular intervals of time, so that we at once recognized their nature, and employed with success the old treatment in all its vigour—employed the lancet, though for many years it had been laid aside.   This is important as showing that there are influences, their nature as yet unknown, which affect the vital character of local disease in an inconstant manner.

During the last few years we have not been without signs of a return to the old sthenic forms of disease.   Even fifteen years ago a typical case of the old form of acute pleuropneumonia occurred in this city in the practice of the late Dr. Croker.   The symptoms were those of the highest inflammatory reaction, attended by violent excitement of the heart.   There was great pain and dyspnœa, a bounding pulse, a burning skin, and the rusty and tenacious sputa which for many years had not been seen in our hospital wards.   This patient was treated by free venesection, copious leeching, and the exhibition of tartarated antimony; and though the lung had passed largely into consolidation, the patient made a complete and rapid recovery.   Cases of a similar kind have reappeared in our wards during the last three

2

years, and the use of the lancet, which for a quarter of a century was
unknown with us, has been on several occasions resumed, and in all
such cases with the very best results. The relief has been always
immediate, the resolution of the disease, as shown by physical examination, generally rapid, and the convalescence, with one exception,
most satisfactory   In three out of four cases the treatment consisted
in one bleeding, which sometimes was followed by the application of
six or eight leeches to the seat of pain. No further treatment beyond
the use of the simplest palliatives was employed.

Must we not, then, agree with Sir Robert Christison that the disuse
of venesection, so remarkable in these countries during a period of
about forty years, is wrongly appealed to as evidence of our advance
in the healing art? We are not to hold that the former practice of
venesection was improper or unscientific; and while we admit that,
under the influence of old custom and the anatomical theory of disease,
blood-letting was abused in many cases, we must be careful not to drift
into the opposite error of neglecting this remedy where it is called for,
nor be guilty of the folly of holding that the physicians of the past
two or three generations were bad observers and harmful practitioners.
That they were men of truth is obvious to every one who understands
disease, and who takes at its proper value the opinion of those who show
such overweening confidence in the present so-called pathological
medicine—so much based upon mere structural and chemical changes
—and such neglect of some important medico-ethical considerations,
as, for example, the modesty of science and the practice of a reve-
rential spirit towards those whose works prove that they were great
and truthful men.

The change of type is to be seen in the character of the symptoms
and, as I have endeavoured to show, in the condition of the pathological changes. But it is to be recognized chiefly by the therapeutical test, by the behaviour of disease, whether general or local, under
treatment. It may be well to repeat that the change seems to date in
the present century from about the time of the first invasion of cholera,
and has continued more or less ever since.

The change from sthenic to asthenic (so far as we at present know)
is one more of the vital than of the structural or chemical characters
of disease. The symptoms indicate, as it were, a lower tension of all
the vital phenomena. The convalescence is less perfect and slower,
as are also the physical signs of the resolution of local disease. The
capability of bearing a reducing treatment is singularly diminished.
Local lesions exhibit a greater latency. The nervous system shows

earlier signs of depression, while tonics or stimulants have been better borne.

So far as medical experience goes, we are forced to admit that the foundation for the healing art must rest on another, if not a broader, basis than that of anatomical and of chemical changes in disease. There are differences—and for want of a better name we may call them *vital*—which more intimately relate to life and health than to the anatomical or chemical changes produced by disease; and these are to be reached by the study of the *living* phenomena of the body, and of the influence of agents upon them. In truth, the fruitless attempt to base medicine upon anatomical or even chemical changes should be a lesson to those who neglect the infinitely varied mutations of vital or of nervous action.

The healing art, whether medicine or surgery, requires a wider field of study than is afforded by the dissecting-room or the laboratory. The anatomists, the histologists, and the chemists of some of the modern schools of medicine would derive a deep practical lesson from the words of Goethe,[1] who says, alluding to the insufficiency of mere anatomy to explain the mysteries of life—

> For he who seeks to learn, or gives
> Descriptions of, a thing that lives,
> Begins with "murdering, to dissect,"
> The lifeless parts he may inspect—
> The limbs are there beneath his knife,
> And all—but that which gave them life!
> Alas! the spirit hath withdrawn—
> That which informed the mass is gone.
> They scrutinize it, when it ceases
> To be itself, and count its pieces,
> Finger and feel them, and call this
> Experiment—analysis.

The study of normal anatomy being then fruitless in solving the problem of healthy life, it might be anticipated that researches as to morbid structure have thrown but a fitful and limited light on disease. In truth, the knowledge of Curative or of Preventive Medicine is not to be learned in the dissecting-room of a medical school, or in the dead-house of a hospital. Until this truth be acted on, many precious years of the best time of the student's life will be wasted. It has been attempted to base medicine on pathological anatomy, as if by its study we could solve the infinitely varied problems of disease and of therapeutics. The explanation of even death through anatomical research

---

[1] *Faustus.* Translated by John Anster, LL.D., of Trinity College, Dublin. 1835. P. 120.

is admissible only in exceptional cases. But it is of value—less as a key to the origin and cause of disease, than to diagnosis and the science or the many changes which attend morbid action.

LECTURE III.

Fever described, but not defined, as "a condition of existence without any known or necessary local anatomical change and subject to new laws, different from those of health"—Error committed by the school of Broussais—The "Law of Periodicity"—Danger to the fever patient due to the primary disease or to its secondary complications—Secondary affections of continued fevers more inconstant than those of the exanthemata—Classification of diseases: (1) Diseases having *an anatomical character*: (2) *neuroses*, having no known anatomical character; (3) *fevers*, subject to the law of periodicity, causing secondary affections, transmissible by contagion.

Fever is a condition more easily described than defined, and it is far easier to declare *what it is not* than *what it actually is*. During the continuance of a fever the system seems, as it were, to enter upon a new and special phase of existence. Most, if not all, functions are liable to be either interrupted or modified in a varying degree, and this possibly without the occurrence of any local anatomical change. We cannot say, I believe, what fever is in its essence, yet one thing appears certain—that it is not symptomatic of the organic changes which may be found combined with it, but is rather the generator and governor of those affections. It is, then, a condition without any known or necessary local anatomical change.

It is true that in certain forms of fever there are secondary manifestations of local disease. The pustulation of the skin in variola, the ulceration of the intestine in the so-called typhoid, and the bronchial congestion in typhus, are examples of these conditions. But looking at fever in a wide sense, we may safely hold that these secondary anatomical changes are inconstant in their amount, in their nature, and even in their seat; inconstant as to their time of appearance, their symptoms, their intensity, and their decadence, and utterly incompetent to explain the phenomena of the disease.

The great fact remains, that in epidemics of fever cases arise in which, after the general symptoms have run their course, so as to present a perfect specimen of the general disease, we may dissect the brain, spinal marrow, nerves, the pulmonary and gastro-intestinal mucous membrane, the liver, every organ you please, and find no anatomical change. I believe we may say that when the fatal diseases of the world are considered, the most destructive are those which have no recognized anatomical character. You may believe that when we speak of fever generally, secondary lesions are either wanting or are inconstant in their amount or in their nature. Upon their incompetence to explain the matter I have already remarked.

It will naturally be asked, If this be so, how did the French school commit the extraordinary error of declaring that a special anatomical change characterized every case of fever? The reason is simply this: they committed two grave errors in medical philosophy: first, in confounding the *effect* with the *cause;* and secondly, in assuming the nature of a disease over the world from its observation in one locality. Had Broussais and his followers studied fever in Ireland, Scotland, or England ; had they gone abroad and examined it in the East or West Indies, or on the coast of Africa, we should have heard little of the doctrine that fever was not essential, but only symptomatic of this or that local inflammation.

Observation has long shown that fever is a state of existence under a law of *periodicity*, and this is more or less true as to the general affection and as to its local results, though this law is more often manifest in the case of the former than in that of the latter. In the disease, I believe under any of its forms, two sources of danger affect the patient. One of these is death from simple depression of all the vital powers; for the poison of fever, like that of the rattle-snake, has a directly depressing influence on the system. Another source of danger is the production of secondary diseases. A general notion of this will be best obtained by considering an ordinary case of small-pox. The patient is taken ill; he has shivering, fever, pain, vomiting, and so on ; and then we observe vesicles on the surface, these vesicles filling with pus, afterwards drying, and then disappearing. No man will say that the fever was symptomatic of the eruption. It is exactly the reverse ; the eruption was the result of the fever. So it is in fever ; the local disease is the product of the general. There is, however, this difference between what we term continued fever, typhus, or typhoid, and the exanthemata, that while in the latter the local affection is almost always accompanied by certain characters, it is not so with respect to the secondary diseases of the fevers specified. However, between the exanthemata and typhus fever there is this point of resemblance, that the secondary affections are utterly incompetent to explain the general phenomena of the disease, while in typhus, and, I believe, in typhoid, they are doubly inconstant in their seat, their nature, and their amount—and this is true even in cases occurring during the same epidemic. But they are of very great importance.

It may be asked, Are they inflammations? I believe they are not inflammations, or, if they be such, they have a specific character. Certainly in their first stages they are not inflammatory; but in many instances, after they have existed in their non-inflammatory state, there comes on a reactive irritation, so that we may then have a mixed condition of essential and symptomatic fever. In my opinion this is the history of the ulcerations of the intestine so common in typhoid fever, for in the beginning—as in variola—we often find tumefaction and infiltration without increased vascularity. It has been proved that in many cases the morbid process goes no further, and we have retrocession of the infiltration, as we see retrocession in the eruption of smallpox.

It may be laid down that while the great majority of separate diseases catalogued in books have an anatomical character, fever is wanting in this particular with regard to the practice of medicine. We may, then, divide diseases into three great classes.

In the first class we have diseases which have an anatomical character—diseases to which we can give an anatomical expression. I need not occupy your time in giving examples of this class.

In the next place, we have a most important class of diseases which, in the present state of our knowledge, cannot be connected with any recognized anatomical character, and yet they are not fevers. I allude to the *neuroses*, or, as they are commonly termed, nervous affections; of these mania, epilepsy, lock-jaw, hydrophobia, hysteria, chorea, convulsions, are familiar instances. Here we have some most remarkable affections, which have not any known anatomical character; that is to say, we cannot yet show that they depend upon any known or ascertained anatomical change of any portion of the system, including the brain, spinal marrow, and nerves. The general character of this singular group of affections, which we call *neuroses*, shows that, whatever be the nature of the disease, the seat of it is in the nervous system; but, in the present state of anatomical knowledge, we are not justified in saying what the condition of the nervous system is to which they owe their origin; whether it is an organic change at all, or whether, supposing such a change to exist, its amount is proportionate to the violence of the symptoms. Even the results hitherto obtained by the microscope have been chiefly negative; the microscope has added but little to what was before known on those subjects. I may state here, lest you should fall into a misapprehension, that I do not wish you to believe **that** organic change is not found in any of these diseases. The fact is, that in many of them such does exist; but when we come to inquire what those organic changes are, we find that they are so inconstant, so variable, frequently so similar in opposite diseases, that they have hitherto altogether failed to throw any positive light upon the subject.

This, then, is the second class of diseases; the first class having an anatomical character, the second having no anatomical character. Now we come to the third class, which comprises fevers. Fevers, as we have already said, have no anatomical character. Then, it will be asked, how do they differ from the *neuroses*? As far as we know, and strictly speaking, they differ very little; but there is this feature connected with them, that fever seems to be a special condition of life which is to exist for a certain time, and then to cease—that is to say, it is under the law of periodicity; and in this respect the phenomena of fevers differ very much from those of the pure neuroses. There are other differences, too, between fevers and neuroses. It is quite true that in a large number of fevers death may take place without any organic change that we can demonstrate anatomically; but it is true, on the other hand, that in a large number of cases there is a tendency to the development of what are to be designated the secondary lesions of the disease. Thus, if we compare these two classes, the neuroses, which are not fevers, and the fevers properly so called, we find this great difference, that among the former (as for example in hydrophobia) we do not see any tendency to the development of ulcers of the intestine; in epilepsy we do not find any tendency to the development of bronchial diseases; in mania we do not see a cutaneous eruption; in convulsions we do not find any of these various organic changes produced. This tendency, then, to generate or produce local anatomical changes secondary to the fever is another remarkable distinction between this class of affections and the pure neuroses.

There is a third very remarkable distinction between them. Fevers —using the term in a general sense, embracing, as I have already pointed out, a great number of essential diseases, as the exanthemata, typhus, plague, and yellow fever—are capable of being transmitted by contact or by vicinity; many of them—I believe almost all—are more or less contagious. So that in their subjection to the law of periodicity, in their liability to generate or produce various organic changes in different parts of the system, and in their transmissibility by contagion, we have three very important distinctive characters, although we cannot reduce them to an anatomical expression.

A great deal has been written on the subject of the proximate cause of fever, and theory upon theory has been promulgated. We are, however, at this moment as ignorant of the proximate cause of fever as we were in the time of Cullen, or even long before him. It may be expected, however, looking at the advance of medical knowledge, that the proximate cause or causes of fever will yet be discovered; but it is a general and justifiable opinion that essential fevers result, in most cases, from the introduction of a poison into the system. The whole of the phenomena of poisoning by organic matter seem to point out a close analogy between fevers and those diseases in which a poison is introduced into the system. If a man who is in perfect health is exposed to the contagion of syphilis, in a short time his system becomes a laboratory for the formation of syphilitic poison, and he is capable of communicating the disease. As far as we can form a judgment on this question we may say that there is a very close analogy indeed between fevers and toxic diseases, whether they be fevers which are the result of contagion or not; and in this way we see a connecting link between fevers, which we call acute diseases, and diseases which are neither acute nor febrile. Thus, for example, we do not say that a patient who is labouring under syphilis, which he has caught by contagion, is in fever; but he is, nevertheless, under a condition which, so far as the chemico-vital state of his body is concerned, is somewhat analogous to fever; that is to say, his system has received a poison, and having received that poison, it seems to work upon it, or the poison to work on the system, and the result is that the system becomes a generator of the same poison that it has received.

Now let us go a little further into this subject. I might give various other illustrations; and, indeed, I think you will find that some unexpected analogies will arise in this matter, and that you will even perceive an analogy between two such opposite diseases—such dissimilar diseases as typhus fever and pulmonary consumption. For there can hardly be a doubt that, under certain circumstances, tubercular matter introduced into the system acts like contagious matter, and that it produces a development of tubercular disease in the system thus infected. Such cases, then, may be considered as examples, if you will, of very chronic fevers, long-continued fevers, and fevers which are not, apparently at least, under the influence of the law of periodicity. I am perfectly persuaded that the more we study that class of diseases, which seems to be general rather than local, we shall find that the possibility of contagion will be more and more exhibited. I am strongly of opinion that the majority of the acute essential diseases are contagious, and I think it certain that there are other diseases also which we do not call fevers that are contagious. It is hardly possible to doubt the contagiousness of cholera; and we may go still further, and extend the possibility of contagiousness even to such diseases as tubercular affections, and perhaps even further.

We know that scarlatina, measles, and smallpox are generally constant in their phenomena, and especially in the phenomena of their secondary changes—so much so that in them the secondary change is taken as a distinctive mark of the disease. These affections are probably, as I said before, more directly contagious; and it becomes a question whether this may arise from the circumstance that the matter of contagion in these cases is more elaborated—is perhaps more perfect according to its kind—or whether greater facilities are afforded for the conveyance of contagious matter during the desquamative processes so common in these diseases. The patient who contracts the disease is very much in the same position as a person who contracts syphilis; that is to say, that an organic poison of a special kind, whose essential characters, however, are so subtle as to escape chemical investigation, has been presented to his system and has affected him. The phenomena of typhus and typhoid are more variable; and this may arise from the want of constancy in the exciting cause. We can hardly suppose a man to get smallpox unless he has been infected by another who has had smallpox. But continued fever, or typhus fever, seems capable of being produced by a great number of causes, or, if I may so speak, by a number of imperfectly developed or imperfectly acting causes, and these, of course, may be infinitely various. We also see this very curious difference between typhus fever and the exanthemata, that while among exanthemata, so far as we know, the one exciting cause produces its own disease—the exciting cause of smallpox producing smallpox, that of scarlatina producing scarlatina, that of measles producing measles—this does not seem to be the case with respect to fever. For here is one of the most important and interesting facts connected with the entire subject, that the same exciting cause—at least as far as we can see of it—is capable of producing different kinds of fever in different persons. This great fact has not been sufficiently dwelt on by the various writers on fever on the Continent and in England, especially by that class of men whose object seems to have been to make themselves classifiers of diseases—makers of classifications—at which nature laughs.

Here is another of the great facts which show the inexpediency of drawing hard and fast lines of distinction between what are termed *typhus* fever and *typhoid* fever—that the one exciting cause will in one person produce one form of fever and in another a different form of fever. Now, we see nothing of this sort in the exanthemata. What may be the reason of this it is difficult to say; and we explain it very often by

. expressing the fact in different words. It is supposed that it may be
due to some variation in the state of *receptivity* of the body at the time.
For in the production of the effect of the poison there are two elements:
first, the nature and composition of the poison which is to act; and,
next, the chemico-vital state of the body which is to be acted on. The
two causes combined produce the result—fever. But if, the cause
being the same, the bodies be in different states, we may expect different kinds of fevers; and this is all that we can say on the subject.

Now let me address especially the junior members of the class, or
those who have hitherto worked exclusively in the surgical wards. I
want them to look on the local acute diseases of fever as they would
look on the pustules of smallpox, the efflorescence of erysipelas, or the
eruption in measles or scarlatina. In these maladies the manifest local
disease most commonly affects the skin, but is clearly secondary to
a specific morbid state of the system. It runs its course and subsides
spontaneously, and unless in exceptional cases the constitutional disturbance subsides with it.

Now, this seems to be the case in the secondary affections of fever,
whether they be attended with anatomical change or be simply neurotic, whether the head, chest, or abdomen shows signs of disease.
This latter is the product of the essential condition—that is, of the
fever—and not its cause. You may meet cases where but one cavity
is affected, even throughout the fever, where the three cavities are
simultaneously engaged, where they are severally attacked, or where,
in the whole course of the fever, there is no anatomical change.

Now, what I want you to believe, and what, when your actual experience of successive epidemics has been obtained, you cannot help
believing, is, that as regards these secondary diseases, there is no constancy in their production—none as to amount, none as to intensity
—and you may add, as to their combination and even their seat. Important though they may be, frequent as certain forms of them are in
certain epidemics or in certain localities, they may be looked on more
in the light of accidents than of constant occurrences.

They may be occasionally so extensive and so intense as that death
may be probably attributed to them; while, on the other hand, their
amount may be very trifling, and have no proportion to the severity
of the general malady. In fact, it is impossible to predicate what
course the secondary disease may take from spontaneous and sometimes sudden retrocession to extreme disorganization. Thus the
affection of the lung may vary from a slight to a dangerous degree of
bronchial irritation, with congestion, causing extensive and rapid
consolidation, and even a fatal sphacelus. Or there may be a great

development of tubercle, either confined to the lung or engaging many other organs. Again, a rapid consolidation may take place—generally, as it were, silently—and attended by a cessation of the fever. We shall return to this when discussing the pulmonary complications. So also you will find great variations in the nature and intensity of the abdominal affections, from slight partial congestion, with or without deposit in the mucous glands of the intestine, to extreme relaxation, softening, and perforation of the tube—it may be in many places with or without general acute peritonitis—or, as certain cases in the epidemic in 1827, there may be numerous intussusceptions, great congestion and enlargement, with softening of the spleen; and, though the intestinal suffering be extreme, even without ulceration or perforation of the tube.

Now, gentlemen, what I wish you to bear in mind is, that the relation between the anatomical states of organs in fevers is a variable one, whether as regards the seat, the combination, the intensity of the affection, or the time of its appearance, or its effect on the general malady. Every great epidemic of fever, of whatever kind, must be studied first separately, and then comparatively, and you will find that the history of fever is a much wider subject than you might infer from books.

LECTURE IV.

CONTAGION—Exclusive doctrines are to be deprecated—Endemic disease arises independently of contact—The numerical system of Louis fails in practical medicine—Evidence in favour of contagion from the *Doctrine of Chances*—Investigations of Dr. Whitley Stokes and the Bishop of Cloyne; with Dr. Paget's remarks thereon—Variation in the degree of contagiousness of acute essential diseases.

As I have said, a striking difference of fevers, compared with the pure neuroses and the structural diseases, is their *contagious* nature.

With regard to this characteristic, medical opinion has been long divided; and I would advise you, as a general rule, not to range yourselves among the advocates of any exclusive doctrine. You are not, therefore, to stand in the false position of men who are fighting for a particular doctrine, whether they be contagionists or non-contagionists. Should you do so, your mind will be occupied with the excitement of controversy rather than with the search for truth. You will become advocates, while you cease to be inquirers, and once this change occurs in the mind of the observer, he loses caste in the ranks of science.

The advocates of an exclusive doctrine on each side of this great question are able to produce many facts in evidence of their particular views. The facts thus brought forward may be, and probably are, in each case true; but the conclusions drawn from them may not be warranted. It would thus be wrong to infer that a disease was not contagious from the failure of evidence of its communication even in many instances. Equally illogical would be the deduction that a disease arose only by contagion, even where multiplied examples of such an origin could be appealed to.

There can be no doubt that disease has originated, and may originate, without contagion. This must be obvious to every man.

Again, we see a vast number of cases in which disease is endemic. I need scarcely allude to the common case of ague. There are certain districts where ague is constantly produced, and where, if a man who has not had ague goes, and is not in contact with any human being whatever, he will, almost certainly, get the disease. Here, then, clearly, there has been disease independently produced, or at least without *human* contagion. There are certain districts in South America and in the West Indies, vast districts on the coast of Africa, forest districts in Hindostan, where, if a man sleeps for a single night —although we will suppose him to be alone, without any companions but the wild beasts of the forest—he will get some form of fever. We see also, if we look at the records of medicine, unquestionably even within the later periods of the world's history, the appearance of new diseases, totally new diseases. So that we cannot at all deny that disease may be generated, and that it may spread without the intervention of human contagion. We must believe, I say, in the origin of diseases under some exciting cause; but that exciting cause need not be human contagion. On the other hand, innumerable facts show that fever existing in the system is capable of being propagated from one man to another; that it is, in fact, a contagious disease in the strictest sense; and this transmission of the disease may not be merely by contact, but by vicinity—within, it is true, a limited space. Now, the facts which we must rely on to impress this doctrine of contagion on your mind, when you come to examine them, will appear less direct than you might suppose. A great number of men who have written on this subject were really but ill-instructed in the rules of logic; they have not been trained to think properly and argue correctly on the subjects they were considering. For instance, it was a great object with a number of the French school, especially with the disciples of

Broussais and advocates of the physiological doctrine, to establish the non-contagiousness of disease. For the doctrine of contagion implies essentiality; and the physiological doctrine was opposed to all essentiality. According to this doctrine, there was no such thing as essential disease. Every disease was local and inflammatory; every fever was symptomatic. Therefore, in their anxiety to overturn essentialism, they found this outwork, as it were, of contagion, which should be carried. And nothing can be more singular, or, I may say, heroical, than the efforts which a number of the French physicians made to establish the non-contagiousness even of the most contagious diseases. Many of them went out to the Levant and exposed themselves purposely to the contagion of plague—put on the clothes of persons who were labouring under it; slept in the beds with plague patients; inoculated themselves with the matter from the buboes of persons labouring under the disease, in some instances actually inoculated themselves with the blood of plague patients. Well, in many cases these experimenters did not take the plague, and this fact is still relied upon as a proof of the non-contagiousness of plague and of fever generally. But you will at once see how very inconsequential these experiments are. Here are four or five cases of failure of contagion, and as well might you argue that corn does not grow from seed because one grain sown in the earth will sometimes fail to produce the plant. I may state here, however, that some of these investigators paid the terrible penalty of death in their zeal for science, for they did take the plague and were lost.

Among the direct facts which satisfy our minds as to the contagious nature of fever are the circumstances attending its spread through large masses of people. I need hardly here allude to the singularly forcible argument in favour of contagion which may be drawn from the frightful mortality of our Irish medical brethren in the years of 1847 and 1848. This subject I have already alluded to in the theatre of the Meath Hospital, and it is one which we can hardly look back upon without shuddering. The simple fact alone of the mortality of that class of individuals who are most exposed to the disease, furnishes an argument in favour of contagion which we would but weaken by any observations upon it.

There is a mode of dealing with the indirect evidence for contagion, to which I shall now draw your attention. You all know that Professor Louis, of Paris, founded what he terms the numerical system of medical investigation; that is to say, he attempted to reduce the facts of medicine to numerical expression; so that we should be able, as he supposed, to make medicine an almost exact science. My opinion,

I may state, generally speaking, on the subject is, that for the establishment of all that part of medicine which consists in fixing the data of physical diagnosis, the frequency or infrequency of certain pathological changes and matters of that kind, the numerical system is infinitely valuable; but that we cannot, or have not yet been able to apply it so as to furnish rules of treatment. For the object of the numerical physician and that of the practical physician—if I may make use of such a distinction—are different. The object of the numerical physician is to ascertain a rule of treatment which will cure the greatest number of cases out of a given number; but that should not be your object, or that of practical physicians. It is very well to know that such results have been obtained; but it does not follow that you are to act on them. Your course is not blindly to adopt the formula founded on numerical data when it is shown that by its use you can cure the greatest number out of a given number; your object is to cure the diseases of A, B, or C, as they may come before you. And you are not to neglect what you believe to be right in the case of A, B, or C, because you have this array of figures declaring to you that such and such a course, different from that you may be about to pursue, is the rule for saving the greatest number of lives out of a given number. But we may safely use numbers in a different way—as, for example, in investigating the data of a particular doctrine.

My father, when Professor of the Practice of Medicine in the Royal College of Surgeons, directed his attention very much to the subject of contagion. He was a strong advocate of the doctrine of contagion. Perhaps he went too far in his belief in the exclusiveness of this doctrine. Perhaps, also, he went too far in denying the views of the epidemists, or of the non-contagionists. However, that has nothing to say to the present question. He thought that, in looking at the general circumstances which attend the spread of an epidemic in this country, the probabilities for or against the doctrine of contagion might be submitted to calculation. One of his most intimate friends was the late Dr. Brinkley, Bishop of Cloyne, who was at one time the Astronomer-Royal of Ireland. He was admittedly one of the very first mathematicians of his day, and especially skilled in that difficult part of mathematical investigation—the *Doctrine of Chances.*

In the progress of an epidemic in Ireland (and doubtless also in other countries) in a family of twelve persons the disease has been known to attack eleven out of the twelve. In some cases, the passing of the fever through so large a proportion as eleven individuals out of twelve has taken a very considerable period of time, as you may readily understand. It has taken about three months to go through them all. Now, my father proposed these two problems to the Bishop of Cloyne for solution:—

1st. An epidemic prevails so severely that one person out of seven sickens. A family of twelve is selected in a particular district before the epidemic has visited it. What is the chance that eleven out of that family will take the disease, supposing the sickness of one of the family does not promote the sickening of another—that is, supposing the disease not to be contagious, and supposing the family to be not unusually liable to the disease?

The answer furnished by Dr. Brinkley was, that the probability against such an event is 189,600,000 to 1. That is a very singular and extraordinary result.

2d. The same general conditions being assumed, and also that the number of inhabitants of a district is 7000, what is the chance that in a family of twelve within the district eleven will sicken?
Answer: The chance then is 300,000 to 1 that no family of twelve persons in a population of 7000 will have eleven persons sick.

These numbers furnish proofs so convincing of the truth of the doctrine of contagion, though by no means in an exclusive sense, that it is hardly necessary to go further. The facts on which they were based are ascertained facts; they have been not uncommon facts in epidemic fever; but, recollecting this, the chances against their happening, if the disease were not contagious, would be 189,600,000 to 1 in the one case, and 300,000 to 1 in the other.

On this subject I have had the honour of receiving a letter from Dr. Paget, of Cambridge; and I would not be doing justice to you, or to the question generally, if I did not state the objection made by this eminent physician, as to the soundness of the conclusions in favour of contagion, which appear deducible from these calculations. Dr. Paget observes that the form in which the problems are stated excludes the consideration of all local influences except contagion; in this he is perfectly correct. He considers that had this element of local influence, besides contagion, been included, it must necessarily have diminished, by whatever was its real value, the overwhelming result which the calculations, as they now stand, give in favour of contagion. But even Dr. Paget himself admits that—taking the case of the second calculation—if the consequence of these deductions on the score of local causes were to reduce the probability of 300,000 to 1 to that of 1000 to 1, yet this latter probability would be sufficient to carry conviction to the mind of any candid person. He, however, observes that we have unhappily no means of estimating numerically the requisite deductions, no means of calculating the effect of noxious exhalations from decomposing organic substances, of bad food and other assignable causes, which have been supposed capable of promoting the spread of fevers; and he properly remarks that Bishop Brinkley's results include, with contagion, the possible effects not only of known but also of all unknown causes which may make an individual household more liable to fever than their neighbours.

While I feel indebted to Dr. Paget for having drawn my attention to this point, and to the importance of noticing it, when the numerical value of these results is considered, I think it well to mention that in my father's "Observations on Contagion" there is nothing which would lead one to believe that he advocated that doctrine in an exclusive sense. His object in proposing the problems was to show the great probability in favour of the doctrine of contagion as one and a principal cause of epidemical disease, and this irrespective of the question whether or not other causes might be held to coexist. The result seems to establish the certainty of the existence of contagion as an important cause of the phenomena in question. The singular array of figures is valuable as establishing the fact that contagion has a real existence. The terms of the questions may be held to embrace all other possible causes of sickness. My opinion, however, is that in Ireland local influences have not that great importance either as generators or promoters of fever which some believe them to have.

We must believe that the causes of fever, independent of mere contagion, are various in the extreme, that they are probably numerous and complicated, acting in combination rather than singly, and varying in their effects not only in consequence of their own properties and combinations, but also as regards the condition of the individual in whom fever is developed. Dr. Paget, in observing that our pathology of fever is not so perfect as to assure us that there are no exciting causes besides those which are commonly allowed, notices the comparative immunity of infants and persons above forty years of age from the typhoid fever with rose spots, and affections of Peyer's glands, etc., indicating that the constitution of the individual is an element in the question.

You are then to understand that, while we believe in the contagious nature of fever as an established fact, we do not go the length of saying that all cases of fever originate by contagion. In the present state of knowledge we must, I think, admit that certain combinations of physical circumstances may produce fever, either in a single case or in masses of men. It is hardly possible to gainsay this; but it is at least as well if not better proved that this fever is capable of being communicated by actual contact, or by vicinity, from one individual to another.

If we look to other diseases which affect the whole economy, we find analogies between them and fever; so far, at least, that in them a morbid condition exists which reveals itself in two ways: one, a state of general ill-health: and the other, the production of local and specific alterations. Take, for example, tubercle and syphilis.

The last of these is, at all events, contagious; and though we can hardly show any mode of its production except by communication from one person to another, yet we must believe that at one time causes independent of such a mode of communication did exist, and were capable of originating the disease: and it may be that, as the world advances, and the general exciting causes of fever are diminished, or perhaps removed, this disease too, like syphilis, may only be produced and exist by means of its communication from one person to another; and we may hope that such a state of things would be a step to the extinction of fever, at least as a disease affecting communities of men.

If it be true that we may admit two phases in the history of acute essential diseases, one in which they are not only communicable, but capable of original production by causes independent of contact with the sick, and the other when these latter causes ceased to operate, and the disease is reduced simply to a special condition, which can be communicated only by contact, it is easy to perceive that, so far as prevention and ultimate extinction are concerned, the difficulties attendant on the matter will be greatly diminished. Let us assume that, so far as the cessation of the operation of general external causes is concerned, variola and syphilis are similarly circumstanced, and we may hope, from what has occurred with respect to the former disease, that a similar diminution of fever may yet be attained, when it has at last passed into the condition of a merely contagious disease.

That almost all cases of acute essential disease are contagious I have long believed. The amount or degree of contagiousness varies according to many circumstances, such as the nature of the malady, the amount of exposure, the physical condition of those so exposed, and the character of the epidemic. There can be no doubt that in different epidemics—apparently of similar diseases—the character of contagiousness varies remarkably, and I am glad to perceive that modern British authorities now admit that even typhoid or enteric fever may be propagated by contagion.

"Some physicians," writes my father,[1] "in arguing against the contagious nature of certain fevers, have ventured on the adoption of a principle which appears to me very untenable—namely, that a dis-

---

[1] Observations on Contagion, p. 25.

ease can have but one cause—and hence they infer that the advocates
of contagion, instead of supposing, as they do at present, that contagion
is the general cause of fevers, with which famine, filth, damp, or cold
co-operate singly or collectively, should suppose that one only of these
causes can be the true cause of every particular disease, and that the
admission that other causes contribute to disease is in fact a confession
that contagion does not."

For contagious disease, such as typhus or typhoid, though it may
occasionally attack individuals of the oppulent classes, runs like wild-
fire through an indigent and unhealthy population. The power of
resistance is lessened, and all the evils of the asthenic conditions are
increased.

LECTURE V.

CAUSES OF FEVER—Preventive and Curative Medicine contrasted—Risk of error in
limiting the number of the cures of disease—The *correlation* and the *convertibility* of
disease two important questions, the answers to which are not as yet fully or satisfactorily determined.

WITH respect to those causes which may be held to be capable of
exciting fever, irrespective of contagion, I have only to say that as yet
we know but little about them; and we have the highest authority
for believing that the origin of epidemics is one of the most obscure
and difficult subjects in the whole range of physical inquiry. But I
cannot help expressing my belief that too much stress has been laid
upon the effects of miasmata resulting from imperfect drainage, or the
want of ventilation and of public cleanliness in general. No one will
for a moment suppose that I wish to teach that these influences do
not act in deteriorating the physical health and moral condition of a
people, and in thus increasing the mortality of any existing epidemic,
and that their removal is not an imperative duty of every government
and community.

For some years past great attention has been paid in England and
on the Continent, especially in Germany, to sanitary science—that is
to say, to Preventive as distinguished from Curative Medicine. If we
compare the relative importance of these two great branches of medical science, it seems true that a greater value should be attached to
the first than to the second branch, and for this reason, that the well-
being of infinitely greater numbers of mankind depends more on
Preventive than on Curative Medicine.

The great end of the former is to preserve the health of the masses of mankind so as to prevent or to diminish the necessity of the latter. The one is a matter to be dealt with by a large and wise legislative code; the other is dependent on the slow advance of medical science, and on the individual character and attainments of those who are to carry it out. The one embraces *everything*, as Dr. Acland has well shown, which relates to the physical and the moral well-being of nations,[1] the grinding of the poor, the consumption of human life, as it were fuel for the production of wealth.

Selfishness, indulgence, unrestrained vice, and every cause which tends to deteriorate the body come within its extended scope. Its object is the health and the happiness of our fellow-creatures. Its rules are plain and patent to all, and depend not on vexed questions of difficult science; so that it promises to be the noblest pursuit open to human beings, and he would be a bold man who dared attempt to predicate its triumphs or to limit its results.

The occurrence and the spreading of epidemical disease have long engaged the attention of advocates of sanitary reform; but it does not appear that as yet the difficulties connected with these questions can be said to have been at all satisfactorily solved, even though the importance of sanitary measures be frankly admitted.

The paramount doctrine which has prevailed in England ascribes epidemics to want of cleanliness, overcrowding, deficient or impure air and water supply, imperfect drainage, and so on; while the cessation of local outbreaks of disease after the adoption of a sanitary reform is appealed to in proof that the evils in question arose solely from removable influences. But the argument is defective—it is like that of the therapeutists as regards essential diseases, which run their appointed course and then spontaneously disappear. Epidemics of fever in this way resemble isolated cases. They also have their periods of invasion, of maturity, and of decadence, and the subsidence of an epidemic is in many instances by no means traceable to the adoption of certain sanitary measures. The experience of all great epidemics establishes this fact.

There is, however, one theory or doctrine which underlies the whole history of British sanitary reform, and this is—that many, if not all, forms of endemical or of epidemical disease can be traced to some preventable or removable cause, and that by putting a stop to overcrowding, and by improving the quality of the water and the air in a locality, we may prevent the occurrence of such afflictions.

[1] National Health. By Henry W. Acland, F.R.S., Regius Professor of Medicine in the University of Oxford, etc. etc. 1871.

I need not here point out to you the tendency which exists in many minds to attribute great phenomena to too limited a cause or causes. Thus, for example, some form of essential disease arises and spreads in a particular locality. This is inspected, imperfect sewerage is discovered, and the evil abated by the adoption of proper measures. Then the sanitarians triumphantly appeal to the circumstances as proving that the outbreak was the direct result of the alleged nuisances, and perhaps of them alone.

By this line of argument many sanitarians of that class who have not received a scientific education, and who know but little of the history of disease, hold that such unwholesome and removable influences may originate diseases which are themselves dissimilar.

But the question before us is, Are those influences in this country the sole or the chief causes of fever? It is difficult to believe that they are, because in Ireland, not only in the isolated dwellings of the poor which are scattered over the face of the country, but in the towns also, all those causes which result from the imperfect drainage of dwellings, from the accumulations of decomposing organic matters in their vicinity, and from imperfect ventilation, are, I regret to say, but too constant and too general; and yet the production of fever, whether sporadically or epidemically, is inconstant and irregular in the highest degree. Why should these causes produce fever at one time and not at another? Why should districts remain for years free, or comparatively free, from fever, while the supposed exciting causes remain in full force? or, again, why if the cause be constant, should the epidemic character of the fever vary? We may say, excluding the consideration of isolated cases, that each epidemic has a special or predominant character; thus, the great epidemic of 1826 and 1827 was very different from the epidemic which preceded it in 1818, and from those which followed it in 1836 and in 1847. It was in the epidemic of 1826-27 that we observed the almost universal prevalence of the secondary disease of the intestine; perforations of the intestinal tube were common; and yet, since that period, such an accident is rarely met with, either in the fever itself or during the period of convalescence. It was at that time, too, that those singular and fatal cases of yellow fever, to which we shall have to allude, occurred intercurrently. In this fever, also, termination by well-marked crisis was commonly observed, a circumstance which is comparatively rare in the epidemics of maculated typhus in this country.

I do not put forward these views as in any way original, for Dr. Graves long held the opinion, and taught it in this theatre, that something more than the effect of local causes, as the term is commonly understood, was necessary to explain the occurrence of epidemics in Ireland. Let me read to you a quotation from his seventh lecture, one of those devoted to the consideration of fever:[1] "That fever, in Ireland at least, depends on some general atmospheric change which affects the whole island simultaneously, independent of situation, aspect, height above the level of the sea, dryness or moisture of the soil, or any other circumstance connected with mere locality, is proved by the fact, that when typhus begins to increase notably in the Dublin hospitals, we may always rest assured that a nearly simultaneous increase of fever will be observed at Cork, Galway, Limerick, and Belfast. For a considerable period there was a great tendency among physicians to refer the origin of typhus, and of almost every variety of fever, to malaria or unwholesome emanations from the soil, produced by the decomposition of vegetable matter. In Ireland facts do not bear out this hypothesis, for, as already stated, when an epidemic of fever has become established it breaks out simultaneously in situations the most different, and in some where no such emanations can be supposed to exist; thus I have seen a whole family affected in the telegraph situated at the summit of Killiney, a mountain formed of hard granite; and, indeed, the granite districts beyond Rathfarnham, Tallaght, and Killikee supply the Meath Hospital with its worst cases of typhus." Further on he observes, "Although ready to allow the general improvement of the health of the public from improved drainage, improved habits of cleanliness, and increased comforts, yet I cannot admit that in Ireland we are to expect any notable diminution of fever from the operation of these causes. In making this statement you are aware that I am opposing the usually prevalent opinion. The grounds for my dissent have been partly explained to you already, for, according to my observation, the increase or diminution of fever in Ireland arises from some unknown general atmospheric or, if you will, climatic influence, quite independent of locality, and consequently the most improved and thoroughly drained towns and country districts are quite as liable to epidemics of typhus as are the most neglected and marshy parts of our island. The causes which occasion these epidemics are, on the other hand, in no way connected with the notable variations of the seasons; for with us the ravages of typhus are observed sometimes in dry, sometimes in rainy seasons, and its epidemics appear quite uninfluenced by the cold of winter or the heat of summer."

In Ireland the habits of the poor as to uncleanliness and over-

---

[1] Clinical Lectures on the Practice of Medicine. Reprinted from the Second Edition, 1864, p. 62.

crowding call for great reform, especially in our towns, where poverty, neglect, and overcrowding so often make them foci of endemical disease. The condition of our country towns and villages is simply deplorable, disgraceful to the local authorities, and in too many instances to the proprietary, frequently heedless as to the social and physical condition of those who live under them. Even the state of the metropolis, possessing a Public Health Committee, is shocking, and has been ably shown by Dr. Grimshaw in a recent communication to the Medical Society of the College of Physicians, Ireland.[1]

What I wish you to believe, gentlemen, is, as I have already stated, that our fever is epidemic, proceeding from general but unknown causes—and also contagious; and no one can deny that causes which would act in depressing the health and moral energy of a people, by rendering them less able to resist the effects of disease, would increase the general mortality. The influence of bad ventilation and overcrowding I need not here dwell on; nor, on the other hand, need I occupy your time with more arguments to establish the truth of the doctrine of contagion. You will find in the writings of Sir Robert Christison, of Dr. Murchison, and of Dr. Graves convincing evidences on these points; and let me again refer to the great argument drawn from the liability to contract fever observed among the medical practitioners of Ireland, especially in the epidemic of 1847.

The occurrence of offensive odours proceeding from the putrescence of organic matter naturally led to the widespread idea that the objectionable smell was the exciting cause of sickness, and that all sanitarians had to do was to remove the sources of air and water pollution. But though the researches of Murchison and of Sir William Jenner go far to connect what has been called typhoid or enteric fever with the existence of noxious emanations from human excreta, other weighty questions remain.

For example, Are these emanations the sole cause of the so-called pythogenic or enteric fever? Is this fever essentially different from typhus? Can it be propagated by contagion, irrespective of exposure to putrescence? Can it originate from the contagion of typhus? Is the relation of the local to the general malady the same as in typhus? And do the principles of treatment materially differ? Again, we must put to ourselves this most important query: Does sanitary reform, in providing a supply of pure air, pure water, sufficient drainage, and so on, act by extinguishing the sources of epidemical disease?

[1] That, notwithstanding, the presence of filth does not itself presuppose the presence of fever will appear from the facts relative to certain places in the country districts of Ireland, which will be found in Appendix A.

Or is it that by the consequent improvement of the health of the population the community is better able to resist illness, be it contagious or non-contagious, and to lessen its severity when it does supervene?

This, I apprehend, is, in the present state of our knowledge, the safe and practical way in which to regard these all-important questions. Civilization demands that all deleterious influences, all that offends the senses, should be removed or checked, and the population of a country placed under the most favourable sanitary conditions, especially as to its supply of air, water, food, and clothing; but the subject is a wide one, and embraces far more than the actual origin of endemical or even epidemical disease.

With reference to the presumed origin of that form of fever called by Dr. Murchison the *Pythogenic Fever*, I would warn you, without in the slightest degree throwing doubt on the value of his researches, not to follow the system of attributing complex phenomena, or states of things, to a single cause, or to a too limited number of causes.

" This supposition of a single cause of the effects we witness is quite unsupported by nature. Every animal, every plant, every rock, requires for its production the co-operation of many causes that we know of, and most probably of many more that we have not yet discovered. All nature depends ultimately upon a single cause, but it has pleased that Almighty Cause that the effects which concern us immediately should arise from the co-operation of several of His creatures."[1]

There is another habit against which I would put you on your guard : the one, namely, of holding that every disease of which a description appears in our nosologies is a peculiar and isolated entity, separated by hard and fast lines from any other either in its nature or in its exciting cause. The attention of physicians has been awakened to the doctrine of the correlation of zymotic diseases,[2] a doctrine which has been long suspected to be true by practical men.

Yet, it may be asked, can we not go a step further, and consider whether essential diseases are not *convertible* as well as correlative ? I think that before the session is over you will meet with instances which will incline you to arrive at both conclusions. Cases will occur to you, especially during the prevalence of an epidemic, where the disease seems to hesitate as to what particular character it will assume, so that it is often a matter of the most extreme difficulty, even

[1] Observations on Contagion. By Whitley Stokes, M.D., p. 25.
[2] Zymotic Diseases, their Correlation and Causation. By A. Wolff, F.R.C.S. Eng. 1872.

when an eruption is well out, to say to which of the exanthemata the individual case belongs. Under such circumstances the public used to regard it as a mark of ignorance if the attendant were unable to give an exact name to the malady, but they are more enlightened now.

APPENDIX A.

The following are some extracts of a letter from a gentleman of great ability and truthfulness, who holds an important public appointment in the South of Ireland. He had been requested by the commissioners of a town in that part of the country to inspect the state of the town and report on the works necessary for sewage improvement.

It was about the year 1865, when there was some apprehension of an epidemic of cholera :—

"I went," says this gentleman, "through every lane and street, and examined all the tenements of every class in the latter end of January or beginning of February. There were no main sewers in any but the principal streets, and none of these had them for their whole length. The lanes and alleys leading off from these streets were mostly very narrow, and had no outfalls for sewerage discharge except surface channels, and very few of the houses had any back entrance; a good many had neither yards nor back entrances. But all had dung-pits. If not behind, they were contrived in the widest parts of the lanes by being sunk and inclosed with walls, so as to hold from 8 to 12 cubic yards of manure each. Where the tenement had not the 'easement' of a dung-pit or yard, or right to part of the common way, the manure was stored *in* the dwelling house. Most of the houses were thatched cabins, but several rows of two-storied houses were built, and a good many one-storied slated houses of small size were to be found containing four apartments. I discovered in one of these rows, which had very small backyards (not half the size of the house in any case), that the whole of the ground-floor, and part of the house, except the staircase and passage leading to it, were filled with manure (the scrapings of the roads and streets) tightly packed to the height of eight feet ; and in the rooms above there were two families living—one in each room. The manure had of course heated, and was steaming up through the chinks of a badly-laid floor, the under side of which was dripping wet from the the fermentation below.

"In several of the rows having backyards the surface water was allowed to run through the whole length of the lane from yard to yard, and the occupier of the lowest tenement was looked upon as having the most valuable holding of the whole lot, and something like the Chinese care of liquid manure was shown by extra mould or refuse being provided to absorb or soak it up. The parts of the town to which this description may apply covered about 25 acres, and almost every part of that surface was teeming with effluvia from such decayed substances of every sort as are admitted to be of the most noxious kind, without any provision whatever for carrying off the putrid water which is always to be seen in so wet a climate as this.

"The population is about 6000, of which two-thirds live in cabins furnished with the inevitable dung-pit. These cabins contain 700 families at the least. The dung-pit averages 10 cubic yards in content, so that on 25 acres we have at least 7000 cubic yards of fetid matter, with 4000 people breathing the exhalation of such an accumulation as could not, I think, be found elsewhere in Ireland.

"But nevertheless this town has always been *a remarkably healthy place.* There is a fever hospital which has not been full since the famine dysentery in 1847–8, and which is very frequently empty. There is no dislike on the part of the poor to go into this hospital, because it is not the workhouse, so that the few fever cases that do occur are quickly removed out of the crowded houses.

"It was asked—'How can such a state of things be? or how can it be accounted for that such good public health can exist amidst all this rottenness giving rise to the miasmata so well known as certain producers of fever and cholera?' I suggested that there were two great advantages in favour of health, namely: an ample supply of the very best water and *smoky houses.* The subsoil of the town is gravel and sand to a great depth, and in this there are many strong springs, the purest water being met with at 6 or 8 feet under the surface. The fuel used is all turf, and the blackened walls of the inside of the houses showed that the inhabitants lived in an atmosphere of peat smoke. I cannot help thinking that such smoke, possessing as we know preserving or antiseptic properties, must act as a deodorizer and preventive against infection or malaria.

"I asked one of the occupiers who lived over his dung-heap in an upper floor how he could expect to escape death by fever or cholera to himself or some of his family (a wife and five children), and his reply was, 'Sure we might as well be dead as never to have a bit of dung for the garden.'

"Some legislator has said that 'Ireland is an anomaly'—may be the sanitary statistics of this town are another proof of this."

The inhabitants of this town escaped the endemical disease so common in other towns of the south of Ireland, perhaps because, in addition to the pure water and turf smoke, an intimacy with malaria for many generations had at last made them insusceptible to it.

Dr. Pratt, in a paper read before the Surgical Society of Ireland, recently touched upon this same question. After alluding to the widely accepted theory of the actual origin of fever, as proceeding from the decomposition of animal and vegetable matter, he observes that "after an experience of nearly a quarter of a century as an Irish dispensary medical officer, it is his firm conviction that these agencies alone considered cannot be productive of fever of any type. Were it otherwise, Ireland would before this have been depopulated from sea to sea."

"Among the Irish agricultural classes," he adds, "the farm yards are simply the open spaces either in the front of their dwellings or close behind, the offices, cow-houses, stables, etc., forming a component part of them: the farm-yard manure carefully heaped, in many instances up to the very door, and in such a way that it often becomes a problem to the perplexed doctor, whose aid is desired within, how to effect an approach (especially when called on in the dead of night) without sticking ankle deep in mire or filth, or, perhaps, coming to a worse grief in the shape of a souse in a slough of despond.

"Such is the state of affairs during the winter months. In the hot weather of summer the pits from which the accumulated manure has been removed to the farm, serve as receptacles for slops and refuse of all sorts thrown from the houses. These slops, fermenting in warm weather, produce a green stagnant pool. The gases generated show themselves as bubbles on the surface, which in due time burst, and, of course, discharge their *supposed* noxious contents in the immediate vicinity of the dwelling, with all its inmates, old and young."

Dr. Pratt observes that, in such places, a case of fever, of any type, rarely occurs; the average length of life is high, and illness, except common colds and infantile diseases, is almost unknown.

Even in instances where the peasantry live in a worse condition, the cattle, pigs, and poultry occupying the same room, and the refuse being swept into a pit close by the fireside, he has found the families hale and sound, and strangers to fever.

LECTURE VI.

VARIETIES OF FEVER as observed (1) in different epidemics, (2) in the same epidemic, and (3) in members of the same family, living under the same conditions—This last-named fact is corroborative of the doctrine of the essentialism of fever—Definition of the term *epidemic character* of fever—Outbreaks of 1818–19, 1826–27, and 1847 contrasted—*Typhus* and *typhoid* or *enteric* fever appear to be but species of the same genus—Contagiousness of typhoid fever—Dr. Flint's memoir—Principles of treatment of fever of any type must be based on an acquaintance with the *law of periodicity*, to which the disease is subject.

THE varieties of fever depend upon diverse circumstances. We may take, for instance, the disease in its epidemic character. It may be laid down as an axiom that no two epidemics of fever have been precisely similar as regards the character and aspect of the disease presented to our observation on the two occasions. No doubt in the history of a series of epidemics, extending over a space of many years, some—nay, many—cases analogous in symptoms, and even similar in their mode of termination and in their result, may come under our notice. Thus, if the outbreak of 1830 is compared with that of 1820, cases will be found recorded in the history of the morbility of the former year the counterparts of which, so far as relates to symptoms, sequelæ, and result, may have been observed ten years before. Apart, however, from individual exceptions, when any two or more epidemics are taken into consideration, they will generally appear to differ widely one from another.

But not only has this diversity of type and character been noticed in distinct epidemics, separated by intervals of time, but even in one and the same epidemic numerous cases have occurred, characterized by symptoms essentially distinct, and marked by as widely varied conditions of the bodily system. In one group of cases there will be present utter prostration of strength, and intense depression of vital energy; in another group we may observe abundant vitality and almost unimpaired muscular and nervous force. In the same epidemic, again, fevers may vary in duration; one lasting but five days, another not terminating till the fortieth or forty-fifth day, or even later. Once more, we find infinite variations as to the period of the essential disease at which secondary complications will show themselves. In some cases the secondary affections in one or more organs may not become developed or apparent until after the twenty-first or even the forty-second day of the disease. The seat, too, of complications may be in one set of cases the brain, in another the thorax, and in a third the abdomen.

We may trace this Protean character of fever even further. That in two epidemics, separated it may be by a wide interval of time from each other, the type of the disease, its attendant phenomena, its complications, its duration, and so on, should vary much was perhaps not to be marvelled at. That even in the same epidemic the disease should present varying forms and characters is more remarkable, though still easy of comprehension. But we can carry our investigations a step further, and we shall meet with still more striking results. When fever appears in a family, living in some confined situation in a large city or town, in a badly ventilated dwelling, perhaps in the midst of an unwholesome and densely populated neighbourhood, several members of that family may be struck down by the disease. They may sicken simultaneously or one after the other, so that we are afforded an opportunity of witnessing the effect of the malady on them individually. Under such circumstances it has been observed that a marked variety is presented in the condition of the several patients. One will have the disease in its severest form, another will experience but a mild attack; some will suffer from protracted fever; others will go through an illness of the briefest duration; one will have petechiæ, another will present no eruption; one will display critical phenomena, whilst another will recover without crisis of any kind ; one will have typhus, another typhoid, or even rheumatic, fever.

Now this is a most remarkable fact, and one strongly corroborative of the doctrine of essentialism in fever. We might à priori suppose that where there existed a certain similarity in the physical and moral characteristics of persons so closely related by consanguinity, so alike in habits from living together, and so uniformly subjected to the same mode of life, those persons when exposed to the influence of one and the same poison or virus of contagious fever would present one and the same type of the disease.

It is of the greatest importance, gentlemen, that you should devote your most attentive consideration to reflections such as these in your study of fever, in order that you may be prepared for any exigency arising from the varied and complex aspects in which the disease will present itself before you—in order that you may be duly armed and fitted to encounter the deadly, the subtle enemy you will have to meet.

The constancy in variability of which I have just spoken in relation to fever applies also to all forms of local epidemics. As in the case of individuals, so of epidemics, one outbreak of fever will be marked by profound prostration of the system, by a loss of strength requiring the exhibition of stimulants, while another will present evidences of a sthenic condition of the patients, calling for an exactly opposite mode of treatment. This is what is termed the *epidemic character* of the disease. I remember the fever of 1818 and 1819, the equally formidable outbreak of 1826 and 1827, and lastly the great epidemic of 1847. If we compare the first with the last of these visitations, we shall find that they possess many points of resemblance. Both were examples of severe typhus fever, both had maculæ in patches, both were petechial. The epidemic of 1826–27 was of a milder but more diffusive type; in it vast numbers were indeed attacked by the fever, but the great and profound sinking of the system which prevailed in the other epidemics I have mentioned was not present in this.

So widely spread was the last-named epidemic (that of 1826–27) that at the Meath Hospital we were obliged to have additional accommodation for patients provided. Sheds were built, canvas tents were erected, their floors covered with hay, on which the crowds of patients conveyed to the hospital in carts were literally *spilled out*. I have seen as many as ten patients lying on the hay awaiting their turn to be attended to. In fact, so immense was the number of sufferers that it became impossible to bestow medical care upon them all ; indeed, a large number of them got no medicine whatever, but all received reasonable care and comfort. Abundance of whey was provided, and on this, without any further treatment, numbers got well through the fever—as Dr. Rutty, speaking of the year 1739, quaintly observed, "abandoned to the use of whey and God's good providence." I doubt not that the mortality among those treated after this primitive fashion was not greater than that among the patients subjected to medical treatment *secundum artem*. It should be observed that there was more of an inflammatory character evinced in this epidemic, the skin being hot and dry, the pulse hard and full, etc.

Fever, you are aware, has been somewhat arbitrarily divided into two classes, or placed under two great heads—*typhus* and *typhoid*. Typhus fever is held to take its origin from the vitiated air and the unhealthy condition of body resulting from the crowding together of masses of human beings, coupled, perhaps, with neglect of cleanliness, absence of proper ventilation, clothing, and food, and the prevalence of indolent and disorderly habits. The emanations arising from over-crowding, or ochlesis, as it is termed, doubtless predispose in an extra-ordinary degree to the outbreak and spread of this form of fever, a form of the disease which has received various titles—some from its connection with ochlesis, as *camp fever*, *jail fever;* others from the peculiar morbid phenomena attending it, as *putrid* fever (when it displays a tendency of the solids to run into decomposition); *spotted* fever (from the maculæ or spots so frequently observed on the surface of the body in this form of disease) ; and others again from its well-known formidable character and too often fatal result, as *typhus gravior*, *malignant fever*, etc.

Typhus also is regarded as being the more dangerous form of the disease, but I am by no means convinced that this opinion is correct. There is, however, one reason why this idea should be entertained by British physicians; the epidemics of fever which have been most fatal in these countries have been of the typhus kind, whilst it may be said that we have had repeated visitations of the typhoid form of fever attended with a comparatively slight mortality. Typhus fever, when it comes, at once assumes the true epidemic character, whereas typhoid more frequently prevails endemically, and with less direct fatal results.

Typhoid, enteric, or pythogenic fever is generally attributed to emanations from putrid matter, or, according to Dr. Budd, to the exposure to contagious matter contained in the evacuations of patients suffering under the disease. This contagious matter may be introduced into the system either through the medium of the air in a gaseous form or by means of contaminated drinking water. Typhoid fever is considered to be essentially an epidemic disease; in other words, it may occur in particular situations. The opinion was almost universally held that this form of fever was non-contagious, but the adherents to this doctrine are becoming less numerous of recent years. If it were a fact that typhoid fever was not a contagious disease, we should have a marked and important distinction at once established between it and typhus, but it is not so. I do not say that typhoid fever is so contagious as typhus, yet I will not admit that the former possesses the attribute of being non-communicable. I would strongly urge you, gentlemen, to be very cautious in admitting the line of distinction which authors have drawn between these forms of disease as regards the question of contagion, and you may depend upon it that the number of diseases propagated by contagion is much greater than what is generally admitted. We can found no distinction between typhus and typhoid upon the circumstance that one of these fevers, as, for instance, typhus, is contagious and the other not. I have long believed in the contagion of the non-petechial, or, if you will, the typhoid fever of this country. In the epidemic of 1826–27, to which I have before referred, and which was essentially an epidemic with the so-called anatomical characters of the typhoid disease, we had abundant proofs of contagion; and in this very hospital many of our most zealous students were at that time attacked with fever.

It may be here observed, that although this epidemic was one essentially of the so-called typhoid form, characterized by absence of the symptoms of putrescence, by frequent relapses, by recovery, by crisis, and in very many cases by evidences of disease of the intestinal glands; yet the attendants on the sick, when they were themselves attacked, presented in many cases the symptoms of genuine typhus. It was during this epidemic that I contracted typhus fever; and shortly afterwards one of my clinical clerks, who had been distinguished for his zeal in his attendance on the sick, fell ill. We both had bad maculated typhus without any symptoms of dothinenteritis; in my case the disease ran a course of fourteen days; and in neither instance was there any relapse.

A very remarkable instance of the contagiousness of typhoid fever has been placed on record by Dr. Austin Flint, of Buffalo, United States, in a memoir "On the Transportation and Diffusion by Contagion of Typhoid Fever," published in 1852. In a small isolated community, consisting of nine families, at North Boston, county of Erie, New York, typhoid fever had been quite unknown up to the autumn of 1843. Indeed, in no part of the county of Erie was the disease known to have occurred up to the time mentioned. On the

21st of September in that year, however, a young man from Warwick, Massachusetts, being on a journey westward, took lodgings at the tavern of North Boston, kept by a man named Fuller. He had been ill for several days, undoubtedly labouring under typhoid fever. He died on the 19th of October at the tavern, which was a place of daily resort for the members of seven families, with one exception living within a few rods of each other. One family, consisting of several persons, was on terms of hostility with the innkeeper, and so all intercourse was precluded. Twenty-three days after the arrival of the stranger, two members of the innkeeper's family were attacked with the disease from which he suffered. Subsequently five other cases occurred in this family. In all the other families, with one exception already noted, cases more or less numerous were observed within the space of about a month from the date of the case first developed after the stranger's arrival; and during this period more than one-half the population became affected. The family in which no case occurred was the only one of the seven which was not brought into direct contact with the disease. The other two families resided at a distance, and seemed to be out of the reach of infection.

So extraordinary was this outbreak that the popular opinion in the neighbourhood was that the head of the family in feud with Fuller the innkeeper had *poisoned* a well used daily by the latter, and by six other families, of which five were attacked. That this opinion was not correct was proved by a careful examination of the water by two leading chemists of Buffalo, when it was found to be *remarkably pure*, "the only foreign ingredient detected being a small proportion of saccharine substance, which was explained by the fact that the vessel in which the water was transported had previously been used as a molasses jug."

Typhus, again, is said to be an *essential* disease, affecting the entire economy; whilst typhoid has been looked on as a *non-essential*, or merely a symptomatic affection. The inadmissibility of this view has already been, I trust, sufficiently indicated in a former lecture. It is a doctrine at variance with practical experience; it is a theory quite incompatible with observed facts. Owing to the ever-varying nature of fever, many of its secondary phenomena may or may not be present—we may have typhus without measly eruption or maculæ; we may have typhoid without diarrhœa, rose-spots, or any other symptom said to be pathognomonic. We are compelled to admit that pathological anatomy has failed as a means of pointing out any essential distinction between these two forms of fever. Anatomy, it is true, may reveal to us certain morbid changes and abnormal conditions in different organs in many cases of either typhus or typhoid. But these alterations are only the results, not even the necessary or constant results, of the primary disease; and so they throw no light upon the object of our search—a vital distinction between the two fevers.

Even as regards the presumed causes of the diseases—ochlesis, civic miasm, poverty, hunger, or cold—are not the conditions supposed to be requisite for the development of typhoid present in cases where typhus is generated by overcrowding? Are not filth, putrescence, impure water, and foul air probably existent in such a state of things? Do these influences produce at one time pythogenic, and at another typhus, fever? Do they excite both diseases at once in the same individual? Does A get typhus, while B, exposed to the very same influences, and under perfectly similar circumstances, contracts typhoid?

The treatment of fever, whether it be typhus or typhoid, is reducible to a simple formula, and is essentially the same in both types of disease. We know of no cure for fever; no man has ever cured it. It is, however, curable spontaneously. If you leave it to its own course, it is capable of curing itself. It will spontaneously subside. Remembering the law of periodicity, the great object of the physician should be to gain time, preserving the patient from the dangers which threaten him, which belong to this special state of life. If he can be kept alive to the 14th day, the 21st, the 36th, or even the 60th day, recovery will probably ensue. Every day, every hour of existence preserved and sustained is a clear gain. The risks that he runs are due to debility or to the influence of the secondary affections. We, so to speak, cure the patient by preventing him from dying. We endeavour to gain our end by combating the exhaustion which threatens to prove fatal to him with food, with stimulants, and with tonics. We seek to obviate or to modify the dangers of the local diseases by meeting them as early as we can discover their presence, bearing in mind the depressing influence of the general malady. Herein lies the secret of the treatment of fever. We watch the progress of the disease throughout its varying phases; we meet by judicious treatment, as they arise, the symptoms of secondary and local malady; we sustain the system as far as practicable; we preserve the sufferer at the least expense to the constitution; and we wait patiently until the hour shall strike when, in accordance with the mysterious law of periodicity, the fever shall have departed and convalescence shall have begun.

LECTURE VII.

POINTS OF RESEMBLANCE in the various forms of fever a more practical subject for investigation than their distinctions—As regards the principles of prognosis, diagnosis, and the management, various forms of fever lose their separate and individual significance—Points of resemblance between typhus and typhoid—The famine fever in 1847—Recapitulation.

REFERRING to the last lecture, it may be observed that in these days the attention of investigators on fever has been directed rather to the distinctions between its various forms than to their points of resemblance, and yet it may be asked whether, looking at the end and object of the study of disease, the latter consideration is not the more important.

Indeed, the more experience of essential disease a man acquires the less value he will attach to the classification of it, at least in these latitudes; for though he will find that the mere nosological distinctions (as given in books) are abundant, yet the grounds of action in practice depend more on the general nature of disease than on its specific characters, which, though sufficiently well marked under certain circumstances, are not so fixed as to warrant the belief that they indicate an absolute speciality in disease.

This seems more certain in those forms of essential disease which are classed under the general head of Continued Fevers, such as typhus, relapsing or famine fever, and the typhoid or enteric—the pythogenic fever of Dr. Murchison.

There can be no doubt that in a fever hospital you will see various cases not presenting the same characters. One patient is prostrated at an early period of his illness, his nervous system much affected, the heart weak, and the skin covered with petechial spots, while in the next bed may be one with comparatively little of the nervous symptoms, without eruption, except a few rose spots on the front of the body, and with less prostration; his condition does not seem so alarming as that of his neighbour, but it may be that *his* disease will prove fatal, while in the other case there will be a perfect recovery.

Between these two cases you may find many other points of difference in the history, the exciting cause, the amount of prostration, and the seat and apparent extent of local change. You may, if you will, call one of them typhus and the other typhoid, pythogenic, or enteric

4

fever. That will do no harm. The name of the disease would be an important question if it implied such a difference in nature as would call for a complete difference in treatment. But as regards the great principles of prognosis, diagnosis, and the management which will assist nature in the effort to throw off the disease, they are the same; and so far these cases, though they may individually differ, yet seem to belong to the same family.

I have said that I hold the study of the resemblances or points of agreement among these diseases, to be of more value than that of their differences, and for this reason, that the former bears on the question of treatment much more than does that of their distinctions.

Now, remembering that fever is a condition of which it cannot be said that there is any certain anatomical character, it may be held, even if we confine ourselves to but two forms—typhus and typhoid :—

First:—that they are both essential fevers, in which the local disease is secondary to, and produced by, the general ailment.

Secondly:—that the general malady is influenced by the laws of periodicity.

Thirdly:—that its symptoms may be modified by the local secondary affections, as to their seat, complications, period of appearance, intensity, retrocession, and behaviour under treatment.

Fourthly:—that in both diseases the local affections are inconstant as to seat, period of appearance, intensity, complication, and subsidence; varying according to the locality, the duration of the malady, the epidemic character, the exciting causes, the habit of body, and the influence of treatment.

Fifthly:—that both may exist, and even run their course, without the production of recognizable local disease. This appears to be more often true in the case of typhus than of the other forms of fever, yet even in the typhoid or enteric fever there is no constancy of relation between the symptoms and the local change, and in both the local diseases are inconstant in seat, amount, and time of appearance, and incompetent to explain the phenomena of the malady.

Sixthly:—that these local diseases are, like the general affections, subject to the law of periodicity—that is, they spontaneously subside, sometimes before the disappearance of the fever, at other times afterwards.

But when reactive irritation sets in, various structural changes may occur, and the fever originally essential may become more or less symptomatic. This we may see in very prolonged cases of typhoid.

There are yet other points of resemblance, of which the most important is that both forms of disease are contagious, though probably in different degrees. This is now admitted by the best observers. Furthermore, there is a species of evidence more often attainable in an Irish than a British hospital. You know that we have not unfrequently in the wards the whole, or nearly the whole, of a family sick of fever. The patients have occupied the same dwelling, too often the same room, and they have sickened successively and within short intervals of time. It is difficult to believe but that there has been a similarity in the exciting cause of disease in all, and there is a strong probability that the sickness of one has promoted that of another. Now, in this group what do we find? Is it that the same character of fever affects them all? Nothing of the kind—one patient may be in maculated typhus; in another there is no eruption; in another the case is typhoid, or the so-called pythogenic or enteric fever; and so on among them. Even cases of rheumatic fever may occur. But this is not all; second attacks arise, but these are not necessarily—not, I might say, even commonly—repetitions of the first ailment or group of symptoms. In the typhus fever patient they may be those of typhoid; in the non-maculated there may be abundant maculæ. In the other cases similar circumstances occur, the second attack presenting types differing from the first; one has a short fever, another a long one; one a complicated, the other a comparatively simple attack; one with predominance of cerebral, another with that of pulmonary symptoms, and another with all those of enteric or pythogenic fever; one requiring stimulants in the second attack, though there was no failure of circulation in the first; and similar differences may be seen as to the remaining complications.

Do not these facts point to the conclusion that there is but a slight tension, so to speak, in the individuality or separate characters of the various forms of fever, and that in their essence and from a practical point of view they may be looked on as species rather than genera— the genus being fever, that condition on which anatomical investigations, in the words of Graves, throw but a negative light? I tell you —not that you are to look at every case of fever as similar in character, in complications—that would be bad teaching, as your experience would soon convince you—but that it is a condition much more various than you would suppose, were you to form your notions of it from books. Its many forms are closely related. The exciting causes of one may produce another; the secondary effects have not the constancy which authors describe in seat, in number, in complications, or in effect on the general malady. These forms of disease have all two great characters in common—essentiality and periodicity. Why they differ in general and local phenomena it is hard to say, but we know little of the receptivity of the living body, the laws of the variations of that receptivity, and those which govern its results. This department of vital chemistry is still to be worked out, nor does the study of the apparent exciting causes of the various forms of fever give us much stronger grounds for belief in their essential differences. Dr. Murchison, in his treatise on the Continued Fevers of Great Britain, a work which is one of the greatest ornaments of English medical literature, enters at length into the distinctions between typhus and the relapsing or famine fever, and labours to show that while the one can be traced to overcrowding, the cause of the other is destitution. Yet he admits the observations of Alison, David Smith, and Henry Kennedy, which show that in one epidemic, in the same family, even from the same bed, both forms of fever have been observed. In wide-spread epidemics, he observes, we may have at first relapsing fever only, then relapsing fever and typhus together, and, last of all, typhus alone. "Whatever be the explanation," he says, "the circumstance is remarkable; but it does not justify the conclusion that the two fevers are identical."[1] And he says further on: "As far as I know, the statement remains uncontroverted, that in all cases where fever can be proved to have been imported into a locality by a single case, typhus has produced typhus; and relapsing fever, relapsing fever."

To a great extent the observations which I have offered as to the relationship between typhus and typhoid seem to apply to that between typhus and the relapsing or famine fever. I think the name of "Famine Fever" one of doubtful fitness. In the epidemic of 1847–48, which followed the disastrous famine of Ireland, the contagious nature of the disease was too well established, as shown by the terrible mortality of the members of the medical profession, and of many of the country gentlemen. Now, if ever the characters of typhus were shown, it was then. Every form of continued fever occurred—in thousands of cases—relapsing fever, typhoid or enteric fever, and the worst form of typhus that could be seen. All the forms were contagious, and this, whether the subjects of the disease had or had not been exposed to destitution or overcrowding. The truth seems to be that, while every separate epidemic has more or less of a common character, all great epidemics (at least in this country) may be called mixed, so far as the occurrence of individual cases is concerned. All the circumstances which we have noted as to the relation of typhus to typhoid may be said to occur as to relapsing fever.

---

[1] A Treatise on the Continued Fevers of Great Britain. Second ed. 1873, p. 342.

Without discussing how much is owing to destitution and how much to the attendant overcrowding, whether two epidemic diseases run their courses *pari passu*, or whether the fever, of whatever form it may be, has been modified by the previous starvation—let us deal with some important facts observed in this hospital in the epidemic of 1847.

Although, as might be expected, the number of deaths from famine within the precincts of Dublin, as compared with the country districts, was trifling, still we had not a few opportunities of observing the effects of famine in these wards. Many sufferers from want of food made their way into the city, and falling down exhausted in the streets, were conveyed by the police to the hospital. They had all a strange resemblance. The face—and indeed the whole of the body—showed a dusky hue, the eyes were sunken and with little expression, the features pinched and marked by a profound melancholy; the surface was cool, either dry and shrivelled, or clammy, and in all cases the body exhaled a heavy earthy smell. These people were as a rule apathetic; they made no complaint, but seemed only anxious to be placed in bed and allowed to rest. They asked for neither food nor drink. There were no symptoms of fever, and the natural desire of all who saw them was to give a generous support. But it was speedily found that such a course was a dangerous—it might be said, a fatal one. In several cases animal food and wine seemed to act like a deadly poison, and even where a more cautious use of nutriment was adopted, the patients being fed as infants for days together until the collapse seemed to be overcome, the system would, as it were, explode into the very worst form of maculated typhus, in which death commonly occurred on the fifth day of the fever, and in some cases even earlier. And this is to be noted in relation to the reports of the relapsing fever as observed at the London Hospital in 1843, where the desire for food was general. Similar observations were made in Glasgow and elsewhere, and this craving appetite, not alone in the remission but in the paroxysm of the fever, is appealed to as evidence that the relapsing form of fever is really a famine fever.

But whether the character of frequent recurrence of short attacks of fever be owing to the previous contamination of the system by starvation or not, we shall not discuss. Certain it is that relapses had been common in our wards after 1830. But to say that the epidemic character observed was that of a relapsing fever—namely, a short fever with intervals of apyrexia—is to give a very imperfect idea of the disease. Since then the typical relapsing fever—the five day fever—has been often met with, sometimes showing an epidemic tendency,.

but in very many instances being apparently unconnected with destitution. I may observe that in such cases enlargement of the spleen
was common, and that in no case did the exhibition of quinine in the
intervals of the fever prevent the relapse.[1]

But in Ireland an interesting circumstance in relation to the terrible famine fever was that, in a few years after the cessation of the
epidemic of 1847, fever, which for so many years seemed rooted
throughout the land, gradually disappeared to a singular degree.
The numerous fever hospitals in the country towns were closed, disposed of, or otherwise utilized, and I remember a period of several
years in which our wards were all but empty. We may leave to
others to speculate on the cause of this.

About this time the level of Lough Neagh, in the County Antrim,
was much reduced by arterial drainage, and a large space of marshy
ground on its shores rendered dry. Fever, which had been long prevalent in this locality, was observed to have become very rare, and
this was attributed to the drainage; yet it is more likely that the subsidence of the *endemic* typhus was but an example of the change
which had occurred over the whole country.

Let me recapitulate some of the leading points as to fever which
cannot be too deeply engraved on your minds:—

Its essentiality.

Its contagiousness in various degrees.

Its existence often independently of local or anatomical change.

The relation of the local to the essential malady.

The influence of the local malady upon the general fever.

The inconstancy as to seat, time of appearance, number, importance, and complication of the local or secondary affections,
and their incompetence to explain or account for the phenomena of fever.

The periodicity of these phenomena, seen not alone in the general
malady, but more or less in the secondary affections.

The occurrence of more than one form of fever in the same epidemic.

The speciality in character according to the epidemic.

The similarity in the principles of treatment of the general malady
and of the local changes.

These characteristics will serve as landmarks to you whether you
have to deal only with an isolated case of fever of any form, or with
a wide-spread epidemic of thousands of cases, and I believe they will

[1] See Murchison, loc. cit. p. 408.

more or less be found to apply to every form of the disease, and in every latitude of the world. Let them be engraved upon your minds. It may be necessary to say to the junior members of the class that I claim no originality in putting them forward. I believe that they existed in the minds of most practical and experienced men from the time of Fordyce to our own, and are based on their recorded observations.

Gentlemen, I speak to you, and I have always endeavored to do so, less as a teacher than as a fellow student—a senior one of course, but still, not as a master, but as a comrade.

We shall find as we advance in the true method of studying medicine—which is mainly, the practice of it—that we shall attach less weight to the distinctions and classifications of essential diseases given in books, instilled into our minds in our student days, and clinging to us in the early years of professional life, than to the facts connected with their history, resemblances, and treatment.

Believe me, we shall find this a better use of our time.

Medical literature and medical teaching give many lessons not written in the book of nature, and, when you stand face to face with disease, all such will have to be ignored or forgotten.

LECTURE VIII.

DIVISION OF FEVERS INTO ESSENTIAL AND SYMPTOMATIC—No anatomical expression for the disease—Secondary affections of fever—These may, and do, frequently produce organic changes—The presence of essential disease invalidates the ordinary rules of diagnosis—Illustrations of the truth of this statement—Local symptoms of fever are (1) *functional* or *nervous ;* (2) *anatomical,* i. e. depending on special anatomical changes ; (3) *secondary inflammatory,* i. e. arising from reactive inflammation, itself due to the typhous infiltration of some part or organ of the body—Similar symptoms may arise from essentially opposite conditions in disease—Illustrations of the proposition that *fever is capable of producing local symptoms without organic change.*

THE division of fevers into essential and symptomatic is admitted by most observers. I showed you that amongst essential fevers we may reckon a great variety of diseases. All the exanthemata are essential fevers; so also are influenza, rheumatic fever, typhus, typhoid, intermittent and remittent fevers, the plague, the yellow fever, and I believe we might also add cholera.

As I have already said, we may describe fever, without defining it, as being a special morbid state or condition of existence subject to the law of periodicity, in which the animal economy is found acting under apparently new laws. In this altered state of life general features common to all or to most cases are observed, but the accompanying secondary phenomena are many and extremely varied.

In my opinion, you may take this with you as the basis of your views on fever—that, in the present state of our knowledge, we possess no anatomical expression for the disease. We do not know why secondary affections are sometimes absent, or at what period they appear in various portions of the system. Even with the assistance of the microscope no anatomical character of fever is as yet discovered.

However, although it is capable of destroying life without the production of any anatomical change, we find that fever does frequently produce such organic changes, and that these in turn influence the symptoms of the malady.

The secondary affections of fever, from which such changes directly arise, are not to be regarded as separate diseases, distinct from the essential malady. It would be just as rational to assert that the various affections of syphilis—the cutaneous disorders, the periostitis, the ulceration of the throat, and so on—were distinct and separate diseases, as to say the same of the secondary and local complications of fever. The secondary affections in fever are not its anatomical character, for it precedes them and exists without them.

If such affections are confined to or predominate in the belly, we may have tympany, thirst, diarrhœa, and a variety of other symptoms. If the chest is engaged, we may have difficult breathing, livid countenance and the other conditions resulting from imperfect arterialization of the blood. A diseased intestine may cause death by exhaustion or by perforation, or a secondary bronchial affection or congestion of the lung may destroy life by asphyxia—not an uncommon case in individuals whose bronchial affection has been taken no note of in the early course of the fever. This secondary disease may have been long progressive ; it is often overlooked and neglected from its latency, and a large number of those cases in which death takes place from what is called effusion into the chest, attributed to debility or exhaustion, are in reality examples of a neglected bronchial affection, recognized only when it is too late.

Yet in essential fever we must be cautious in arriving at a just estimate of the value of symptoms, referable to either the brain, chest, or abdomen.

The existence of the state or condition of fever invalidates those rules of diagnosis which are so important where the essential disease is not present. Many sad mistakes in the treatment of fever are attributable to ignorance of this fact.

Suppose you find a man who is not the subject of essential fever suffering acute pain in the head, with delirium, injected eyes, rapid, hard pulse, and so on; the chances are that the man has arachnitis. But let him have such a fever, and this group of symptoms cannot be taken as indicative of the existence of local inflammation. You would commit a grave error were you to treat this man for a disease the presence of which it is impossible to assume from the symptoms, just because the man has essential fever.

Again, symptoms may arise indicating an affection of some part of the intestinal canal, and yet the stomach or intestines may be perfectly free from disease. Thus in nosological books we read that a hot, dry tongue, preternaturally red and parched, is a symptom of gastritis. So it might be if the patient had not fever. But we know that in many cases the treatment which would be proper were there no fever will not answer now. On the contrary, stimulants will probably be required. We give the man brandy, wine, and food, and the tongue becomes pale and moist.

The foregoing remarks lead me to speak more fully of the local symptoms in fever. These we find to be of several kinds. One class of them may be termed *functional* or *nervous;* that is to say, singular phenomena of functional alteration occurring without necessary or corresponding organic changes. I believe that there are none of the great organs of the body which in fever may not exhibit this curious class of symptoms. In connection with the brain we have delirium constantly as a functional condition in fever; pain also, convulsions, coma, and so on. If we go to the thorax we often find cough and accelerated breathing without any anatomical change of the lung. If we turn to the abdomen, we find many of the symptoms which are attributed to anatomical change, yet they may exist altogether independent of it. We find tenderness of the epigastrium, and yet no gastritis, no peritonitis, no inflammation of the liver; we find swelling of the abdomen, or diarrhœa, without any anatomical change; and so we observe that there are none of the great organs that may not occasionally exhibit symptoms depending, so far as we can ascertain, solely upon functional disturbance. This is the first class of symptoms.

The next class includes those which are connected with special anatomical change. We may have this change in the brain, lungs, heart, spleen, or in the glands of the intestine. In the lungs we recognize it by râle, cough, expectoration, the filling up of the tubes with muco-puriform matter, and on dissection, by tumefaction of the mucous membrane, attended by lividity, vascularity, softening, or even ulceration. In the heart we find it accompanied by signs of softening of this organ, generally speaking at first confined to the arterial or systemic heart. Many of you are, no doubt, familiar with the local changes which occur in the spleen and in the intestine.

Then we come to the third class of local affections in fever, and this is a very curious and important one. The condition of the parts here is, as it were, a compound one. The organ is supposed to have suffered infiltration of what is termed the typhous matter; it has become swollen and enlarged. This is a condition which is capable of retrocession, without any consequent injury to the part; but in certain cases this retrocession does not take place, or is interrupted by actual inflammation of the tissues which are thus infiltrated.

Thus we have three important classes of local affections, two of which, though organic at first, are not inflammatory, but may become complicated with secondary or reactive inflammation.

There is, I believe, a fourth set of local symptoms, or of local affections if you will, in fever, which has not, perhaps, received sufficient attention. I think it is extremely likely that, in certain cases, we have organs suffering from want of a natural supply of blood, and that this is extremely likely to take place as far as the nervous system, at all events, is concerned. Any of you that have turned your attention to the subject of the fatty degeneration of the heart—so often brought before the Pathological Society of Dublin—will recollect that one of the most remarkable symptoms of this affection is, that the patient is liable to repeated and extraordinary attacks of nervous disease, shown by a frequent threatening of syncope, or by apoplectic seizures continually repeated, sometimes without consequent paralysis, but in other cases with a temporary paralysis. This is an illustration of the development of important nervous symptoms, not from fulness or congestion of the brain, but from anæmia; and it is one of many illustrations of the great pathological proposition—that similar, or nearly similar symptoms, may arise from essentially opposite conditions. We know that apoplexy and paralysis frequently arise from hemorrhage into the brain; we find that they also arise from anæmia of the brain. In the disease to which I so long directed the attention of the classes in this hospital—the typhous softening of the heart—there is a probability that the brain, under those circumstances, suffers from anæmia; and it may be—though this is a point which has not been sufficiently worked out—that some of the extraordinary nervous symptoms in fever, to which we can assign no anatomical cause, really proceed from an anæmic condition of the brain, the result of a temporary softening or weakening of the left ventricle—in fact, that in typhoid or in typhus fever there is produced, for a certain number of days, the condition which is seen as a chronic state in the fatty degeneration of the heart. It requires very little acumen to perceive that if the brain is liable to this fourth and curious set of local disturbances, other organs may suffer in the same way. I merely throw out this for your consideration. But we might inquire whether the tolerance of wine in fevers is in any way to be explained by an anæmic state of the brain. There are few things more curious than the power which is shown by patients in fever of bearing a quantity of wine or brandy without intoxication. They will often swallow many times more wine than would make them drunk if they had not fever, and wine becomes a sedative rather than a stimulant so far as symptoms are concerned. Does not this indicate a state of the brain the opposite in some respects to that of health? I do not want you to believe that all the good effect of wine is derived from its action on the weakened heart, for it may be that the direct influence of the stimulant itself on the nervous matter is the cause; but, whether we take one or both modes of action, its effect indicates a condition of the circulating and nervous systems the opposite to that of inflammation, as we understand the term.

We come now to think on this important proposition, that the condition of fever, or, if you will, the poison of fever, is capable of producing local symptoms without organic change. We can easily understand the poison of fever producing a general fever without any local symptoms, but it requires a good deal of teaching and observation to persuade men that the poison of fever is capable of producing local symptoms without any organic change. It is quite impossible to exaggerate the importance of this proposition as a guide in the practice of medicine, for it is because it has not been sufficiently accepted—because it has not been engraved upon the minds of medical and surgical students—that so much mischief is done in the treatment of fever.

Remember the grand rule—and if you did nothing else for the whole of the session but learn it, your time would be well spent—that those rules of diagnosis of local diseases which are to be accepted as true in cases which are not essential fever lose their value to a great degree when the primary disease is such. This applies to the local symptoms in connection with the three great cavities. You are not to apply the rules of diagnosis drawn from the observation of diseases which are not fever to the symptoms in fever, because fever is a special, essential state, and has its own conditions and its own rules. And this confirms the observation which I made in the introductory lecture, that the student, no matter how extensive his education may have been in surgery and in medicine outside a fever hospital, has really learned only half of his business if he has not studied fever at the bedside. In consequence of ignorance of this rule, men having a case of fever, with symptoms which, they had been led to believe, in cases not essential fever, were indicative of local inflammation, at once proceeded to treat the case as one of local inflammation.

The patient on the tenth or twelfth day of typhus fever is watchful, delirious, violent, complains of great distress in his head, and so on. Well, what does the practitioner do who has not learned this rule? He shaves the head; he applies ice to it; puts on a dozen or two of leeches; and what is the result? The result too frequently is, that the patient sinks rapidly. The symptoms in this case were not the result of inflammation of the brain; they were not from hyperæmia of the brain. There was, perhaps, an exactly opposite state: at all events it was not such as to require depletion; the patient was suffering under general debility, and he sank under the treatment. This is still a common case. I have seen applications of leeches to the head in an advanced stage of fever with delirium, almost as certainly fatal as a pistol shot through the brain would be. Here let me give you the observations of Louis illustrative of the actual value of the symptom of delirium as an indication of inflammation of the brain in fever; and I may mention here that as Louis' observations were drawn from the Continental typhoid fever, they must be considered as still more applicable to typhus, because in typhoid fever there seems to be a greater probability that the local symptom is more closely connected with the local irritation than it is here. He took, in the first place, twelve fatal cases of typhoid fever which did not present the symptom of delirium. In four of these cases he found redness of the brain, in six the brain was perfectly healthy, and in two there was slight cerebral softening. Now let us take his twelve other cases, in which delirium was an extremely prominent symptom. In many of them the patients were violently delirious. In five of these cases there was redness of the brain, in five it was perfectly healthy, in one there was slight softening, and in one slight injection.

Now compare these two sets of results. Where there was no delirium four patients presented redness of the brain; where there was delirium five presented redness of the brain. Where there was no delirium in six the brain was perfectly healthy; where there was violent delirium in five it was free from disease. The other cases may go for nothing. This result is extremely valuable, as showing how very little we can depend upon the symptoms of excitement of the brain as an indication of inflammation when the patient is in essential fever.

Now let us go to some other organ—take the heart. " Well," you will say, " the heart need not be taken, because in most of our cases the heart shows a depressed and not an irritated state." But there are many cases of fever in which the heart is violently excited, as you will have frequent occasion to see. What is the result of dissection in these cases of excited heart in fever? There are two conditions which, according to ordinarily received notions, should lead you to expect irritation or inflammation of an organ: first, that the patient has fever, and next that you have an organ in a state of great excitement. If the patient had not typhus or typhoid fever, but had rheumatic fever and an excited heart, the chance would be that that organ would be found in a condition of inflammation. If a man has typhus or typhoid fever, and his lungs are excited, we find bronchitis or pneumonia; if his pleura is excited, we find pleuritis, and so on. But here is a case of typhus fever with extraordinary excitement of the organ, and when you come to dissect the parts you find the heart perfectly healthy—not the slightest sign of disease is found—and the same observation will frequently apply to the digestive system. You will have tenderness on pressure of the abdomen, extreme thirst, nausea, and vomiting. Yet on dissection the mucous membrane will be found pale, and there will be no sign of disease.

Again, take the eye. Delirium ferox with an injected eye is the expression of inflammation of the brain where the patient has not essential fever. But take a case of typhus or of typoid fever, and is the injected eye a sign of cerebritis? Certainly not. It is merely to be looked on as a local affection under the dominion of the general disease. The truth is that disease of a really inflammatory character is the rarest thing possible in typhus or typhoid fever; it is so rare that many do not believe that it ever occurs. Apply this axiom, then, to treatment, and see what becomes of that doctrine which advocates bleeding in fever, which advocates starvation and purging, and forbids the use of wine and other stimulants. There is another very important view or argument to be referred to here, which all practical men will understand. If fever was a group of inflammations, or if it was symptomatic of any one inflammation—in other words, if it was an inflammatory disease—we ought to expect that in the larger number of patients who had gone through the process of fever chronic diseases of organs would be developed. If a patient has acute rheumatism, we find that his heart may become engaged. He recovers from the rheumatism, and then he often has a progressive organic disease of his heart. When you reflect upon the extent of fever, the great number of persons that have been at some time in their lives attacked with fever, you should at once come to the conclusion that if those fevers were examples of groups of local inflammations, we should have a much greater quantity of organic local diseases consequent upon them: but what is the fact? The fact is that such accidents are extremely rare. How few cases can be adduced of confirmed mania as a consequence of fever. How few cases can be adduced of paralysis, of apoplexy, or of hydrocephalus as a consequence of fever. Surely if in this enormous number of cases of fever with violent head symptoms there had been inflammation of the brain, in some of them, at all events, we should have as a consequence progressive disorganization of the part.

Again, take the thorax. How few instances are there on record of chronic progressive pneumonia after fever; how few of chronic pleuritis; how few cases of atrophy of the lung; how few of anatomical changes which end in progressive organic disease, which has started from an inflammatory disease that took its origin pending a fever. Go to the heart. We have two classes of heart affections in fever—one a softening and weakening of the heart, and the other an excitement of the heart. I do not care which of them you take. Do we find that, after a recovery from fever, in persons who have had either of these affections of the heart during fever, there is a liability to valvular disease, that there is a liability to hypertrophy of the heart, that there is an adhesion of the pericardium? Nothing of the kind. The fact is that those organs have never been in a state of inflammation. They have suffered pending the fever, and the fever having terminated, the organs are restored to their normal condition. This is a very important consideration, and you may extend it still further. If fever was an inflammation of the bloodvessels, it is not to be supposed but that we should have many cases of disease of the aorta in the thousands of persons who have gone through fever. Yet we find no such results. If we go to the digestive system (and this is, perhaps, the system of all others which is most liable to organic change—at least in the Continental fevers), how few cases do we find—or have we any case to show—of chronic peritonitis as the result of fever? Not one that I know or ever read of; and yet the patient may have had symptoms of severe irritation of the abdomen pending his fever. In fact, all that we know of disease of the peritoneum in connection with fever is simply that, in certain cases of ulceration of the intestine, a solution of continuity of the peritoneum takes place, the fecal matter is effused into the cavity, and the patient dies of acute peritonitis. But that does not touch the argument. Where are the cases of chronic diseases of the liver springing out of typhus fever? It has been long a portion of medical doctrine—it has become traditional—and everything that is traditional in medicine is to be respected—that fever has a depuratory effect on the system. Now, whether it has such an effect or not we shall not here inquire; but the very fact of the existence of that doctrine, which is much older than pathological anatomy, implies, at all events, a general belief that fever does not necessarily lay the foundation of permanent damage to organs; for if it did damage the various organs that exhibit local symptoms in the course of the affection, we should not have the doctrine of its depuratory effects established. The cases of a chronic ulcerative condition of the intestinal tube might be adduced in opposition to these views, but I do not place very much weight upon them. We may divide them into two classes; in the one diarrhœa or some other symptom is established during the fever, which latter runs on indefinitely—here the typhous disease of the mucous glands has been attended with reactive irritation, and this has interfered with the action of the law of periodicity—so that the fever runs on indefinitely. In the next case the fever may be supposed to have ceased, but so much disorganization has occurred that the ulcerative process seems to go on as it might be supposed to do in another case where no typhus had preceded it.[1]

[1] The cases related by Dr. Cheyne in the first and second volumes of the *Dublin Hospital Reports* appear to be examples of this form of disease. He describes them as follows (vol. i. page 29): "In these cases the distress of the patient often bore no proportion to the danger he was in; the former was very little, while the latter was extreme. The disease would proceed without violent symptoms—nay, a patient would seem to be recovering, although without any critical discharge: he would call for full or middle diet, and for days would take his food regularly. The only circumstance in his situation which demanded attention was that he regained neither flesh nor strength; he expressed no desire to leave his bed. Then his pulse became quick and his tongue dry, and he would complain of dull pain or uneasiness in his belly, attended with soreness on pressure, and a degree of fulness in the upper part of the abdomen; the fulness was not elastic nor hard, nor indeed was it considerable. Then came on a loose state of the bowels and great weakness: probably at the next visit the patient was lying upon his back, with a pale, sunk countenance and a very quick, feeble pulse, his mind without energy. Then the stools (mucous) passed from him in bed, and the urine also; perhaps a hiccup came on; next his breathing became very frequent, in which case death was at no very great distance."

LECTURE IX.

LOCAL CHANGES IN FEVER are symptomatic, subject to *law of periodicity*, and probably depend on the presence of a specific typhous deposit—This deposit possesses a *vital*, specific character—Illustrations of this statement—The principal pathological conditions in fever are (1) *functional*, (2) *intercurrent*, and *secondary irritations* of (*a*) mucous membranes, (*b*) parenchymatous structures, (*c*) serous membranes, (3) *secondary irritations associated with typhous deposits*, (4) *independent typhous deposits*, (5) *reactive inflammations*, due to these deposits, (6) *softening of organs*— Effect of *locality* in determining the seat of secondary affections of fever—Effects of *social rank* in the same direction—Prognosis unfavourable and treatment by stimulation so far contra-indicated in cases where nervous symptoms preponderate.

IN the immediately preceding lecture we have seen that the presence of local symptoms during the course of an attack of fever does not necessarily imply or foreshadow the occurrence of any known anatomical change. To learn this point is to advance a great way in our knowledge of fever and of its treatment. On the other hand, observation during life and *post-mortem* inspection prove that local diseases involving alterations of structures—such as thickening, softening, vascularity, effusions, ulcerations, and gangrene—may be produced in various organs during the course of a fever.

Now, the great point in practice relating to these changes is, that they are symptomatic of the fever, secondary to the fever, and, in all probability, under the same law of periodic action as the general malady itself, at least so long as they remain uncomplicated with inflammatory reaction. They do not appear to begin with the fever, but they arise after it has existed for a certain time. There is the greatest variety in the period of their occurrence, and in their combinations; they may, as I have just now said, spontaneously subside with the fever; they may interfere with its critical termination; and, in certain cases where this does not occur, and when the general character of typhus disappears, progressive disorganization may go on in the structures which have been already affected.

In what way are we to consider the nature of these secondary affections in fever? It appears now pretty well established that in the follicular intestinal disease of the Continental fevers there is a special typhous deposit which, at least in the cases of recovery, is under the law, first of a progressive, and then of a retrogressive influence; just as in variola we observe the progressive maturation and absorption of the pustule. Recent pathologists have applied this principle to many other of the local diseases in fever; and although the existence of a special deposit is not yet so well or so fully established in the case of thoracic and cerebral complications, or at least in the case of parenchymatous as compared with membranous structures, still we may believe that an action analogous to that which occurs in the glands of Peyer and Brünner, though perhaps not so apparent, is developed in all the secondary diseases of fever which are not purely functional.

In speaking of a specific deposit in the secondary diseases of fever, I do not wish to convey to you the impression that this deposit presents any definite characters whereby it can be distinguished from other morbid products; for, even with the aid of the microscope, we cannot discover any special distinctive characters in the deposit found in the follicles of the intestine, or in other forms of the secondary affections of fever. It was at one time believed that the so-called " massa typhosa" did present special histological elements; but more recent research has shown that these views are erroneous. Still it is possible that, although we cannot determine the existence in it of any specific *physical* character, it yet possesses a *vital* specificism. Let us illustrate this by referring to two specimens of pus—one taken from the pustule of variola, the other from an ordinary abscess; histologically they will appear similar, yet that they have different vital characters no one can doubt. But other conditions are found associated with this typhous deposit, or occurring when we cannot demonstrate its existence. Under this head we class many of those appearances described as inflammatory—such as redness, softening, tumefaction, and so on.

Some have supposed that these states indicate a reactive inflammation, and that such does often occur, especially in the intestine, is abundantly proved by the researches of Rokitansky and various authors. I think it, however, extremely probable that in certain structures or organs—as, for example, the lung—these appearances of inflammation may precede or accompany the typhous deposit, or that they may occur even without such a deposit at all; and I think it likely that the liability to actual deposit is much less in the lung than in the intestinal glands, and greatly less in the brain and nerves than in either the thoracic or the digestive systems. Were it otherwise, typhous and typhoid fever would be more fatal diseases than they are, death being produced in the one case by coma, and in the other by asphyxia.

But, even though upon a close dissection we may not find anything

5

beyond the recognized appearances of inflammatory action of the mucous membrane, we are to believe that this condition, just like the typhous deposit, is secondary to the fever, and partakes of its specific character. It is not a simple idiopathic inflammation, nor is its existence to lead us into the errors of the antiphlogistic school. This condition, however, although specific and secondary, has still some characters of irritation, or inflammation if you will; and this fact points to the adoption, in certain cases, of a practice which, to the mere theorist, appears inconsistent—namely, the use of local depletion to relieve the suffering organ, while at the same time we employ a general tonic and stimulating medication.

Let me now indicate to you the principal pathological conditions with which, in the treatment of a case of fever, the physician has to deal.

First. We have those remarkable functional derangements which are unaccompanied by any known anatomical changes. They may occur in relation to any of the organs; but they are, perhaps, more important and certainly more frequent in the nervous than in the respiratory or digestive systems, at all events in typhus.

Secondly. We meet with intercurrent and secondary irritations or inflammations affecting principally the mucous membranes, less frequently the parenchymatous structures, and still less frequently the serous surfaces. These irritations, although not associated, so far at least as we can discover, with any special deposit, are nevertheless of a specific character, and under the influence of the laws which govern the general disease.

Thirdly. We have the conditions now specified associated with, though probably for a short time preceding, the typhous deposit, just as we see in variola the vascularity of the skin often preceding and accompanying the vesicular eruption.

Fourthly. We may observe the typhous deposit occurring independently of any other alteration, and apparently not associated with any irritative process.

Fifthly. We observe the reactive inflammation supervening on the typhous deposit—a condition which has been so well described by Rokitansky, and which may produce progressive ulcerations, abscess, or even sphacelus of the affected parts.

Lastly. There is a condition of softening of organs, upon the nature of which we have as yet no very definite ideas. In some instances it seems to be produced by an interstitial deposit of typhous matter, while in others it is difficult or impossible to prove the existence of such a deposit. This state of softening, as we shall presently see, is one of great practical importance. Its influence upon the heart, as you all know, is most remarkable. Its existence in that organ demands special attention, and there is good reason to believe that the same state, when affecting others of the involuntary muscles—such as those of the air tubes, and perhaps of the intestinal canal—has an important influence on the symptoms and progress of the disease.

I trust that, having followed me in the foregoing considerations as to a few of the pathological conditions of fever, you are now in a position to examine more closely some of the most remarkable local or secondary affections that may occur in the course of an attack of essential fever.

In their seat, if not in their nature, these affections are observed to vary in different countries. On the Continent—at least in France, and throughout a large portion of Germany—the frequency, and probably the preponderance, of the secondary disease of the intestines is a fact that must be admitted. So remarkable, indeed, is the predominance of the tumefaction and ulceration of the mucous glands of the intestine in France, that Andral, in the first edition of the *Clinique Médicale*, described fevers under the general head of diseases of the digestive system ; and yet Andral was no blind follower of Broussais. In Ireland, however, we do not find this remarkable preponderance of the secondary diseases of the digestive system ; but when I make this statement I wish you to understand and to adopt this principle that all descriptions of the anatomical characters of fever, as it prevails here or elsewhere, are to be accepted only so far as they apply to the prevailing epidemic. And although it is true that, on comparing the French typhoid fever with our typhus, the existence of follicular disease of the intestine appears to be almost the rule, and its absence the exception in the former affection, while in the Irish typhus this condition of the intestine is rare, you must bear in mind that in Ireland, in our own time, we have had a great epidemic of what was certainly typhus fever, in which the condition of the intestine accurately represented that which is found to prevail on the Continent. This is an important fact, and one which some of the Continental writers on pathology do not seem to be aware of, or they would not be so apt to adopt arbitrary distinctions and positive opinions on the matter. In the epidemic of the years 1826, 1827, and part of 1828, disease of the mucous glands of the intestine was so frequent that its existence might be held to be the rule, and its absence the exception ; and it is also true that intestinal ulcerations have been repeatedly observed in maculated typhus of Ireland, their amount and frequency varying with the epidemic influence. Let me refer you again to

Dr. Cheyne's papers in the first and second volumes of the *Dublin Hospital Reports.*

Similar observations have been made in Scotland also. What, then, shall we say of that doctrine which declares that there is an essential distinction or difference, marked by pathologico-anatomical characters, between the Continental fever and our typhus, or between the continued fever of Great Britain and fever as we have it in Ireland?—a difference to be expressed in this way, that in the Continental or in the British continued fever there is extensive ulceration of the intestine, while in the Irish fever this condition is wanting. Dr. Lombard, of Geneva, whose experience of fever in this country was manifestly insufficient to justify his coming to any decided opinion on the subject, holds that we have in Great Britain and Ireland two different fevers, one highly contagious, which he calls the Irish typhus, and in which cephalic symptoms predominate to the exclusion of abdominal ulcerations ; the other sporadic, and most likely not so infectious, in which the abdominal symptoms are more pronounced, so much so that the follicular disease and consequent ulceration are always present. These two fevers are, in the opinion of this writer, to be found in most parts of Great Britain ; but the first is most prevalent in Ireland, and in places whither the Irish come in great numbers ; the other, similar to the European sporadic fever, is met with in all places, varies with the seasons, and is not necessarily produced by, or under the influence of, contagion. Had Dr. Lombard been aware that ulcerations of the intestine are frequently met with in our petechial typhus, and, again, that the typhoid fever, or at least a fever with extensive dothinenteritis, has raged epidemically for two years in this country, he would have been slow in venturing to settle the question in so decided a manner ; and I have before mentioned to you that during the prevalence of any particular epidemic in this country we meet with cases agreeing in all their general characteristics, and having the distinctive marks of typhus ; in one set of which follicular ulceration is met with, while in another it is absent.

If, however, we inquire what are the diseases secondary to typhus, for the removal or modification of which we are most often called on in the wards of a fever hospital, especially in the worst cases of petechial typhus, I would say that it is the pulmonary rather than the gastro-intestinal complications. Certainly the secondary disease of the bronchial surface is often the most formidable of the local affections in our Irish typhus. So great, indeed, is the frequency of this complication, that long before I was aware of the opinions of Rokitansky on this point I frequently suggested in my lectures whether the secondary bronchial disease might not be held to stand in the same relation to the Irish typhus that the follicular disease of the intestines in France bears to the fever in that country. Let me read to you a passage from Rokitansky's work, translated by Dr. Day for the original Sydenham Society, bearing on the points before us. He speaks as follows of the effect of the typhous process on the mucous membrane of the air passages : "In primary bronco-typhus the general disease originally localizes itself here, avoiding all other mucous membranes, even that of the intestine, for which in general the typhous process shows the most decided preference. The latter mucous membrane exhibits, however, in many cases a recognizable though always subordinate and secondary development of the follicles, in which the adjacent mesenteric glands participate, and in such cases it is very often a difficult matter to distinguish the typhous element in the above-named affection of the bronchial mucous membrane. The peculiar stasis of the spleen and of the great *cul de sac* of the stomach, the remarkable intumescence of the former, and the singular character of the blood, the typhous nature of the general disease, and especially the altered condition of the bronchial glands invariably serve, together with other symptoms, to indicate the typhous nature of the bronchial affection. The alteration occurring in the bronchial glands is of the same character as that affecting the mesenteric glands in abdominal typhus. They become swollen to the size of a pigeon's or even of a hen's egg, are of a dark violet colour, which afterwards becomes lighter, present a relaxed and friable appearence, and are infiltrated with a medullary typhous matter. Like typhous mesenteric glands, they may become the seat of a tumultuous metamorphosis, and thus, either with or without perforation of the adjacent mediastinum, may give rise to pleurisy. This form is often combined with pneumo-typhus and typhous pleurisy, and is beyond all doubt the basis of the spotted contagious typhus, and very probably also of the Irish and North American typhus, forms of the disease which in the majority of cases run their course without any intestinal affection. With us this affection is rare, and in point of frequency is not to be compared with abdominal typhus."

I may here observe that by the term "tumultuous metamorphosis" is implied the occurrence of violent symptoms with suddenness and rapidity of progress. Dr. Day remarks that Rokitansky has used the term in a new sense, but it means generally—as I understand it—that a violent and reactive inflammation occurs in the parts altered by the typhous process, which may cause great congestion, turgescence, perforation, or even gangrene. As Rokitansky does not indicate any distinctive features between the spotted contagious typhus and the Irish and American typhus, we may safely hold them to be the same disease.

With respect to the question of the comparative frequency and importance of the pulmonary as contrasted with the nervous symptoms in fever, as it affects the lower and upper classes in this country, my impression is—taking the experience of a long series of years— that the secondary bronchial or, to speak more generally, the pulmonary complications are much more frequent and dangerous in hospital than in private practice. It is not easy to explain why this should be so, but certainly we find a greater preponderance of nervous symptoms in the typhus fever as it affects the upper classes of society than in cases of the disease as we meet with it in hospital; while in hospital practice the nervous symptoms, though we cannot say that they are absent, less frequently require special interference. No doubt we meet with coma, delirium, and subsultus tendinum occasionally, but the predominance of nervous symptoms in the early periods of typhus which is so common in the upper classes of society is less often seen in our wards; and if you will reflect on the simple fact that we so rarely have to shave the head among our hospital patients, you will see the truth of what I say. Remember, too, how many cases we have had in which, while all the symptoms of typhus —such as prostration, weakness of the heart, eruptions of maculæ and petechiæ, and well-marked secondary diseases of the mucous membrane of the intestines—were present, the patients' minds remained nearly unclouded, and no symptom occurred calling for any special measures directed to the head. The typhus of Ireland, then, is not characterized, as Dr. Lombard has described it, by a preponderance of cephalic symptoms, at least when it occurs in that class from which he supposes the best specimens of the disease to be drawn. He is as incorrect in his statements about the predominance of cephalic symptoms as when he says that the absence of follicular ulcerations of the intestines is a distinctive mark of Irish typhus.

In the typhus fever of the upper classes in this country the nervous symptoms are generally much more aggravated and developed at an earlier period; and it may be that this preponderance of the nervous symptoms, this tendency to affections of the brain in one class, even though these affections be principally toxic and functional, is a cause of the comparative exemption of such cases from the secondary bronchial disease. As you advance in the study of general pathology, you will find plenty of examples in which diseases of structure or of deposition are suspended or replaced by purely nervous affections. Explain it as we will, the general proposition appears true that the nervous symptoms, comparatively speaking, are less developed in the fever of the lower classes, while those indicative of disease of the mucous membranes are much more prominent; and conversely that in the upper ranks symptoms indicative of irritation of the mucous surfaces are less prominent, while the nervous symptoms are severe; and this, perhaps, may throw some light upon the doctrine, which has been long held by many, that the mortality of fever is greater in proportion as we ascend in the scale of society.

I have already told you that, as regards prognosis, the preponderance of any of the nervous symptoms of fever should cause us more apprehension than that of any other class of symptoms, and especially when this preponderance is observed in an early period of the disease. This greater susceptibility of the nervous system in the higher classes may itself be a cause why we cannot use wine with as great liberality in this class as with ordinary hospital patients. And this, again, may explain the greater fatality in private practice, inasmuch as, in consequence of the excitement of the nervous system and the frequent incapability to bear stimulants largely, we are debarred from the use of that which is the great medicine in fever.

I think we may lay it down as a principle that the more the secondary affections of fever are anatomical, the greater will be the utility of stimulants; and conversely the more they are functional, and especially in cases where these symptoms are more closely related to the cerebro-spinal centres, the less will be the efficacy of wine. It might be supposed, from à priori considerations, that the man in the higher classes of life who has been accustomed to the use of wine would require it more and derive greater benefit from it in the course of a fever, which—it must be remembered—is a disease of debility and prostration, than the peasant who has not been habituated to the regular use of stimulants; but I believe that the very reverse is the fact, and that the greatest triumphs of the stimulant treatment in fever are to be found when it affects the agricultural peasant, whose nervous system has not been excited either by the use of stimulants or by intellectual exertion. I know that some will object to this on the ground that our Irish peasantry are habitually intemperate, but this charge of intemperance is only one of the many erroneous statements put forth with reference to our countrymen.

The Irish peasant is not habitually intemperate—neither do his means permit nor his inclinations lead him to be so. When he does indulge it is on special occasions, but in hospital we seldom meet a case of injury to the general health produced by a course of intem-

perance in the peasant. The case is no doubt different in the class of
artisans who are the inhabitants of our large cities and towns. In
this class we find that when fever attacks an individual we can neither
use stimulants with the same boldness nor reckon on their success
with the same confidence as among the more sober classes of the population. In this respect the Irish are not peculiar.

LECTURE X.

Secondary Bronchial Affection of Fever—*Pneumotyphus* of Rokitansky—Views of
this author as to the *anatomical expression* of typhus and typhoid respectively—
Description of the bronchial affection of fever; frequent absence of symptoms
therein—Râles sonorous, mucous, or crepitating; no increased sonority—This
affection is not ordinary "bronchitis;" it comes on silently and subsides spontaneously—Argument from the effects of treatment by stimulation—Modes of termination of the affection.

In our inquiry into the secondary affections of fever we shall have
to consider manifestations of disease in the lungs, which have so strong
a claim on our attention from the frequency of their occurrence and
the important results by which they are followed. We will take up
the subject of the bronchial affection of fever in the present lecture.

This affection is so frequent and common in maculated typhus that
Rokitansky proposed to found a nomenclature for the various forms
of fever in accordance with the most striking secondary diseases
characteristic of them. Thus he designated typhoid as *typhus abdominalis*, and maculated typhus as *pneumotyphus*. He considered that,
whilst typhoid affected the intestinal mucous membrane as its secondary anatomical result, typhus, on the other hand, engaged the pulmonary tissues; that "as the anatomical expression of typhoid fever was
intestinal ulceration, so the anatomical expression of typhus was disease of the mucous membrane of the chest."

Now, in making statements such as these the great German patholo-
gist seems to me to have gone too far. I believe him to be in error
in his assumption respecting typhoid, as he equally is at fault in his
conclusion touching the bronchial affection of typhus. If he had
said, "In the cases of typhoid which have come under my cognizance
and treatment I invariably found disease of the intestinal canal to be
present, and in all my cases of *typhus gravior* the bronchial tubes and
mucous membrane of the chest were diseased," he would have been

correct. But cases both of typhoid and typhus of the severest character and most prolonged continuance may occur unattended by the symptoms of local disease which have been regarded as so constant in their appearance, and which have even been asserted to constitute the disease of which the fever is merely symptomatic.

At the same time we must not repudiate Rokitansky's views simply because they differ from those based on the study of fever in this country. The German observations have been made in good faith, and are of value so far as they are pathological records of the phenomena of fever as observed in a different country and as affecting a distinct race of people. In the typhus fever of our own land we often meet with serious engagement of the bronchial tubes. We not infrequently see a similar morbid affection in cases of typhoid; but in typhus this local disease always makes its appearance at a comparatively early stage of the fever, whilst in typhoid it usually comes on at a later period. Again, we have had in this country a form of disease strangely opposed to all such artificial distinctions as those of fever under the headings of typhus abdominalis and pneumotyphus; it was called *gastro-catarrhal typhus*, a term which sufficiently indicates the character of the disease.

To a person who is not in the habit of examining patients in fever very closely, the frequency and importance of the bronchial disease would not appear very evident or striking as he walks round the wards of an Irish fever hospital. We find the patient, perhaps, in a state of stupor, but from this he is easily roused. He is covered with petechial spots, red or livid, as the case may be. There is nothing remarkable about his breathing; he is not reported to have any cough; his pulse is probably 120 or 130, and his heart is weak. That patient, with but little hurry of breathing, not complaining of any distress, and without cough, may be, and frequently is, at that very time in an advanced stage of the secondary bronchial disease. When you apply the stethoscope, and make the patient draw a deep breath, you are surprised at the great amount of disease that is revealed, although the symptoms of the important affection are absent. One would expect that in such a case there would be lividity of the countenance from the non-arterialization of the blood; but here is one of the curious things connected with fever which it is extremely difficult to explain —that you will often see but little lividity in such cases. At all events it is not sufficient to draw attention to the condition of the patient's lung. In most patients labouring under bad typhus there is a peculiar dusky hue of the face, and this whether the bronchial disease were present or not. But I have over and over again seen the most extensive bronchial disease, where every tube seemed to be half-filled, and yet where little of that kind of lividity which we see in a case of asthma or of bad suffocative catarrh existed. Let us consider this fact for a moment, for it is full of matter for reflection. What does it tell us? It announces this highly important principle, that in their formation, and in their progress, the secondary diseases of fever are, as it were, silent. They occur without the usual symptoms which are observed in idiopathic inflammations. They are not idiopathic inflammations, and therefore they have not the symptoms of them. Let us omit no opportunity of impressing on our minds the fact that these diseases are not inflammations. They form silently; they advance silently; they subside silently, generally along with the fever, but sometimes before it has ceased. Consider for a moment the formation of a pustule in an ordinary case of smallpox. The pustule gives no notice of its formation. You turn down the clothes, and you find the arm covered with vesicles; the patient has not complained, but you find there is the eruption. So it is with respect to the bronchial disease in typhus; so it is with respect to the intestinal disease in typhoid. We see the bronchial disease forming in this singular and latent manner, without excitement or suffering of the patient. We see the same in the intestine and in the heart. The softening of the heart, so commonly noticed in fever, is in its commencement and all through a silent process. The process of change up to its maximal intensity, and that of retrocession to the period of recovery, considered simply, when they are not interfered with by accidental irritation, go on silently. Thus the disease may proceed to its maximum without symptoms, and retrocede without symptoms. Now, under these circumstances, I have said that, when you apply the stethoscope, you very often find extensive râles. These râles may be sonorous, mucous, or crepitating; the degree of each of those characteristics varying in every case, and in different portions of the lung, in the same individual. When you use percussion, you find that there is no dulness anywhere. I have not observed, in the bronchial affection of typhus fever, the curious result of percussion which we see in cases of primary bronchial disease. I allude to increase of sonority of the chest. This is a very remarkable fact. In a large number of cases of acute inflammatory bronchitis, it is remarked that, so far from the chest being dull, it is actually clearer than natural; and this is explained by the circumstance that there is a great accummulation of air in the air-cells of the lung—that, in fact, every little air-cell of the lung is in a condition of distension; it is full of air, which cannot find a ready egress during expiration, in consequence of the tumefied state of the bronchial tubes;

and hence we have the increase of sonority. I have not observed this in cases of typhus fever where there was no consolidation of the lung; but, at the same time, it is to be noted that we have not specially studied this point in fever cases. When the patient draws a deep breath we frequently find that the râles go on increasing up to the very end of the inspiratory act; and in certain cases, the following curious circumstance is noticed, and it is one of those which illustrate what I have termed the silent action of the disease. On applying the stethoscope, you may hear but little, or a loose, râle in the larger bronchial tubes, or in some of their secondary ramifications—that is, during ordinary breathing. If you contented yourself with such an examination, you might come to the conclusion that there was very little the matter with the patient's lung—slight mucous disease in the lower part of the trachea, or in the very large tubes. But you might be altogether wrong; for, under these circumstances, it frequently happens that when the patient is made to draw a deep breath, you are startled with the extent and intensity of the râles running to the very end of the inspiratory act. It is in this condition that the patient's life is seriously endangered; for if this bronchial disease does not retrocede, but continues to advance, it may happen that the sufferer falls suddenly into a condition of asphyxia, tracheal rattle comes on, and he dies a mechanical death—in fact, he dies suffocated. You may leave your patient apparently going on very well, and be summoned to him in the course of a few hours, to find him *in articulo mortis*. This is a common occurrence, as I mentioned to you before, in persons in whom the bronchial disease has been overlooked or neglected.

You will commonly hear it said that this or that patient in typhus has got bronchitis; and, if we were to be guided by physical signs alone, such a statement would seem to be correct. But I wish you to believe that the essence of this affection is not bronchitis, but rather a special condition of the air-passages, secondary to the fever, the result either of the typhous deposit or of the vascularity with turgescence to which I have already alluded. If bronchitis—that is to say, if inflammatory action supervenes—it must yet be considered as reactive and specific. I am anxious to lay stress upon this, because there are still many practitioners who hold that the physical signs of bronchitis are sufficient to establish the existence of primary inflammation. Now, I do not know any characteristic difference between the physical signs which may occur in ordinary idiopathic bronchitis and those which present themselves in typhus when the air-tubes are engaged. In both there may be sonorous, sibilant, mucous, and crepitating râles; and yet the two diseases are pathologically distinct. Observe that whatever diminishes the calibre of the tubes, whether it be deposit, typhous congestion, or true inflammation, will give râle; whatever causes secretion, whether it be true inflammation or something the very opposite of inflammation, will give râle. We have, as I said before, in typhus the physical signs which are observed in true bronchitis; but beware how, in any given case of fever, you conclude from their presence that the patient has true bronchitis. In certain cases there may be reactive irritation; but never forget that the typhous disease alone, without any inflammation whatever, is competent to produce all the signs of bronchitis. Why do I urge this so much on you? Because I wish to avail myself of every opportunity of removing from your minds the erroneous doctrines of inflammation which have been so long in vogue. We are greatly influenced by names; and though I do not suppose that there are many who would treat a case of the bronchial affection in fever with the same reducing measures which they would employ in the idiopathic disease, yet I am sure that the idea of these signs proceeding from inflammation makes many of us, who have not yet unlearned our early teachings, timid in the use of stimulants.

We find that this bronchial disease runs a course exactly analogous to that of the other secondary affections of fever. It comes on insidiously, or, as I said before, silently; it gradually advances to its maximum, and sometimes increases to that degree that the patient dies by asphyxia. This is often the case when the disease has not been recognized at an early period. It is in almost all cases preceded by the symptoms of fever for several days. I think in the best marked cases it first shows itself about the fourth or fifth day of the disease, but it may supervene at any period of the case. It subsides spontaneously. You will have abundant opportunities of observing the following curious circumstance in the subsidence of this disease, either when the affection runs its natural course or when it has been necessary to treat it specially. In the true idiopathic bronchitis, when a patient is placed under treatment, we observe the disappearance of the râles to be gradual; they are less intense and less complicated day by day; and this goes on probably for a week or ten days, or it may be a fortnight or more, before the last shade of râle disappears. In the typhous affection, on the contrary, you will often observe that the most extensive, intense, and complicated râles disappear as if by enchantment, leaving the respiratory murmur perfectly pure. This sudden disappearance of the physical signs is only an argument among many to show their non-inflammatory origin. Nothing can be more remarkable than this; it seems analogous to the sudden disappearance of the eruption of scarlatina from the skin. You may often see this eruption lasting for three or four days, and then suddenly disappearing, leaving the skin white and pure. Consider the case of the lung in the same way, and in place of the scarlatina eruption take the secondary bronchial disease—or eruption, if you will—and you can understand the occurrence of a similar change. Mind, I do not say this happens in all cases; and I suppose that for its occurrence it is necessary that there shall have been little, if any, reactive irritation. And, as I said before, we see it in cases not only where the disease has been little, if at all, interfered with by treatment, but in others in which we have used such remedies as dry cupping, counter-irritation, and various stimulant medicines. Here the practitioner is often surprised at the rapid and complete success of his treatment, and may take credit to himself for bringing about a change which was to a great degree, at all events, induced by the operation of the law of periodicity, to which the secondary local effects, as well as the essential disease, are subject.

In the next place we find that the best treatment in such cases is the stimulant. The mere circumstance of a patient having or presenting the most intense signs of bronchitis in typhus fever does not by any means warrant us in bleeding him, in reducing him, in exhibiting tartar emetic, or in withholding wine. Nothing of the kind; the best treatment for such cases is the free use of wine, ammonia, turpentine, bark, dry-cupping, and so on.

Another argument is drawn from the interesting fact, that in a large number of cases of softened heart in typhus we find a combination with the bronchial disease, and it is quite fair to conclude that the conditions of the lung and heart, as regards the influence of typhous poison on the muscular structure of both these organs, are similar. We have long held the opinion that what is called "effusion into the chest" in catarrhal typhus is a consequence of the weakening of the muscular structures of the bronchial tubes. The practical conclusion, then, to be drawn is, that the physical signs of bronchitis in a case of maculated typhus fever should not make you conclude that the patient had bronchial inflammation; and therefore you should not treat the case as such.

I have just stated that the bronchial affection of fever does not always disappear with extreme rapidity. Cases frequently occur where that affection subsides as an attack of ordinary bronchitis does —the râles become more scattered and less intense, and they finally cease. In a third class of cases, even after the essential disease has departed, the patient may be placed in imminent danger from effusion on the chest; or, again, while he may not be exactly threatened with asphyxia, yet his aspect and general condition may become eminently suggestive of the presence of pulmonary consumption. He loses strength, and grows pallid and emaciated. A loose cough sets in sometimes, with profuse expectoration. In short, the bronchial affection simulates phthisis. Under these circumstances a quack sees the patient and pronounces him to be far gone in consumption. After a time the bronchial affection subsides, the sufferer rapidly improves—in fact, gets well—and the quack wins all the credit of having cured a case of confirmed phthisis.

So important do I regard this subject of imperfect or protracted recovery from the bronchial disease of typhus to be, that I purpose to devote our next lecture to its further investigation, and to a consideration of the kindred topic of tubercle as a sequela of fever.

LECTURE XI.

BRONCHIAL AFFECTION OF FEVER *continued*—Alternating secondary affections—Imperfect convalescence due to reactive bronchitis—Cases resembling phthisis—Three forms of tubercular disease, as a sequela of fever, (1) *coexisting tubercle*, (2) *acute consequent tubercle*, (3) *consequent softened tubercle*—Diagnosis based on the *want of accordance between physical signs and symptoms* in suspected phthisis after fever—Expectoration of small calculi some months after bronchial typhus—*Tubercular fever* in the typhus epidemic of 1826-27—This fever may be contagious.

THERE is a remarkable type of fever, incidentally referred to in a former lecture and not at all uncommon in this country, in which we have an alternating disease, as it were, between the abdominal and the pulmonary organs in continued fever. This is a very bad form of fever—one of the worst. We find that to-day—we shall say—the chest is greatly loaded, that we get no good respiratory murmur; there are most intense râles, and all the symptoms of extensive disease of the lung are present. At this time the belly is soft; it is not tender on pressure; and there is no diarrhœa. Things go on for two or three days, when we find the belly to be swollen, tympanitic, tender on pressure; there is diarrhœa; and on applying the stethoscope to the chest we find it comparatively free, and the râles either gone or almost altogether gone.

We turn our attention to the abdomen, and, on relieving the symptoms there to a certain degree, the chest again shows signs of disease; and in this way the affection alternates as it were between the two great cavities, and forms a combination which is extremely difficult of management. And I think that these cases of gastro-catarrhal typhus—that is to say, of typhus with secondary disease in the two cavities, that disease meanwhile alternately varying in its severity—are more likely to be followed by the development of tubercle after the disease has subsided than the catarrhal typhus without abdominal complication. But on this point I do not wish you to believe that my mind is completely made up. My opinion is one of those that men form gradually and unknowingly, without being able to refer the sources of that opinion to any particular observation. But it does not happen in every case that the bronchial disease of typhus either subsides in that sudden manner we have been speaking of or advances to such a height as to destroy the patient's life.

There is another case, and a very important one, where we observe an imperfect convalescence, the chest remaining very much engaged. That is to say, after all the general symptoms of fever have subsided, the petechiæ have disappeared, the typhous expression has vanished, and the patient is anxious for food, we find that the phenomena of the chest remain but little altered; that there is extensive bronchial râle. In this case it appears to me that what has happened is, that a reactive inflammation has occurred, and that a form of bronchitis has been added to the typhous disease. Something very similar to this occurs in the case of disease of the intestine in fever. This has been indicated by Dr. Cheyne as one of the cases of imperfect convalescence in fever. It would appear as if a secondary inflammation supervened upon the typhous alteration of the intestine, and this caused the convalescence to be imperfect. It is extremely probable that the same thing occurs in the lung. There is nothing more important, gentlemen, in the study of diseases than to keep analogy continually before us; and you may expect that the processes of disease observed in one cavity of the body will be repeated in the others. The case in the wards to which we gave the turpentine was a good example of this.

These cases are frequently mistaken for phthisis—and this is not to be wondered at, for the patients have a very phthisical aspect: they are emaciated by fever; they have often a species of semi-hectic upon them; they have cough; their respiration is difficult; and they have frequently profuse expectoration. You will say, then, Is there any difference between the symptoms in these cases at this stage and those in cases of phthisis? I do not know of any difference but this, that in the patients labouring under phthisis there is often a very copious muco-puriform expectoration—a thing rarely seen during the presence of the disease in fever. It is very natural, then, that, under these circumstances, a practitioner seeing a patient for the first time might come to the conclusion that he was phthisical; and it is quite proper that all physicians in this state of things should be apprehensive of such a condition, because it is certain that in some instances of typhus fever a disposition to permanent organic change in the lung seems to have been created by the disturbance of the system in consequence of the fever.

We have three forms of tubercular disease induced in this way. The first is what I may term *acute coexisting tubercle.* This is a most curious form, in which, while the petechiæ are still on the surface, the lung becomes full of soft cheesy matter.

Let me call your attention particularly to this disease. We have not seen many instances of it, and but on one occasion had we a post-mortem examination; but this was a very well-marked case. It occured several years back in our wards, and was one of those cases which we do not easily forget. The patient, a man between 30 and 40 years of age, had enjoyed perfect health up to the time when he was attacked with fever; he was not subject to any form of chronic bronchitis, or of pulmonary irritation; so that there is not the slightest reason to believe that tubercular matter existed in his lungs before he was attacked with the fever. He came here at the end of the first week of his illness with the usual symptoms of maculated typhus, complicated by the secondary bronchial disease. So far there was nothing unusual about the case. It was observed, however, that the râles were more intense in the right than in the left lung; that there was a greater amount of large crepitus than we commonly see in the typhous disease, indicating that the minute tubes were much engaged. The chest was perfectly clear on percussion, but I took alarm at the great amount of bronchial râle which had become developed at so early a period. The patient was treated by dry-cupping, blistering, and the use of senega with carbonate of ammonia; but yet we did not observe that these measures produced any sensible effect on the physical signs—a circumstance which should have still further increased our apprehensions, but at that time we had no suspicion of what the result was to be. There was no remarkable suffering; the patient did not complain of dyspnœa, his breathing was not much accelerated, and, in short, he had no symptom which would distinguish his case from ordinary typhus with severe bronchial disease. We now, however, observed that day by day, with nothing but a bronchial râle, the anterior portion of the chest, especially on the right side, became equably yet progressively dull, although there was little if any change in the character of the large but crepitating râle, nor was there any indication of hepatization—the lung always continued permeable to air. The petechiæ remained remarkably stationary. About the eighth or ninth day the patient began to sweat profusely. And this sweating appeared to occur in two paroxysms within the twenty-four hours, so that he seemed to have a combination of severe hectic and of typhus fever. He died on or about the twelfth or thirteenth day of his disease, the front of the right side having become very dull, but not absolutely so, and the large crepitus remaining with singular constancy all through. On the day of his death the petechial eruption had scarcely faded.

Although we had never had any instance of the acute development of cheesy degeneration pending the typhous state, yet I ventured to make the diagnosis of the disease here, for the physical phenomena were precisely those which occur in ordinary acute inflammatory cheesy infiltration of the lung. The right lung was found to contain a great quantity of soft, gray, cheesy matter, deposited in isolated patches, varying from the size of half a pea to that of a hazel-nut. The masses were not encysted; they were soft, but yet showed no appearance of suppuration. A few deposits of the same kind were found on the left side.

The great amount of this deposit is in itself sufficient to prove that it was one of the secondary affections of the typhus fever; for although a man may live with a certain amount of chronic tubercle developed in his lung, it is quite impossible to conceive that he could have had such a quantity of soft cheesy matter, nearly filling up one lung, while his health and respiratory function remained unaffected, as was the case in this man until the occurrence of the typhus fever.

I believe that this was but the extreme degree of what often occurs in fever; and we shall just now see that there are strong grounds for holding that cheesy matter is formed, though in smaller quantities, during the secondary bronchial disease of fever, and yet the patient recovers without having the symptoms of phthisis.

The next form we term *acute consequent tubercle;* that is to say, when the patient has passed through his fever, and has had an interval of repose, everything apparently promising a perfect recovery, there is a sudden explosion of tubercular disease, with symptoms of high irritation, and with a rapid development of miliary and granular tubercle.

The last form, which is not by any means so frequent as the others, is the *consequent softened tubercle*, in which, when a patient who has had catarrhal disease in the early periods of his fever has recovered, although with an imperfect convalescence, the disease passes, some-

6

times rapidly, into the ordinary pulmonary phthisis, and is followed by the same result.

I spoke to-day in the wards of a practical question, as to your diagnosis, when called to a patient who has gone through typhus fever, and in whom the chest is very much engaged; this is a case to which you will be often called in consultation. The patient has been under the care of another person; he has gone through severe fever; he is on the 25th, or the 30th, or the 36th day of his illness, and appearances of his being consumptive occur. It is possible that the patient may be of a consumptive family, and an alarm is excited. He has wasted in flesh; he has quick pulse; he may have had some sweats; he has cough and muco-puriform expectoration. Well, such is his position. You are called on then to say, in the common phrase, whether his lungs are affected or not. You examine the chest carefully; and, if you find the following circumstances present, you may in most instances be able to assure the patient's friends that as yet the patient is not phthisical. If you find that the physical signs of bronchitis are universal, that in no part of the chest you fail in discovering sonorous, mucous, or muco-crepitating râles, in various degrees of combination —in other words, stethoscopic indications that *every portion* of the bronchial tree is equably affected—if, then, with this universality and intensity of bronchial signs, you find that the patient's respiration is not much excited, that he is not complaining of dyspnœa, or that his respiration is not rapid, you may be almost certain that the patient is labouring only under the remains of typhous bronchial disease, and that he has not yet passed into a phthisical condition. You make the diagnosis here, gentlemen, from a source which you will find of great importance: *it is a diagnosis from the want of accordance of phenomena.* What do you find here? Signs of universal bronchial affection. Now, we know that in ninety-nine cases out of a hundred of the development of tubercle after fever, where there is universality of deposit there is extreme constitutional suffering—there is great dyspnœa—there is extraordinary acceleration of breathing, so that in the case above specified the want of accordance between the extent of disease and the amount of suffering leads you to a negative diagnosis, and enables you to declare that as yet the patient is not the subject of consumption. If, on the other hand, this patient had, with the physical signs which I have described, any hurried or difficult breathing, and the signs and symptoms of great irritation of the lung, it would be quite impossible to say that he had not consumption. In a very large number of cases you will find that this rule will apply. In bronchial disease following not only typhus fever, but a variety of other affections, you can apply this rule of diagnosis very commonly indeed; in the remittent fever of children you can apply it; in cases of the bronchial disease which follows measles or scarlatina, and in a variety of other affections, the diagnosis from the want of accordance of the phenomena is applicable. It is very important, indeed, to study carefully those means of diagnosis which are available where you have not an opportunity of repeated observation. In most cases of consultation the consulting physician sees the patient but once. If you should be able to see him three or four times, at intervals of two or three days, you would not be under this difficulty; but by this weapon of diagnosis, if I may make use of such a phrase, you will be able—even by seeing the patient but once—to give a satisfactory diagnosis.

I have drawn your attention to the great probability that exists that in many cases of fever, with the secondary bronchial disease, there is developed not merely the affection of the mucous membrane, but more or less of actual organic change, consisting in a local deposition of tubercle; and yet it does not follow that the patient will ever have the symptoms of phthisis. He may recover, and often does recover completely, with a perfectly pure respiratory murmur, without any cough, or without any symptoms whatever of disease, but after a period varying from three months to nine months he expectorates a few calculi. There cannot be any doubt, when all the circumstances of the case are considered, that those calculi were petrifactions of deposits which were formed pending the fever, and which, from their being small and isolated, without any consolidation of the surrounding tissue, and from their having been unaccompanied by cavities, altogether escaped observation. The number of individuals who have gone through this bronchial typhus, and at some subsequent period are observed to expectorate small calculi, is quite sufficient to warrant this conclusion.

Now, looking at the entire subject, I think it more than probable that, in many cases, even where this proof of the previous occurrence of tubercular deposit has not existed, such deposit has gone through a process of calcification, and the patient has not afterwards passed into phthisis. The cure may be effected either by calcareous transformation, absorption, or suppuration at a number of points so minute as to elude detection by physical means, the signs being lost or confounded with those of ordinary bronchial disease. I think that this occurs in many cases in which we have a doubtful convalescence, with a quick pulse and a hectic state, in those who have had fever with severe bronchial disease.

How are we to look on this tubercular deposit as a result of the

typhous state? Were these patients already subjects of the phthisical
diathesis, although no actual deposit had taken place at the time of
their being attacked with fever? Or are we to look upon tubercular
matter as occasionally one of the secondary secretions of fever? I
strongly incline to the latter view. This much, at all events, is certain,
that in a large number of cases there were, previously to the attack
of contagious typhus, no existing symptoms or physical signs of
phthisis, nor did the patients present those characteristics which indicate a tendency to this affection. Tubercular deposit, as one of the
secondary products of fever, is probably to be looked upon as among
the rarer consequences of the disease; for although we have seen
many instances of it, yet in the great majority of cases of fever with
bronchial disease there is no evidence of its having occurred. Why
it should occur in one case, and not in another, we do not know; but
it is very probable that there are great varieties in the nature of the
typhous deposit in different patients and in different epidemics. It is
not unreasonable to suppose that the inconstancy which we observe
with respect to the seat, amount, periods, and complications of the
secondary diseases of fever should be also repeated as to their
chemico-pathological characters. And thus one patient may have a
secretion or deposit which is not tubercular, while another exhibits
this alteration to a greater or less degree. All this, you will see,
bears strongly on the question of the specific or non-specific nature
of tubercle after fever; and the facts which we have just now been
examining seem to point to the conclusion that the doctrine of tubercle
being a purely heterologous product, resulting from a specific contamination of the system, is one which we must be cautious in accept-
ing. But there are other circumstances in relation to this matter
with which you should be acquainted.

Hitherto we have been dealing with cases in which the tubercular
formation seemed to be, as it were, an accident in the chain of typhous
phenomena; cases in the majority of which, at all events, the actual
amount of the deposit was generally inconsiderable. I have already
spoken of one case in which a great quantity of cheesy matter was
formed during the existence of a genuine and well-marked typhus fever,
but in the instances hitherto under consideration we may hold that the
deposit was but a superaddition to the ordinary secondary bronchial
disease. Let us now inquire whether there is any evidence of a
fever closely allied to, if not identical with, typhus or typhoid fever, and
in which the secondary lesion is purely the deposit of tubercle—the
tubercular matter and the fever standing in the same relation one to
the other as the matter of the smallpox pustule does to the essential

disease of variola. I cannot pretend to give you any extended information on this point, but the following circumstances are important.

In the epidemic of typhus fever of 1826 and 1827 the two most remarkable circumstances were the great prevalence of the follicular disease of the intestines and the liability to relapse. In a good many instances it was found that the fever in the relapse was of a more severe character than in the first seizure. You may have observed something of the same sort during the present season; for we have had several instances in which, while the first attack ran a period of only from, five to eight days, with the comparatively mild symptoms of what is called typhoid fever, the patients, on relapsing, had severe, long-continued, and maculated fever. In some of them, too, the bronchial system, which had escaped in the first illness, was profoundly engaged during the second attack. It was found that in several instances in which the patients had gone through the first attack of fever, and relapsed, they presented a group of symptoms very different from those in the primary illness. The fever was much more violent, the sufferings greater, and the local symptoms more numerous and decided. One case I shall never forget. A young woman had gone through the usual primary attack of fever, and recovered satisfactorily. There was nothing either in her previous history or in the symptoms of her fever to distinguish this case from that of hundreds that had passed through our wards. After remaining a few days in a state of convalescence, this girl was reported to me as having relapsed. As there was nothing unusual in this, we merely directed the ordinary expectorant and cooling treatment; but on the second or third day it was plain that the disease was taking on a new character. The patient had symptoms of local suffering, or irritation, if you will, in all the cavities. The head was hot and painful, she was delirious; the heart was excited, and the pulse was rapid and wiry, the skin was burning hot, and the general symptoms were those of the most severe ataxic fever, with the greatest agitation and distress.

But I have not yet enumerated all the symptoms of this singular case. In addition to the high fever and cerebral excitement, the patient suffered from unceasing and extreme dyspnœa, running into orthopnœa. The countenace was swollen and livid. There was a constant cough, with a scanty bronchitic expectoration, and pain of both sides. Then the symptoms of irritation in the belly were as well marked. It was greatly swollen, tympanitic, hot, and painful on pressure. The tongue was red, dry, and cracked; the thirst immoderate, and she had frequent diarrhœa. Now, observe that no effort of ours produced the slightest alleviation of any of her symptoms; and under this

storm of disease she sank on the seventh day from the commencement
of the relapse. We found, on dissection, an almost universal deposit of
miliary and granular tubercle. I never saw anything similar before,
nor have I seen anything like it since. The lungs, liver, spleen, uterus,
kidneys, as well as all the serous membranes, were implicated; and
the amount of the disease, particularly in the lungs, liver, spleen, and
arachnoid, was beyond anything that you can imagine. The deposit
was of the same character everywhere. It was the disseminated tubercle, not the infiltrated, consisting of gray semi-transparent granules,
the size of mustard seeds or smaller. In the lungs no one portion was
less engaged then another. The little tubercles, some semi-transparent,
others white, or yellow, and opaque, were so closely packed that they
all but touched one another; yet each was distinct. There was no in-
osculation, or running of one into the other ; nor was there one among
these myriads of deposits that showed any trace of suppuration. The
bronchial membrane was of a deep red colour, and the pulmonary
structure, which was nowhere hepatized, presented a bright scarlet hue.
In the spleen, which was enlarged, the deposits were nearly as abundant as in the lung ; a few of them had attained a larger size and a
more granular structure. The pericardium, peritoneum, and arachnoid membrane were all studded as closely as possibly with the miliary
tubercles.

Now, reflect on this case. Who can doubt this extraordinary
deposit was the result of the second attack? The very quantity of it
is sufficient to prove this; for, if we take even the lung, no one could
believe that this amount of disease existed, either before the first
attack or during the period of convalescence, when there were apyrexia and quiet breathing; again, remember that all these deposits
were in the same or very nearly the same degree of development,
and that this disease occurred in a patient who had gone through her
first fever without any remarkable symptoms—during an epidemic
when relapse was so frequent as to be considered almost the rule.

Gentlemen, this might be called a tubercular fever. Call it, however, what you will, it was a fever, with secondary lesion of a peculiar kind. This change, or local disease, was in one sense anatomical,
no doubt, in that there was tangible visible alteration; but it set the
local anatomical divisions of fever at nought, from the fact of its being
universal. The disease was, indeed, as essential as the malady or
fever which produced it. Why tubercular matter was produced here
in such incredible quantities, and in so short a time, we do not know.
Why, in the same epidemic, this patient, in common with many
others, suffered in this way, while the great majority of the sick reco-

vered, we cannot tell—any more than why one patient in fever, and in the same epidemic, shall have disease in the mucous glands of his intestine; a second, congestion and typhous deposit in his lungs; a third, an enlargement of his spleen; a fourth, a softened heart; a fifth, presenting all these changes combined; and so on, with an endless variety.

In this singular case it is probable that the immediate cause of death was asphyxia, for the lungs were almost completely filled with the deposits; but there was so much local disease of the same kind elsewhere that it is difficult to say how much or how little the deposit in the lungs acted in causing death, especially when we recollect that the fever alone, from its very virulence and malignity, might have destroyed the patient. Had there been a smaller amount of tubercle in the lungs, she might have thrown off the fever, and afterwards died with the symptoms of rapid phthisis. This occurrence was observed by us in several instances during that very epidemic; and in some the period which elapsed between the cessation of the fever and death, with all the symptoms and physical signs of suppurative tubercle, was not more than from ten days to a fortnight. On dissection the lungs were found everywhere filled with softened tubercle, which in many places had formed small anfractuosities.

The observations which I have now made to you refer to the connection between fever and the occasional production of cheesy or of tubercular matter, as one of its secondary effects, and I think I have said enough to show you that tubercular deposit and the typhous state frequently stand to one another in the relation of effect and cause. We might now inquire whether there are other forms of essential fevers in which the tubercular deposit is a necessary consequence —in which, to use the language at present in vogue, it becomes the anatomical character of the fever. You know that I am not fond of discussing the distinctions of fever. The cases which I have laid before you were examples of tubercular deposit developed in the relapse period of fever; and although in this relapse certain anatomical characters were developed, we are not on that account to say that the essence of the fever in its relapse was different from that in its first period. You all know that typhus fever may relapse into typhoid fever, and typhoid into typhus. I am compelled to use the expression of one fever relapsing into another, which is an inaccurate one, for want of a better, and you all must know my meaning. But is there any form of fever in which the tendency to produce tubercle, or the actual production of it, is from the very commencement a distinctive character? The following circumstances occurred in the practice of the late Mr. Cusack, and, as far as they go, they seem to prove that there may be a true, essential, and tubercular fever, which also may be contagious, affecting many members of one family.

An infant at the breast, eight weeks old, was attacked with fever. The principal local symptoms were oppression of breathing and fulness of the abdomen. The child refused its food, and death took place at the end of the third week. On dissection the lungs were found filled with miliary tubercle, and the same deposit was extensively exhibited upon both pleuræ and peritoneum.

The next case, which occurred in this family, was that of a girl seven years of age. She took ill just at the period of the death of her sister, and her symptoms were closely similar to those of the infant just spoken of. She had fever, oppression of breathing, and swelling of the abdomen. It was thought that the origin of this disease might be from malaria, and on this account she was removed to the country ; but she died within six weeks from the invasion of the fever. On dissection a precisely similar state of parts was discovered, the viscera being extensively filled with disseminated tubercle, and yet without any suppuration of the deposit.

Now comes the most important fact connected with this history. The two brothers of this girl, who had been at school, arrived to spend their vacation just at the time of her death. They came to the country house in which she had died. Their ages were respectively eight and nine years. Within the first week the elder sickened ; he had fever ; oppression of breathing, soon followed by cerebral symptoms ; he also died with signs of effusion on the brain ; and on dissection the pia mater, arachnoid, lungs, and peritoneum all presented the tubercular deposit, with the same character as in the preceding cases. Upon his death his younger brother sickened ; in this case, in addition to the symptoms of fever, the local suffering was principally referred to the head. The child, after going through a tedious illness, recovered without showing any symptoms of phthisis. During his illness his eldest sister, aged twelve, became affected with fever having the same general character as that which was presented in the other cases, but without any decided local symptoms ; she also recovered.

It might, perhaps, be better were I to leave these facts before you without comment, but I cannot avoid expressing my opinion that they go far to establish not only the existence of a form of fever of which the anatomical result is often tubercle, but also that this fever may be, under certain circumstances, contagious.

The essentiality, also, of this species of fever is indicated in the history of the foregoing cases; for we observe the same want of constancy as to the appearance, amount, and seat of the secondary deposit which is so striking a characteristic of the secondary local affections of other essential diseases. The fourth and fifth cases probably illustrate the want of constancy observed in fevers in relation to the secondary affections and their results.

LECTURE XII.

SECONDARY PNEUMONIC COMPLICATIONS OF FEVER—Secondary *congestion or consolidation* of lung—The term "typhoid pneumonia" is incorrect—"Acute asthenic pulmonary disease," or "typhoid pneumonia," appears under *seven* forms—"*Aborted* typhus" in connection with the occurrence of lung consolidation—Local disease may assume a *sthenic* type even in the presence of a general *asthenic* condition—Description of the secondary pulmonary affection of fever under its *three* principal forms—Differential diagnosis between this disease and *acute primary pneumonia,* based on both pathological and anatomical grounds.

THE study of the affections of the lungs in fever leads us next to examine a class of cases in which a congestion more or less severe, or it may be a consolidation of the lung, takes place in connection with the typhous state. You have already witnessed several cases of this kind. In some there have been signs only of a congestive state, affecting a portion of one or both lungs; a state stopping short of consolidation, and indicated by a crepitus with large bubbles—a muco-crepitating râle, without much dulness, or the other signs of impermeability of the pulmonary tissue. In other instances, however, we have observed the occurrence of decided dulness. Between these extremes we meet with a number of cases varying in the degree or amount of the diseased action.

To these cases the general term of "typhoid pneumonia" has been given. But you will be convinced, when your experience has been enlarged, that under this term many different forms of disease have been classed; and it is very doubtful whether a true pneumonia is ever developed in the course of a fever. You will meet with the physical signs which attend pneumonia; but these, as you all must know, are insufficient to establish the existence of the disease; and even these very physical signs are seldom so well marked, so complete as it were, as in simple inflammation of the lung. Nor, again, do they follow in the regular succession which we find in true pneumonia.

I am not fond of fine-drawn distinctions in disease, especially when these distinctions are based on some anatomical speciality, and do not lead to any differences in our principles of treatment; and I think we shall arrive at practical results sooner by reviewing some of the more striking cases—I will not say of typhoid pneumonia—but of the acute asthenic diseases of the lung which tend to consolidate that organ. I mean, when using the terms "acute asthenic," to imply a disease which forms more or less rapidly, and is associated with, or secondary to, a condition of the system in which, with fever of some kind, we find evident signs of debility. Leaving refined shades of distinction aside, we may then recognize the following forms of the affection we are now considering:—

1. Congestion, with more or less consolidation in cases of what is called "diffuse inflammation," "erysipelatous inflammation," or, by some, phlebitis.

2. Similar or nearly similar conditions (so far, at least, as we are taught by pathological anatomy) in cases of purulent absorption, with or without manifest phlebitis.

3. The intercurrent disease of the lung in cases of the eruptive fevers, when they are of the low, putrid, or malignant type.

4. Congestion and semi-consolidations of the lung, as intercurrent affections in fever, and more especially in typhus fever.

5. Analogous conditions arising in the course of the non-maculated and the so-called typhoid fever.

6. The disease occurring in connection with delirium tremens from excess. In such cases we will often find a group of asthenic local diseases, which are generally seated in the stomach, heart, the bronchial membrane, the parenchyma of the lung, and even the pleura and pericardium. In some instances we find that the patient has also typhus fever.

7. Rapid, extensive, and complete consolidation of the lung occurring in the course of a malignant typhus. In some instances the patient dies asphyxiated, while in others a portion of the pulmonary structures falls into sphacelus, and death takes place with the symptoms of acute gangrene of the lung.

Such are some of the more prominent cases which have been classed under the head of typhoid pneumonia. There is another division of which we have had many examples, and yet I do not wish you to take what I am going to say about it in any other way than in the light of suggestions. The case, as I said before, is by no means uncommon. The patient is attacked with the usual symptoms of typhus fever, and he comes into hospital after two or three days' illness. There is nothing about him to make one think that his disease will not run the usual course of the epidemic of the day, and we are prepared to expect a fever of at least a fortnight's duration. On admission he may have no symptom which would call attention to his chest; but, as early in some cases as the beginning of the fourth, and in others of the fifth day, it is discovered that the upper lobe of one lung is solid, or nearly so. The clavicle is quite dull on percussion, so is the scapular spine, and the dulness extends to the line of the mamma, with well-marked tubular breathing. This discovery has been so often made accidentally that I am sure many of such cases have passed unnoticed, at least where the attendant is not well informed as to the insidious nature of typhous local diseases, and does not make it a practice and a duty to examine daily, as far as he can, the condition of every organ.

But the most remarkable circumstance in these cases is that the constitutional disease seems to be cut short. The expression of fever leaves the countenance, the peculiar colour or hue of typhus disappears, the eye becomes bright and intelligent, the tongue cleans, and the pulse comes down to a natural state. And thus we have seen patients so altered in the course of twenty-four hours that one had some difficulty in recognizing them. All the symptoms of typhus were gone, and nothing remained but the consolidation of the lung. And this, too, is not attended with any notable suffering. There may be a little cough, some dull pain, or an inability to lie on one side ; but that is all. The respiration is scarcely, if at all, accelerated ; in fact, it would seem that there was no irritation or excitement of the organ ; and the case is another proof of how much less the sufferings in disease are connected with the mechanical than with the vital conditions of organs.

By the operation of some law, which we do not as yet understand, there seems to exist a connection between the cessation of the essential disease and this consolidation of the lung ; the fever appears to *abort*, and the pulmonary change is critical. Under such circumstances our prognosis is favourable, the fever having ceased by a well-marked and peculiar mode of crisis.

This local disease, too, is generally easily managed. Indeed, the cure is often so rapid that I have thought that our remedies had little to do with the result. How are we to look at such cases? That they are not examples of inflammation of the lung is plain ; and it appears probable that, if this local disease had not occurred, the patient would have gone through the course of the fever of the day. Does it not seem as if the constitutional disease exhausted itself, as it were, in the production of the local affection, just as, in certain cases of simple variola, we see the fever to subside on the appearance of the pustule? I do not know whether such cases have been observed elsewhere, but of their existence we have had here abundant proofs. It is worthy of remark, too, that when we compare these cases with the ordinary forms of typhus, attended with secondary disease of the lung, the local affection is developed at an unusally early period; and it may be that, in the more protracted cases of fevers, the nature of which is to develop local affections, the periods of this development and of the cessation of the fever may also be coincident. We do not, however, find that this is so common as to establish a rule. Let us, assuming that these curious cases were really examples of typhus with a secondary deposit, again compare them with the more ordinary forms of the disease, and we shall find that they want two important characteristics of the longer fevers; one the successive or simultaneous production of various local diseases; and the other, the occurrence of that secondary inflammation or irritation of the parts in which the deposit takes place. That the latter circumstance is one of great weight in relation to the preventing or delaying of crisis, it is impossible to doubt. As to the case of successive or simultaneous production of local diseases, this, at all events, marks a more severe and complicated disease.

Gentlemen, I will not here enter into the wide subject of crisis in fever; yet I may point out to you, as a matter well worthy of investigation, the possibility of the occurrence of crisis by other modes than those which are generally enumerated; thus we may have a crisis without sweating, diuresis, hemorrhage, or diarrhœa, but which takes place by a silent change in the condition of an organ, and yet a change which will, or may, itself spontaneously disappear.

Here let me warn you against a common error with respect to cases of disease of the lung arising in the course of some form of constitutional malady or fever. They are usually set down as pneumonia, typhoid pneumonia by some. Now, the name itself would be of little moment if its adoption did not lead to errors in practice. And although it cannot be affirmed with certainty that in none of these cases is there pneumonia, yet we have good grounds for believing that, in many of them, inflammation, as the term is commonly understood, is either absent from the first, or, if it occurs, that it is only secondary to a special lesion induced by some form of essential disease.

It is difficult to give any well-defined classification of the various forms of diseases described under the head of typhoid pneumonia, or to draw the line between simple asthenic inflammation of the lungs and those conditions described from an early period under the terms of bilious, putrid, or typhoid pneumonia. And observe that when I make use of the term asthenic pneumonia I refer more to the condition of the general system than to the activity or inactivity of the local disease. For so far as local inflammatory action is concerned, there is proof that it may originate and proceed with rapidity, and even with vehemence, in the very last periods of life, so that the disease may be sthenic *quoad* the local condition, and yet the case itself be asthenic in reference to the general state of the economy. Much of the confusion with regard to this subject has arisen from the circumstance that too great weight was attached to the presence of certain physical signs, which were taken as always indicating similar vital conditions. The succession of the signs of crepitus, dulness, cessation of vesicular breathing, and its replacement by bronchial respiration, is too often held to indicate a simple pneumonia, in which the local disease is the principal condition, and the fever only a secondary one. But it is certain that this train of phenomena, or some modification of them, may occur under exactly opposite circumstances—the local disease being symptomatic of the fever, and not the fever of the local disease. And there is the strongest reason for believing that even though the mere anatomical condition of the lung in the two cases be similar, yet there is an essential, a vital difference, and that practically we cannot deal with the local disease in the latter case as if it were an original affection. This applies to all those cases with the physical signs of pneumonia, which are secondary to any form of fever, whether it be typhus or typhoid, whether it be variola or erysipelas, purulent poisoning of the blood, glanders, malignant scarlatina, or malignant measles. In these cases, even though the physical signs accurately correspond with those of the typical pneumonia— which, by the way, is by no means always the case—we must believe that we are dealing with a special condition of parts, a condition special not only as compared with ordinary pneumonia, but inasmuch as it is derived from the parent malady.

In the present state of our knowledge, gentlemen, we cannot declare that any special pathological condition exists by which we can distinguish these secondary diseases one from the other. We may say this much, that practically they appear to agree in being indicative of an asthenic state of the system, and therefore, the supervention of their physical signs at any period of those various diseases must not be permitted to divert your attention from the general condition of the patient, or to make you proceed to treat a case as one of sthenic pneumonia because it has some, or even all, of the physical signs of that condition. Do not suppose that I am taking up your time unnecessarily by insisting on these points, for they lead us directly to deal with one of the greatest, if not the greatest and most wide-spread error in the practice of medicine—namely, the treatment of all local acute diseases with feverish symptoms as inflammations. Here is a group of acute local diseases with feverish symptoms, and not only this, but a set of cases exhibiting some or all of the physical phenomena of acute pneumonia; and yet if we subjected them to the ordinary treatment of inflammation, the worst consequences would almost certainly follow. You must learn to look at the antecedents and the accompanying general phenomena of these diseases, and set your face against the adoption of any treatment which is based on the doctrine that they are original inflammations.

I have good reason to believe, and I rejoice at it, that the erroneous views to which I allude are every day becoming less and less frequent, thanks to our improved system of clinical instruction and to the independent spirit of investigation which now animates so many of our students. Notwithstanding, they are still too often acted upon, and over and over again patients who have enough to contend with as the victims of some fell fever or other constitutional disease are lost, or assisted to their death, by the adoption of a local or general antiphlogistic treatment, in consequence of the physical signs of a pneumonia being discovered. Their stimulants are withheld or withdrawn; tartar emetic, or mercury, or even blood-letting is rashly resorted to; and it often happens that, even though the physical signs of the pneumonia are removed or modified, the patient sinks from the combined effect of the original disease and the exhaustion produced by this treatment. I do not think that any of you will fall into these or similar errors, after what I have so often said; it will, at least, not be my fault if you do.

Let us now consider the parenchymatous affections of the lung in fever, or, if you will, the typhous disease of the pulmonary structure. It may be stated generally that whatever be the differences in the various cases of this affection in fever, the local disease follows the general law of other lesions secondary to the fever; that is to say, it agrees with them in its frequent absence, mode of invasion, latency in the earlier periods of its development, spontaneous retrocession, and, lastly, pathological effects. It is quite true that, as compared with the best marked examples of acute sthenic pneumonia, it is not wanting in any of the physical signs of that disease taken singly, but it is generally different from it in the order or arrangement, as it were, of these physical signs. And, indeed, I think the rise, progress, and retrocession of a pneumonia which has passed into hepatization, as we so continually see in ordinary cases of the disease, is rarely observed in the course of a typhus fever. I have already drawn your attention to those curious cases of consolidation of the upper lobe of the lung. Now, whether these be genuine examples of an arrested typhus, or not, it is difficult to say, but their whole history and progress is very different from those of ordinary pneumonia; and I repeat that there is nothing rarer than to see in the course of a typhus fever that regular succession of phenomena with which Laennec has made us so familiar, so indicating the several successive stages of an idiopathic acute pneumonia.

The most common case is the occurrence, generally at an early period, especially in the maculated forms, and often at a later period in the non maculated and so-called typhoid fevers, of a well-marked crepitating râle in the lower lobes of one or both lungs; it is generally much more extensive and distinctly marked in one lung than in the other. The amount of dulness is seldom very great, and we find the disease, as it were, to linger, and for days together to show no disposition either to produce solidity of the lung on the one hand, or to proceed to resolution on the other. It is often quite latent, and recognizable only by careful physical examination; and its discovery, as you will readily understand from what I have said before, is sometimes an unfortunate circumstance for the patient. In the present state of our knowledge we must believe this condition of the organ to be either the result of a certain amount of typhous deposit into the lung, or of a special state—an inflammation, if you will—which is, however, under the general law of the fever, partaking of its specific character and capable of spontaneous retrocession. It is seldom attended by pain or by hæmoptysis, and constantly exists without any important modification of the general symptoms of the case.

The second form of the disease is of a more serious character, and seems to be connected either with an original pyogenic disposition, itself secondary to fever, or we may suppose that the typhous deposit undergoes a rapid purulent transformation, so that in this way a condition of the lung is established, having some resemblance to the third stage of pneumonia, as described by Laennec. I have not myself seen a sufficient number of these cases to justify me in speaking very decidedly as to their physical signs; but I think I have seen enough of them to warrant me in believing that the course of the disease is different from that of ordinary suppurative pneumonia. We have not observed the intermediate stage of well-marked hepatization between that which is characterized by the occurrence of early râle on the one hand, and the signs of interstitial suppuration on the other. The complete dulness and the bronchial respiration which accompany the third stage of pneumonia as described by Laennec we have not observed, the physical signs being principally a persisting râle passing from a fine into a large crepitus, and semi-dulness on percussion. On dissection the lung is found soft, friable, of a grayish-red colour, but still very permeable to air, though infiltrated with purulent matter. It is as if the purulent secretion took place coincidently with, or immediately after, the first or congestive stage. Some of the patients have had sweatings and a sanguinolent and somewhat sanious expectoration; but we have not hitherto observed the ordinary adhesive prune-juice sputa in these cases. I have seen this disease in connection with purulent deposits in the neck and posterior mediastinum, but it may occur without the formation of purulent matter in any situation other than the lung; it may supervene in the advanced periods of the case, and at a time when the patient seems about to recover, or it may come on much earlier, and when the skin is thickly covered with the petechial eruption. The last case is the most formidable; but though it is attended with the greatest danger, the disease in it is, however, not always fatal, and we have had several instances in which recovery took place. I need not say that they were all treated upon a tonic and stimulating plan, in addition to which we employed dry cupping and blisters.

The last case of which I shall speak at present is by far the most acute and formidable of the pulmonary affections of fever; it is characterized by a sudden, complete, and singularly extensive consolidation of the lung. In the course of twenty-four, or even sometimes of twelve, hours the most extensive and complete dulness may be produced in a lung which had been previously free from physical signs or at most had only exhibited some ordinary bronchial râles. We have thus the signs of complete hepatization, not preceded by the crepitating râle; the disease begins by consolidation, and then one of two results follows—either the patient dies speedily, generally with loose râles in the opposite lung, combined with tracheal effusion; or after a day or two he begins to expectorate a horribly fetid matter, and we discover by the stethoscope that a large cavity has formed in the lung. This is a true gangrenous cavity in the very centre of the solidified mass, and the disease has a close pathological analogy to the process of acute mortification which has been described as occurring in some of the worst cases of the typhous disease of the intestinal glands.

Let us now pass in review the circumstances in which these forms of disease occur; for when we compare them with the ordinary conditions of acute primary pneumonia, we cannot but admit that they indicate a lesion of a very different nature.

In the first place, the physical signs are preceded by fever; and it may not be until days have elapsed that the symptoms of lung affection as it were spontaneously arise. Secondly, the fever is obviously an essential fever; it may occur with or without petechiæ, and other complications may or may not be present. Thirdly, the disease sets in without any apparent external cause. Fourthly, when the purulent form is observed, it appears to be, not the third, but the second stage of the affection; and I may here remark that, on dissection, we rarely, if ever, find what we may term perfectly concocted purulent matter. Lastly, the invasion of one form of the affection may be sudden, and the signs of extensive and complete consolidation be among its earliest phenomena. It is in this case, too, that if time be allowed, large eschars, forming cavities which may communicate with the bronchial tubes, are liable to occur.

I may remark here that in two cases of this rapid consolidation the gangrenous eschar did not communicate with the bronchial tubes. One was a case of severe typhus, in a man who had long before suffered from gangrene of the opposite lung; the other occurred in a case of what is termed the erysipelatous or diffuse inflammation.

The first patient had no gangrenous expectoration. The lower lobe of the left lung presented a very large non-encysted and recent cavity, of a dark colour, filled with fetid grumous fluid. In the opposite lung was found an old cavity, lined with strong fibrous membrane, and containing a quantity of a substance like putrid flax. It had three hollow projections, and communicated with the bronchus.

In the second patient there was complete and recent solidity throughout the lower anterior part of the right lung. A cavity, the size of a large walnut, without bronchial communication, was found filled with fetid purulent sanies.

7

LECTURE XIII.

PNEUMONIC COMPLICATIONS OF FEVER, *continued*—"Typhoid pneumonia," so called, is not dependent on a coexistent gastritis—Correct view is that both pulmonary and intestinal lesions spring from the one parent condition, that of fever—Physical signs of ordinary pneumonia are often found, but in an irregular succession, in the secondary pneumonic affection—Sign of *tympanitic resonance* in latter, first described by Dr. Hudson—Probable causes of the production of this percussion sound—The author's views—Dr. Lyon's views—Three explanations of the production of the sign—Frequent absence of *crepitus redux* in resolution of secondary typhous disease—When inflammatory affections do occur in fever, they are reactive or tertiary in their nature—Typhous affection of the larynx—Rokitansky's "laryngo-typhus."

I ENDEAVOURED to convey to you, at our last lecture, that the conditions which have been described under the head of typhoid pneumonia were probably examples not only of a pathological but of an anatomical state of parts different from that which is found in the simple original inflammation of the lung. And it is a great deal easier to say what they are not than what they are—to state their negative rather than their positive characters.

Now, I wish to mention here that a certain change has occurred in our opinions as to the origin of the so-called typhoid inflammation of the lung. We at one time held that it was the coexistence of gastritis which gave to the pneumonia the typhoid character. This view was held by us before we had, by that imperceptible power of conviction which arises from experience, admitted the two following principles in their entirety :—

1st. That symptoms which are diagnostic of local disease, where the patient has not an essential fever, are either altogether valueless or much lessened in value when such a condition exists; and

2d. That the gastric lesion is rare even as a secondary disease in fever ; so that when irritation of the structures of the stomach occurs it is a tertiary and accidental phenomenon.

Our present opinion on this matter is in general the following: that in cases in which there are, in connection with the signs of typhoid lesion of the lung, evidences of gastro-intestinal disease, both the pulmonary and abdominal lesions spring from the one parent condition, and that, so far from the specialities of the pulmonary being derived from the accidental complication with the abdominal disease, both have a common character originating in the same source. I am quite sure that a large proportion of those cases described as examples of asthenic pneumonia depending on gastric complication have been examples of essential fever, with the two affections coexisting as secondary lesions.

We have seen that in these cases, I will not say of typhoid pneumonia, but of typhous or typhoid affections of the lung, the various physical signs of pneumonia, singly considered, may be present, and are actually often to be found. They fail, however, very frequently to present themselves in that regular order or succession which is observed in true acute pneumonia.

Now let us inquire whether there is any physical sign peculiar to these cases of typhous pulmonary affections which does not occur, at least as the rule, in idiopathic inflammation of the lung. I do not know of the existence of any such, unless it be the sign of tympanitic resonance over the diseased lung—a condition first noticed by Dr. Hudson, of this city, and to which much importance is to be attached. Dr. Hudson states that in certain cases of typhous consolidation of the lung the sound on percussion is sometimes very different from that observable in the ordinary condition of hepatization. He describes it as " a tympanitic clearness over the solidified lung without air being present in the pleura;" indeed, he goes so far as to say that in one case the tympanitic resonance on percussion existed fully to the same degree and was of the same kind as in pneumo-thorax. Here the lung was found perfectly solid throughout, with the exception of a small extent over the anterior and postero-inferior parts which was still crepitating.

It is very difficult to understand what condition of parts could have caused this singular tympanitic resonance over a solidified lung. When we speak of tympanitic resonance, it must be always borne in mind that the tympanitic sound does not always imply clearness on percussion. When a cavity exists in the centre of a solidified lung, or when hepatization of the left lung is present in connection with flatulent distension of the stomach, the sound on percussion, though dull as compared with that of the healthy lung, has a distinctly tympanitic character; to this we have long been in the habit of giving the name of tympanitic dulness. I have never found it, however, to simulate the tympanitic resonance which occurs in pneumo-thorax, or in dilatation of the air cells; it is inferior in degree and different in character. It is probable that in cases in which the sound on percussion resembled that in pneumo-thorax, there was an actual secretion of air to some extent between the pulmonary and costal pleuræ. Dr.

Hudson met with four cases, in which the observation of tympanitic dulness was followed by dissection. One was that of a man who died of extensive inflammation of the left lung in the Meath Hospital in the spring of 1832. At the close of the case, from the hollow sound on percussion at the lower part of the left side—it had been previously quite dull—a pretty general opinion existed that a pneumonic abscess had formed and burst into the pleura. On dissection, the side having been punctured, no air escaped; the lung was red and solid, but without abscess, and the pleura was adherent over two-thirds of its extent.

I am quite prepared to admit that, with extensive solidification of the lung, the dull sound on percussion may yet have a tympanitic character; but I have seen no case in which this sound could be confounded with that of pneumo-thorax, or of dilatation of the air cells. With reference to the bearings of this question upon the signs of typhous pneumonia, I can at this moment remember only two cases which are worth detailing to you. In one tympanitic dulness did occur over the diseased portion of the lung, without our being able to account for it by any accumulation of air either in the pleura or in the stomach. The case was of a low putrid character, and I remember suggesting it as just possible that there might have been a typhous pneumatosis developed in the diseased lung; but I am sure that we were not able to establish the existence of such a condition on dissection; the case occurred a good many years ago.

In the second case, which was one of manifest typhus, the posterior portion of the right lung became solid or nearly so, while the anterior face of the organ preserved its vesicular respiration. Now, we found that over this portion of the chest—that is, over the front of the thorax on the right side—the sound, as compared with that over the opposite lung, was morbidly clear; it was true tympanitic clearness, not dulness, and it continued for three or four days, and gradually disappeared with the resolution of the posterior solidity: this case occurred in the Meath Hospital, and was seen by Dr. Hudson himself. I confess I am quite at a loss to explain the nature or mode of production of this phenomenon. Dr. Lyons mentioned to me that in a case of asthenic pneumonia occurring in a patient of intemperate habits, whom we saw in consultation, the anterior superior part of the left lung presented for a couple of days a condition of morbid clearness, but subsequently became engaged in the general consolidation of the organ.

Dr. Lyons is disposed to regard the abnormal clearness which occurs in these cases as the result of the increased pressure of the respiratory column of air in the still permeable portions of the pulmonary cells, which he considers in certain cases become from this cause expanded beyond their natural volume. His views are that the inspired air presses with a certain force on the whole pulmonary surface, and that if a portion of this surface becomes impermeable to air from solid deposit, occlusion of the tubes, or other cause, the remaining portion of the pulmonary tissue is acted on by the whole of the inspiratory force, before which it is thus made to expand. This portion of the lung may thus be considered to be in a condition of temporary dilatation of the cells, and so gives a correspondingly clear sound on percussion.

Dr. Hudson's discovery of this sign is of great value in many points of view, but, I think, chiefly as leading not only to the clearer distinction between ordinary pneumonia and the secondary disease of fever, but as a diagnostic of the essential character of the entire malady in the latter instance. In Dr. Hudson's cases the disease seemed to be the typhous affection of the lung, and the facts you will find in his lectures on the "Study of Fever." Many times since his memoir first appeared we have met with cases in our wards presenting this sign in various degrees of intensity and extent. All these cases were examples of typhous or asthenic consolidations of the lung. His observations are confirmed by Dr. Hayden, in one of whose cases the solidified lung, though it sank in water, gave the same sound on percussion that had been given by the chest during life.

Now, there seem to be but three explanations of this remarkable sign: first, the secretion of air into the pleura under the influence of the general disease; secondly, compression of the lung while it still is permeable to air; thirdly, an interstitial pneumatosis in connection with the typhous processes.

Dr. Graves has shown that a temporary pneumo-thorax without pulmonary fistula, and yet sufficient to displace organs, may occur in pneumonia. We know that a compression of the lung while it still continues permeable—as from liquid effusion into the pericardium or pleura—may cause a partial tympanitic resonance. But looking at Dr. Hudson's cases, at those recorded by Dr. Hayden, and at our own experience, it seems most probable that in the typhous consolidations of the lung there may occur an interstitial secretion of air, recognized by local resonance, and which may disappear with the subsidence of the pulmonary lesion.

It is not unlikely that this condition is often overlooked in consequence of the frequent latency of the pulmonary complications in fever, and that the formation of air in the vessels is sometimes a result of fever we have direct proof. It is now some years since a middle-aged man was a patient in the fever ward with maculated typhus of the most severe kind. I cannot now say whether the lungs were greatly engaged, but it was the nervous system which seemed chiefly to suffer. Muttering delirium and deepening coma appeared early. These symptoms were followed by a universal subsultus, which increased to an extraordinary degree, and for the last two or three days of life affected, as it were, every little muscular fibre in the face, the incessant twitching of which produced an influence on the expression of the countenance and an appearance I had never before witnessed. This continued up to the time of death. On dissection every vein in the pia mater and in the substance of the brain was found to contain innumerable bubbles of air, which were also present in the sinuses.

There is a circumstance in connection with the resolution of these typhous diseases of the lung different from what is commonly observed in sthenic pneumonia. The true inflammatory hepatization rarely disappears suddenly. It subsides gradually, and the transition state between dulness and clearness on percussion is generally marked by the "crepitus redux." In the cases before us the resolution is often singularly rapid, and unattended by the crepitus of resolution. If, then, we consider the state of solidification simply, we find it on the one hand forming without the crepitus of the first stage of pneumonia, and on the other disappearing rapidly, and without the râle of resolution. Thus we are permitted, as it were, to witness the silent and spontaneous development and retrocession of one of the secondary internal diseases of fever.

This rapid change from the state of consolidation to that of permeability to air, unattended by the crepitus of resolution, probably shows that the disease was unconnected with inflammation either as a primary or as a reactive condition.

You will remember that I suggested to you that some of the cases which have been described as typhoid pneumonia might be held as examples of an aborted typhus. These were characterized by early consolidation, early disappearance of the typhous state, and a rapid and often spontaneous subsidence of the local disease. I cannot help thinking that between such cases and those in which the general disease runs its usual course there is another class in which the progress of the merely pulmonary disease is marked, more or less, by signs of irritation or inflammation of the lung, which is either reactive or specific, or both reactive and specific. I apprehend, too, that these cases which, as it were, float between the aborted and the perfect typhus, are more numerous than might be supposed; and in such instances the malady is often treated throughout without a suspicion of its being really an example of typhous disease.

What has been now said should impress on your minds the principle I have urged upon you—that the rules of diagnosis of local inflammatory disease which are good in ordinary cases lose their value in a great measure when the patient has fever. This was long ago proved by the researches of Louis on the condition of the brain in fever, and it was the non-recognition of this fact which constituted one of the greatest errors of Broussais. I have told you that if you gained nothing during the session but the knowledge of this principle, your time would have been well spent. How many cases have we not had of headache, delirium, watchfulness, or its opposite, coma, yet without encephalitis? And so it is with the remaining cavities—symptoms of functional alteration are met with in connection with the cerebral, pulmonary, circulating, and digestive systems in fever. They may or may not be attended by organic change, and that organic change, when it does exist, is not necessarily inflammation. We cannot, I believe, lay down any satisfactory rule of diagnosis which would show that in one case of local functional disturbance there was organic change, and in another there was not.

I do not seek to teach you that inflammation, with prominent symptoms, and calling for local antiphlogistic treatment, never occurs in fever. You must be cautious in using the word "never" in medicine. That true cerebritis has been met with in fever is certain, especially in the form of meningeal inflammation. But it seems probable that this occurs less frequently in the head than in the chest or abdomen, and it is almost certain that when it does exist it is not a primary but a reactive inflammation.

It becomes one of the most difficult problems in practice to distinguish between the functional and organic affections of the nervous system in fever. The secondary lesions of the brain vary as to their frequency according to the character of the epidemic, as we have seen in the late prevalence of the black fever, or—as it has been called—the cerebro-spinal fever. But the great point to be remembered is that these cerebral lesions have all the characters of the secondary affections—namely, their inconstancy in amount, seat, period of appearance, their mode of retrocession, intensity, and incompetence to account for the characters of the general malady. Let this principle be ever present to your minds, for it is impossible to exaggerate its value. Long ago it was acted on empirically by the best physicians, who refused to adopt antiphlogistic measures in treating the local symptoms in fever, and who employed stimulants irrespective of them, when the general condition seemed to demand such treatment. It now comes before you as the result of an extended observation, and the study of the pulmonary phenomena, as we have seen, enables us to go a step further, and to declare that not only are the symptoms of local irritation often doubtful or illusive, but that even the physical signs of pneumonia, when occurring in a case of fever, are not to be taken as proof that a local inflammation has occurred.

If these things be true so far as essential fever is concerned, it would appear probable that in other acute diseases under the influence of a law of periodicity, and, perhaps, in many that arise from the operation of an introduced poison, the same circumstances may be found, so that we might apply to a much larger circle of diseases those principles, as to the secondary local affections, which belong to fever.

In speaking of the bronchial membrane in fever, we said nothing with respect to lesions of the larynx or trachea as a result of the fever. Taken as a localized disease, I would say that this lesion is not very commonly met with; and we may safely hold that it is by no means so frequent in the petechial fever of these countries as it appears to be in the fevers of the Continent.

This is the condition to which Rokitansky has given the name of laryngo-typhus, by which he means a secondary lesion of the mucous membrane of the larynx and trachea, analogous to that of the bronchial membrane. It is, then, a secondary affection of the fever developed in the windpipe, and either confined to that part or predominating in it. I think it probable that in most cases of this disease there is an associated affection of the bronchial membrane. But, so far as the fever of this country is concerned, the converse of the proposition does not hold good; for we constantly see the most profound bronchial affection without tracheal or laryngeal symptoms.

We have met a few cases which would answer to the description of Rokitansky's laryngo-typhus. A more proper name for this disease would clearly be "a typhous affection of the larynx." In those cases which we have seen, the symptoms were loss of voice, or a certain degree of hoarseness; the cough never was the so-called *tussis clangosa*, although it often partook of the laryngeal character, and I do not remember any instance of stridor but one in connection with the other laryngeal symptoms. In some cases the weakness or hoarseness of voice continued for a considerable time, and did not disappear until convalescence was far advanced.

I have often thought that, in these cases, the lesion of voice was to be attributed more to the weakness or paralysis of the laryngeal muscles than to any form of irritation or inflammation of the mucous surface. For although we cannot bring any observations from dissection to throw light on this point, we may fairly believe that the laryngeal muscles are liable to be affected in fever, just as the muscular fibres of the heart are often found to be; that the same process which causes a typhous deposit in the mucous surface may be repeated in the vocal muscles; and that a certain time must elapse before these organs recover their healthy condition. They may also be weakened quite independently of any structural change, just as occurs in the heart; for in this latter organ there are doubtless two forms of debility in connection with fever—in the one, we have weakness with actual softening of structure; in the other, a debility which appears to be purely nervous.

This leads me further to draw your attention to the probable existence of similar conditions in the circular, and perhaps also in the longitudinal, fibres of the bronchial tubes in this secondary disease. I have little doubt that such a condition exists in many instances, and that a weakness, with or without softening of these structures, becomes an important element in the bronchial disease of fever. If, as some modern authorities have urged, these circular fibres are really the expectorating muscles, we can readily see how any weakness or paralysis affecting them would greatly increase the danger of a patient already suffering under copious secretion into the bronchial tubes. We can further understand not only how this condition would superinduce what is termed "effusion into the chest," but also why it is that in the treatment of the bronchial disease of fever there is such danger from the employment of the antiphlogistic method, and how, on the other hand, such admirable results follow from the bold use of tonics and stimulants.

When we come to speak of the heart in fever, I will draw your attention to the fact that in many of our most remarkable examples of typhous softening of that organ there was a great amount of the secondary bronchial disease; and in such cases you will constantly see the associated diseases of the heart and the lung progressing or retrograding simultaneously, the treatment adapted to the one being suitable also to the other. In the heart, so far as we know, we have to deal with an affection only of the muscular structure; in the lung we have at least two different forms of anatomical structure affected —the muscular and the mucous tissues. But the existence of the essential typhous state so far affects these tissues that their vital condition is depressed in a similar manner; and it happens that what-ever is tonic and stimulant to the one is equally so to the other, and so by supporting and augmenting the vital energy of both structures we can add the assistance of art to the efforts of nature in throwing off the disease.

In connection with the subject of laryngo-typhus, I remember a case of complete aphonia without any other laryngeal symptom in a patient suffering from fever for some days. There were no signs of any disease in the upper portions of either lung, and we were at a loss to explain the symptom. After a few days the chest was again examined, when it was discovered that the postero-inferior portions of both lungs had passed into complete consolidation. For this the patient was treated, and resolution was established in the ordinary way. Simultaneously the voice began to improve, and was shortly quite restored. The explanation of the occurrence of aphonia in this case is difficult, but it may be that the symptom was due to reflex irritation of the pneumo-gastric nerve, dependent on the condition of consolidation in a portion of the lungs.

LECTURE XIV.

THE HEART IN FEVER—The state of the pulse, especially in typhus, not always a reliable guide—Weakening of the heart may coexist with a full, bounding pulse —*Slow* pulse in convalescence is consequent on a typhous weakening of the heart —*Rapid* pulse in convalescence is of unfavourable import, pointing to (1) *tubercu-losis*, or (2) secondary *reactive inflammation of the mucous glands of the intestine,* or (3) *phlegmasia dolens*—In such cases the local malady assumes the prominence hitherto presented by the essential disease—Illustrative case of hepatic abscess in convalescence from the yellow fever in 1826-27—Intermittent fever at close of epidemic of 1827—Frequency of phlegmasia dolens—Bleedings in cold stage, after Dr. Mackintosh—Failure of quinine in cases of simulative ague, arising from (1) phlegmasia dolens, (2) urinary disease, and (3) the puerperal state.

NEXT in order I shall speak of the conditions of the heart in fever —a topic which calls for our most attentive consideration.

From the earliest times physicians have been in the habit of rely-ing on the pulse as a guide for the administration or the withholding of stimulants in fever. Now, I must tell you that in typhus at least the pulse is not always to be depended on as a truthful indication. In true typhus one of the most unreliable and illusory symptoms is the state of the pulse, especially in the earlier stages of the disease.

For instance, in a case of the true petechial character you may find the patient, even on the fourth day, with a full and bounding pulse, while within 24 hours the whole condition will have changed. Now, this state of pulse has too often led to errors in practice both of commission and omission—of commission, from the adoption of general or local depletion; and of omission, from the postponement of the necessary treatment, owing to the apparent inflammatory condition of the system. The opportunity is lost of employing nutrient and stimulant remedies in time. You, gentlemen, educated as you have been, and taught to look on fever with an eye rather to the general aspect of the disease that to its local accompaniments, will not, I trust, fall into this error. I tell you that in typhus fever, at the very time when the pulse has that full, bounding, and seemingly inflammatory character, debility of the heart, with or without softening, may already have set in. As regards the circulatory system, I will say to you: Examine closely the state of the pulse, and then the character of the heart's action. If both coincide in vigour, so far so well; but you must be prepared to find very often a full and bounding radial pulse coinciding with a feebly acting heart—a condition probably progressive. Here we have evidence of the necessity of anticipative treatment, and commonly of its good effects.

We have now passed in review some of the important typhous affections of the lung. I have told you that in cases of this kind there have been frequently signs of an analogous condition in the muscles of the heart, and to this subject I now crave your attention.

Long ago Laennec stated that in certain cases of low fever he found the heart in a softened condition—in what he termed *l'état poisseux* of the muscles of that organ. He did not recognize the real nature of this condition, but held it to be evidence of the degeneration of the muscular structure of both the voluntary and the involuntary systems, resulting from the dissolution of the fluids in putrid fever. He suggested whether in those cases of fever which exhibit rapidity of pulse during convalescence this symptom is to be attributed to a softening of the heart. This opinion is not well founded, the true typhous softening of the heart, so far from being followed by rapidity of pulse during convalescence, has much more frequently the effect of making it slow—slow not only as considered with reference to the condition of health, but actually falling below the ordinary standard. That rapidity of pulse is commonly associated with typhous affections of the heart, in which there is a weakening of the organs while the fever continues, must be admitted. But this is a different proposition from that advanced by Laennec, who speaks of the symptom during convalescence. Many of the greatest triumphs of the stimulant treatment in our wards have been seen in cases where the pulse was as high as 140 in the minute, the effect being to lessen its frequency from day to day until the period of convalescence was reached.

I have little doubt that Laennec met with the true typhous softening of the heart, although he misinterpreted its nature. You may take it as an established fact that in typhus the heart may be softened to the most extreme degree, while the voluntary muscles remain intact. And you may further rest assured that rapidity of pulse in convalescence, so far from indicating any remains of the typhous disease in the muscular structure of the heart, is in most cases a proof of the existence of some lurking disease of some important organ or organs. I say in *most* cases, for we sometimes meet with instances in which this state of things cannot be discovered, and where the quickness of pulse shows that the heart had contracted a habit of rapid action, which it requires time to get rid of. But these cases are exceptional; and whenever you find rapidity of pulse in a patient who has thrown off his fever, you are to take alarm.

These cases of quickness of pulse are of two kinds. In one class the pulse has never lost the rapidity it attained during the fever; or it has, perhaps, come down fifteen or twenty beats in the minute, and its rate then remains stationary. In the other cases the pulse, which had become quiet, again rises to 100 or 120, or even higher, and remains at that increased rate for days together, without our being able to detect any cause for this rapidity. The latter is, I think, the worse case of the two; at least it appears oftener to indicate a new pathological change.

The local diseases which most frequently attend this condition are of two kinds—one of them is tuberculosis in the lungs and other parts; the other is the existence of a secondary reactive inflammation in the mucous glands of the intestines.

But now suppose that you examine a patient having a quick pulse in convalescence with great care. You percuss his chest; you examine the state of his respiration in every way; yet you cannot satisfy yourself that there is any disease in his lung; and you will recollect what I mentioned in a former lecture, that in most cases of this tuberculosis after fever there is great local and constitutional suffering. Well, you may make up your mind, from the absence of all these signs, that the patient is not becoming tuberculous at all events. On proceeding to examine the abdomen, you will find, perhaps, that he has a good appetite; that his thirst is gone; that the belly is soft, without any tumefaction; that there is no tenderness on pressure

anywhere, no throbbing of the abdominal aorta, no tendency to diarrhœa—in fact, no symptom whatever of disease of the mucous membrane of the intestine. And yet, as in the case in the small fever
ward, you have a pulse with this unpleasant degree of quickness.
Although this patient has convalesced after a long fever, and is now
gaining flesh and strength, we have found that the pulse continues
rapid. I rather think that it is now quicker than on the 21st day of
his illness, and it makes me extremely uneasy about him.

Now, gentlemen, suppose that under such circumstances you did
not find disease either of the lung or of the abdomen—in this patient
the signs of abdominal and pulmonary lesion have disappeared, as
well as the characteristic expression of what may be termed the condition of fever—what should you suspect? Generally you may look
for phlegmasia dolens; for we have seen many cases in which, after
fever, the pulse continuing rapid, this disease exploded. This is, I
think, more likely to occur in the non-petechial than in the petechial
cases, in the long than in the short fevers; it is very liable to arise in
patients who have had a fever running on beyond twenty-one, thirty,
or forty days. These patients, after the true symptoms of fever have
subsided, remain with a rapid pulse, and probably in a week or so
symptoms of phlegmasia dolens come on. The disposition to this
complication is sometimes remarkable, for you will very often find
that the patients have two or three distinct attacks of it. It may
affect one leg, and the patient may pass through that attack; still the
pulse does not regain its natural rate. After a week or ten days the
other extremity will be attacked; nay, it is even possible that a third
seizure may occur—a relapse, as it were, of the disease in the part
first affected. In this way patients will go on labouring under the
affection and its consequences for months together, although recovery
ultimately takes place.

In most of the cases I have seen there was distinct notice of the
invasion of the disease—that is to say, the patient was attacked with
pain in the calf of the leg. He is seized, say, in the course of the
night, and in the morning he exhibits all the characteristics of the
disease—a large swelling, pain on pressure, and all the other symptoms. Sometimes you find a cordy state of the superficial veins; at
other times, not. When you can feel a deep-seated vein, you will
occasionally find it in a hard and cordy state.

I think it right to warn you of these contingencies, for I am sure
that in the course of your practice you will often have a patient recovering from fever, and going on in every respect well, except that
the pulse does not come down. The rule then is, that, if the most

minute examination fails to detect disease in the great viscera, the occurrence of this complication may be looked for.

The term phlegmasia dolens is not always applied correctly, for the disease is not necessarily painful. We have seen a few instances in which the discovery of the local affection was entirely accidental. Of course you will not suppose that I am confident that the patient in the ward will have phlegmasia dolens; all I say is, that he is in that state which would justify you in suspecting something of the kind.

I have mentioned the rapid deposition of tubercle, ulceration of the intestines, and phlegmasia dolens of the lower extremities, as the diseases we have found to occur most commonly in these instances of apparently unaccountable quickness of the pulse after fever. Doubtless there are many more examples of local disease arising under these circumstances; but the general rule will hold good, that this symptom foreshadows a disease which, although at first latent, will before long become manifest.

These diseases are generally attended with much irritation, and the condition of the patient is one rather of irritation, or inflammation if you will, than of essential fever. And this is one of many illustrations of a circumstance often observed by the clinical investigator—namely, the change of character of disease, locally and constitutionally in the same patient, and within a not very extended period. The typhous condition, generally considered, changes into a different state. The essential state disappears, and a local irritation, with its symptomatic fever, becomes the prominent malady. Nay, you will find that the very condition of a local disease, formed during the first—the typhous or essential—period, will itself change, and take on the characters of what is termed by some a "healthy inflammation."

You may sometimes see this well illustrated in that terrible disease, accompanied by purulent deposits in many of the articulations, which may be called "idiopathic pyæmia." The patients may throw off the typhoid state which attends the earlier periods of the disease, and then the affection of the joints seems to change in its nature, and to take on the characters of ordinary arthritis. I have, however, seen this only where one or two of the larger joints had been affected with the primary disease; and it was most remarkable to witness the changes both in the constitutional state and in the local affection. It was no longer necessary to use general stimulation; it was no longer improper to employ local antiphlogistic measures.

You will see in the article on "Hepatic Abscess," in the "Cyclopædia of Practical Medicine," a case which we may well study in connection with this subject. The patient was a middle-aged man, who was attacked with the yellow fever, of which we had such striking examples in the epidemic of 1826 and 1827. A valuable account of this disease is to be met with in Dr. Graves' "Clinical Medicine." This patient was the first who was saved. The treatment which I adopted on the appearance of the jaundice and the spasms of the belly was the free application of leeches to the abdomen, the use of calomel and opium in full doses, and a liberal allowance of wine. The man recovered, to our great surprise; but whether from the measures employed, or from the circumstance that the epidemic was then losing its malignity, it is difficult to say. However, his recovery seemed perfect; the pulse became natural; the yellowness rapidly disappeared; no gangrene of the limbs or nose had occurred; and he was finally discharged, to all appearance quite recovered.

Within a fortnight he again applied for admission. He was evidently very ill. The pulse was rapid. He had copious sweats. The breathing was hurried, but not laboured, and he had a hacking dry cough. I at first suspected that his case was one of the acute consequent tubercle which I have already described to you. I could discover no sign of abdominal disease, and the physical examination of the chest, repeated with great care from day to day, gave results very different from those observed in the acute deposition of tubercle after fever. There were neither the intense and persisting bronchial râles nor the progressive dulness; and so I remained in the most unhappy of all positions to which a physician can be exposed—namely, that of having to treat an acute disease of which he knows neither the seat nor the nature. However, the suspense did not last long. In a few days, at the time of visit with the class, I found him coughing up purulent matter, and the nurse showed us a vessel which held more than a quart of the same fluid, which the patient had coughed up during the night. The expectoration had come on suddenly. On the day before I had made a most minute examination of the chest, both anteriorly, and posteriorly, and had failed to discover any sign of disease. Yet we now found that the posterior portion of the left side, as far as the scapular spine, was absolutely dull. There was no bronchial respiration, no resonance of the voice, and, I think, no râle. We came to the conclusion that an abscess, probably of the liver, had opened into the chest. I will not go into the details of our treatment, which was that usually employed in cases of internal suppuration. The patient rapidly recovered, and left the hospital without the slightest physical sign of disease in either the chest or belly. During the next ten years I had repeated opportunities of seeing this man, who continued to enjoy the most perfect health.

This case is well worthy of your careful study. It shows, in the first place, that rapidity of pulse, after convalescence, probably indicates some profound lesion; next, that we were right to pause before making the diagnosis of acute tubercle, when there was a want of correspondence between the physical signs and the constitutional symptoms. It is an additional illustration of the possible existence of hepatic abscess, without perceptible hepatic tumour; and, lastly, it is remarkable as being the only instance during that singular epidemic tendency to yellow fever, in which organic change of the liver seemed to occur. Dr. Graves dwells strongly on the point that in none of our dissections did we find hepatitis; and it is quite possible that, even in this case, during the violence of the first attack—that is, when the patient had the yellow fever—the liver was not inflamed, and that its subsequent suppuration may have been owing either to abdominal phlebitis or to a pyogenic diathesis. I assume that the abscess was in the liver; but even this is not absolutely certain. It assuredly was not originally in the chest. Whether the purulent matter made its way into the lung by a perforation of the diaphragm, or whether the case was an example of vicarious action of the lung, thus removing the purulent matter from the liver, are questions which can never be answered.

As I have alluded to the invasion of phlegmasia dolens after fever, I may mention a case which occurred many years ago in this hospital. You all know that intermittent fever is a rare disease in this country. It is not endemic in our vast mountain districts, nor in our level boggy plains; and, indeed, for many years we never had a case of ague in hospital that did not occur in the person of one of the labourers who went to the fenny districts of England to cut the harvest. These men were often attacked with ague on their way home, the disease being immediately excited by the cold, wet, and fatigue to which they were exposed on their journey. At the close of the epidemic of 1828, intermittent fever became very general; in fact, it was epidemic, and for a time almost every case in our wards was an example of some form of ague.

It was at that time that I tried the treatment of bleeding, in the cold stage, as recommended by Dr. Mackintosh. Our results, in a very large number of cases, were decidedly opposed to the practice.

Now, at the time when the wards were filled with intermittent fever, a patient was admitted with symptoms of tertian ague. As was natural when so many cases of the same form of disease were in the house, this did not excite any special attention, and the man was ordered quinine in the usual doses. But the disease did not yield to the specific; on the contrary, the paroxysms became more severe, and the type of the fever changed to quotidian. I then became alarmed. I stopped the use of bark, and proceeded to make a careful examination of the patient. No signs of disease were found in the chest or belly, but it happened that in throwing off the bed-clothes for the purpose of examining the lower part of the abdomen I accidentally exposed the lower extremities. The thigh and leg at one side proved to be greatly enlarged. The whole extremity was white and elastic, and the saphena vein in a cordy state. Now, this man had never complained of any local pain or uneasiness, and was as much surprised as I was at the state of his limb. He was treated by leeching and the use of calomel and opium, and speedily recovered. He had no paroxysm of the fever after the change of treatment.

I have hardly a doubt that this patient's life would have been lost but for the circumstance that we omitted the quinine in time. Not that I wish you to suppose that the swollen leg after fever is itself a very dangerous disease; for we have no reason to think it more so than ordinary phlegmasia dolens; but I believe that the persistence in the use of bark in cases of *simulative* ague is fraught with danger. Indeed, there is here a double danger, for we thus not only neglect but exasperate the acute disease.

You are all familiar with the intermittent fever, which is symptomatic of urinary disease. On this subject, and on the danger of mistaking the affection for ague, and treating the case with bark, the late Mr. Abraham Colles used to dwell with great force in his lectures on surgery.

There are, doubtless, many other instances where a local irritation excites a fever, which, for a time at least, has all the characters of a true intermittent. Puerperal women are liable to this disease; I do not allude to the true puerperal fever, but I have often known women soon after child-birth to be attacked with well marked tertian or quotidian fever, in whom it was difficult, or impossible, to discover any local disease of importance. In some there had been an abortive irritation as it were: perhaps some tenderness of the uterus which had been removed by treatment; or in others a tendency to inflammation of the breast—but these had subsided, and the intermittent fever persisted. I have over and over seen bark administered in such cases, and always with bad results. The tertian was changed into quotidian or double tertian, the quotidian into double quotidian, and in one case, where the use of bark was persevered in for a length of

8

time, the patient sank with symptoms of inflammation in the abdomen and lungs. I believe that for the treatment of this condition we should trust to change of air, good diet, opium, and nervines. I have known one case in which the practitioner had given bark to a great extent, with the effect of exasperating all the symptoms, in which, when the medicine was omitted, draughts of valerian, ether and opium used, and the air changed, the disease rapidly disappeared.

***

LECTURE XV.

THE HEART IN FEVER, *continued*—Louis' conclusions, based on *post-mortem* observations —Typhous softening of the heart *during life* first studied at the Meath Hospital in epidemic of 1837-39—As regards state of the heart, fever cases fall into *three* categories : those accompanied by (1) *no alteration in heart's action*, except of rate ; (2) *weakness after a few days*, consequent on depressed vital power ; (3) *cardiac excitement*—Neither a depressed nor an excited state of the heart in fever necessarily implies organic change—*Dynamic* condition of the heart a more important indication for treatment than presence or absence of any structural change—True carditis very rare in fever—Typhous weakening predominates in left side of the heart— State of involuntary muscular fibre in acute essential disease is of great importance —Laennec's theory as to typhous softening of heart erroneous, for there is no correspondence between the softening of voluntary and involuntary muscular structures—Illustrations from yellow fever of 1826-27—Exemption of heart from typhous affection is a ground for a favourable prognosis—Continued excitement of heart equally a ground for a bad prognosis—Excited heart with compressible pulse most unfavourable—Transfusion of blood under these circumstances—Absence of red blood after death, the only noteworthy pathological appearance in this case—Blood-waste in fever to be met by administration of nourishment.

IT may be taken for granted that most, if not all, internal organs of the body are liable to become the seat of the secondary affections of fever ; and the symptoms having a more or less common character, varying only according to the seat of the disease and the liability to reactive irritation, it would be strange if the heart formed an exception to the rule.

I have shown you that Laennec occasionally observed a softened state of the heart in persons who had died of fever, but that he did not recognize this muscular change as distinct from that general condition of the voluntary muscles held to proceed from the dissolution of the fluids.

Louis, in his great work on the pathological anatomy of fever, corrects the doctrine of Laennec, and shows that in his cases where softening of the heart was met with after death "no similar lesion was found in any muscular organ, as all the muscles which preside over voluntary motion preserved amid the general disorder their natural colour and consistence." He established the following points as the result of his dissections: First, that the softening he observed was not the consequence of putrefaction; secondly, that it was often partial, affecting more the systemic than the pulmonary heart; thirdly, that it was to be met with apart from any analogous condition of the voluntary muscles; and fourthly, that it was not inflammation, but, to use his own words, "something the reverse of inflammation." He further found that the disease was best marked in proportion as the fever was earlier fatal, being much more frequent in those which died from the eighth to the twentieth day than in cases in which life was more prolonged.

It is to be remarked that neither by Laennec nor by Louis are any observations recorded which would lead to the discovery of this typhous condition during life. I have pointed out that the suggestion of Laennec with reference to a rapidity of pulse during convalescence from fever is not to be accepted. With a view of determining whether, pending the existence of this typhous change in the heart, we could establish its diagnosis—and in the hope of attaining some degree of precision in treatment as regards the employment of stimulants, a series of researches was commenced in the wards of the Meath Hospital during the epidemic of 1837–39. These were continued more or less for the next ten or fifteen years. You will see the original memoir in the *Dublin Medical Journal*,[1] in which it is, I think, sufficiently proved that the typhous secondary condition of the heart is not difficult of diagnosis; that it is, like the other local conditions of fever, inconstant in its occurrence and amount; that its advance and retrocession often follow the corresponding changes in the general malady; and that by its recognition and study we are greatly assisted in the use of stimulants and of nourishment in the treatment of many cases of fever.

Now, as regards the state of the heart in fever, you may divide the cases roughly into three categories. In the first there appears to be no alteration whatever in the heart's action beyond the usual increase of rate which belongs to fever. This is a condition which we have found most often in cases of what may be called benign, though they may be well-marked fevers. They are not malignant fevers, and so far as the impulse of the heart and the character of its sounds are concerned, little or no alteration occurs. These cases run a compara-

[1] First series, vol. xv. No. 44, 1839, p. 1.

tively regular course, unforeseen accidents and complications are rare, and the subservience of the disease to the law of periodicity and to judicious treatment are remarkable. The second is that wherein, after a few days, we have weakness of the heart consequent on depressed vital power. The third and worst of all is that in which we find cardiac excitement of more or less violence existing through the entire or a considerable portion of the illness.

Even in the case of the two last-named categories—that wherein there is depression of the heart's action, often attended with softening of its substance, and that in which violent excitement of the organ is met with—you must bear in mind that neither the depressed nor the excited condition of the heart in fever is enough to justify the inference that any organic mischief is present. It is true that we not infrequently find a softened state of the muscular structure, yet without marks of inflammatory action, in cases where well-marked depression and feeble action of the heart have existed. But where intense excitement of the heart's action has prevailed, we may meet with no evidence of anatomical change, with no sign of inflammation. The softened state which is associated with the weakened dynamic condition is wanting, and the heart has a perfectly normal and healthy aspect.

What I wish to convey to you is this, that as regards prognosis and treatment we have to look rather to the dynamic condition of the heart than to any structural change in its tissues. Thus we may have all the signs of extreme weakness of the heart without the occurrence of any softening; and, on the other hand, the heart's action may be excited to an extreme degree where inflammation will be completely absent. You are, therefore, not to have recourse to antiphlogistic measures merely because the heart is excited; and, again, you are not to infer that there is actual softening where the heart's action is depressed. It is true that feebleness of sounds and impulse attends softening of the heart, yet in certain cases their rapid reappearance under stimulants seems to show that a depressed innervation may exist for a time independent of the softening of the organ.

As regards the use of stimulants in fever, you are to look more to the vital than to the organic changes of the organ. We have determined that signs of a well-marked and continued depression of the heart's energy are commonly associated with actual softening—at least it was so in one epidemic—and, on the other hand, that even a continuous excitement in fever may occur without any carditis. In fact, true carditis seems to be extremely rare in fever; and this might be expected when we remember how seldom the serous membranes are affected in the disease. I have before spoken of the rarity of organic disease of the heart traceable to an attack of typhus or typhoid fever —which contrasts so remarkably with what is seen in rheumatic fever. This will prepare you for believing that the excited state of the heart in fever, when it does occur, rarely calls for any interference. And experience shows that we must be very cautious in the use of stimulants in such cases, not from their exciting influence on the heart itself, but from their disagreement with the nervous system.

In cases of convalescence, where the heart has been depressed, and probably softened, the returning vigour of the organ is an indication that the stimulants should be lessened or given up.

It is, then, with the depressed condition of the heart that we have principally to do. As I have said to you already, this state is commonly associated with a softening of the muscular structure due to the secondary influence of the fever poison. It arises, as it were, silently in the course of the fever, and it subsides spontaneously, leaving the structure—organically at least—in a state of health.

In regard to the weakening with or without softening, we find that it predominates in the left side of the heart, so that our researches confirm those of Louis. We have, it is true, found a very few cases in which, both the ventricles being engaged, the right appeared more softened than the left, but this was entirely exceptional. Although in our typhus fever debility and softening of the heart predominate in the left ventricle, yet—when it is more accurately compared with the fever of the Continent—future observations may show that the softening of the right ventricle is of more frequent occurrence than in the cases observed by Louis.

The investigations as to the state of the heart in typhus may be said to belong to our own time. The pathological anatomists of the Continent, although they investigated so closely the *post-mortem* appearances in fever, neglected the examination of certain portions of the system, the reason being that they were seeking rather to establish a theory than to arrive at the whole truth. Hence the condition of the muscular fibre in a number of diseases has been much neglected. Even at the present day the best works give us very imperfect information as to the abnormal conditions of muscular fibre, whether of the voluntary or of the involuntary systems. Much remains to be discovered upon this point.

In connection with acute disease of the internal parts the state of the voluntary muscles is, probably, not of much importance, but with regard to the involuntary muscles it is far otherwise.

The larynx, trachea, and lung are muscular organs, so also is the digestive tube, and there is reason to believe that muscular fibre exists in other places where it has not as yet been described. But of all the involuntary muscles the heart is the most remarkable, both from a physiological point of view and in the manifest changes which it may exhibit in the course of an essential fever.

I have mentioned that Laennec considered the softening of the heart in fever an example of general muscular softening depending on the dissolution of the fluids. Now, you may believe that neither in fever nor, I apprehend, in any other disease, acute or chronic, is there any necessary connection between the state of the voluntary and that of the involuntary muscles. Louis has shown that the softening of the left ventricle and its friability were sometimes so great as to cause the heart to break down on the slightest pressure, while the voluntary muscles preserved their firmness, and were in a perfectly healthy state.

Our observations are strikingly confirmatory of this. We have seen patients with every one of the conditions termed putrescent— with black petechiæ, gangrenous sores on the back, sordes on the teeth, and fetid and bloody discharges—and nevertheless when we came to examine the voluntary muscular system after death, it appeared perfectly red and firm, exhibiting well-marked cadaveric rigidity. I remember very well that when those frightful cases of yellow fever occurred in this hospital, the disease commonly attacked the strongest young men—models of muscular development. In these subjects, notwithstanding the malignity of the disease, the black vomit, and the gangrene of the extremities, the condition of cadaveric rigidity was most remarkable and long continued.

In a very small proportion of cases in which we found the typhous softening of the heart, we did observe something analogous to such a change in a class of muscles which may be termed "mixed" or "semi-involuntary." Thus in two or three instances where the heart was softened we found a certain amount of softening of the pectoral muscles, but except in this portion of the voluntary system there was no departure from health.

Now, looking at the action of the heart in fever, you will see cases in which, for a time at least, nothing abnormal exists; even the rate of the pulse may be long unaffected, though this is rare. This often varies, being sometimes quicker and sometimes slower, but with this exception there is nothing abnormal observed in the whole course of the case. There is neither increase nor loss of impulse, no lessening of either sound of the heart, no unusual preponderance of one sound over the other; in fact, if you except the alteration of rate, there is nothing abnormal as regards the heart; yet, though this condition may continue all through the case, and is a ground of a good prognosis, there are examples where it has continued for three weeks, and then a complication of bad symptoms has appeared. This we have observed more in typhoid than in maculated typhus.

That this occasional escape or exemption of the heart from mischief is a favourable circumstance there can be no doubt; it shows that, like other organs in fever, it may be untouched in certain cases by the secondary processes of the disease. This bears on the point we have so often insisted on—the variableness of all local affections as to seat, intensity, and time of appearance in essential disease. One patient may have the heart engaged; in another with the same character of fever it escapes. That is all we can say.

In the next category we place the cases of excitement of the heart —a condition justifying an unfavourable prognosis, especially when it is a continued one. It may exist in the earlier periods of the fever, and continue after the symptoms of prostration have set in, when the heat of the body falls and the pulse becomes feeble, contrasting strongly with the force or vivacity of the heart's action. This is a very strange condition, but one full of danger. It is not yet understood, and we have failed to connect it with any anatomical change in the heart. In some patients it may continue all through the case; in others it is ephemeral—that is to say, it exists for two or three days and then subsides, though it may return.

In others, and these seem to be the worst cases, the heart during the early and even the middle period of the fever has not been affected with depression or the signs of softening, when we observe the terrible symptom of an increasing excitement of the organ with an increasing weakness of the patient. When you apply your hand over the heart you find it acting violently and with a jerking character, similar to that of ordinary nervous palpitation—a quick, sudden, violent action —while both sounds are loud, sharp, and distinct. Any of you not accustomed to such cases would expect to find a strong resisting pulse, but it is not so; you may find it extremely small; it may be just perceptible and easily compressible, and it is a fact that this excited action of the heart may continue for days when every trace of pulse at the wrist has disappeared. This condition of the heart, whether it has existed all through, whether it is intercurrent or ephemeral, or, as we say, terminal—coming on at the close of the case—or lasting many days, is, I need not tell you, of the worst augury.

You will ask, What is this affection? Is it inflammation? We have every reason for believing that it is not so. Is it an example of that functional state of organs in fever of which I have spoken ? Certain it is that in our dissections in these cases we do not find anything abnormal in the heart—no vascularity, no lymph, no alteration of the valves, no inflammation of the aorta, not a single anatomical evidence of inflammation.

A good many years ago we had a case of excited action of the heart with progressive failure of the pulse. A woman had been employed in washing the clothes and bed linen in a case of severe maculated typhus. She was admitted in a bad form of fever, with great prostration. The heart soon assumed the excited and jerking action ; the pulse was rapid and weak. Wine had no good effect, and about the twelfth day her condition seemed hopeless. N pulse could be found at the wrist, and the skin was cool, as was also the breath. None of the ordinary local diseases could be detected, though the excitement of the heart continued. Under these circumstances I determined to try the transfusion of blood, and the operation was performed by the late Mr. Smyly. About twelve ounces of freshly drawn blood, not defibrinated, were thrown in, with the effect of restoring the pulse, so that it could be reckoned, and of making the breath warm. The action of the heart remained unchanged, but the patient sank in about thirty hours after the operation.

On dissection, conducted with great care, no anatomical change or lesion whatever could be detected in any of the cavities. The heart was empty and the ventricles firm, while the posterior portions of the lung presented nothing of the congested state common in fever. The whole lung posteriorly as well as anteriorly was perfectly white, dry, and apparently bloodless. It seemed as if all the blood, at least the red blood of the body, had disappeared in the course of the fever, a condition which I believe was first noticed by Laennec.[1]

----

[1] It is now some years since Dr. George Harley was led to believe that in certain cases the colouring matter of the blood was to be found in the urine, under the guise of what he termed *urohœmatin*. This substance closely resembles the hæmatin of the blood in appearance and properties, and especially in the fact that it contains iron. If the quantity of urohæmatin is in excess, its presence is readily detected by a deepening of the colour of the urine on the addition of some nitric acid, the effect being heightened when the mixture is heated. From his investigations, Dr. Harley is inclined to regard urohæmatin as the *débris* or the product of the colouring matter of the red blood corpuscles, and he considers the amount of the substance present to be to some extent a gauge of the destruction of red blood corpuscles in health or in disease. I need scarcely say how interesting the examination of the urine would be in a case similar to the one just detailed. The discovery of a very marked excess of urohæmatin under such circumstances would have supplied a missing link in the diagnosis of an extreme blood-waste.

It has ever since been a cause of sorrow to me, remembering the law of periodicity in fever, that in this case we did not repeat the transfusion. The restoration of the pulse in the radial artery, and of the warmth of the breath, showed that by the operation we had gained time.

I have little doubt that this lessening of the quantity of the blood in fever occurs more or less in many cases independent of local disease or excessive discharges, and this you will at once see bears strongly on the point of the careful and continuous giving of nourishment in the course of fevers. I believe that this is beside the question of the use of wine or other stimulants in fever.

LECTURE XVI.

THE HEART IN FEVER, *continued*—Depression of the heart, more marked in typhus than in typhoid—Signs of the change connected with (*A*) the impulse, (*B*) the sounds—The phenomena attending depression are variable—Description of their development, generally from the *fourth* day.

A. IMPULSE:—Possible sources of error in diagnosis: (1) constitutionally feeble impulse, (2) emphysema of lungs—Necessity for comparison of condition of heart from day to day—Peculiar modification of impulse in certain cases—Vermicular action—Effect of *position* on impulse of heart—Loss of impulse generally progressive, sometimes rapid—" Where differential diagnosis is difficult or impossible it is often unnecessary as a guide to immediate practice"—Retrocession of the local malady is gradual.

B. SOUNDS:—*First phase of lesion:* second sound becomes relatively, but not positively, augmented. *Second phase:* disappearance of first sound. *Third phase:* disappearance of both sounds (a condition of most unhopeful augury)—Fœtal character of the sounds in some cases—Speculations as to failure of *second* sound —Loss of impulse and failure of sounds generally advance *pari passu*, but not invaribly so—As failure of sounds begins at the left side, so in recovery the phenomena follow the inverse course.

WE must now speak of the third and most important condition— as regards treatment—of the heart in continued fever. We have spoken of its quiescence and its excitement, and we are now to study, first, the signs of depression of the heart in fever; secondly, how far those signs are diagnostic of the softened state described by Louis; and, thirdly, the general nature of that change.

The phenomena attending depression of the heart are of more importance in the maculated typhus than in the typhoid fever; at least they appear earlier—often much earlier—and seem to be more connected with softening in the former. As you might expect, the state of depression is recognized by the characters of impulse and of sounds. Now, after what I have so often impressed on you in the wards, I need not urge the importance of the principle that, in deducting practical conclusions from the phenomena of the heart, their value will be derived not from the comparison or contrast of one patient's case with that of another, but rather from the study of each case with itself at different stages of the disease from its commencement to its termination.

Now, as regards the action of the heart in fever there are many interesting phenomena to be studied. You will, of course, understand that they will not prove to be constant in future epidemics or in all countries. I have no doubt that the secondary affections of the heart are under the same rule of variability as to occurrence and intensity as are the other lesions in fever. Now, I suppose that you have a case of maculated typhus, in which this secondary affection sets in. You will often find after the third or fourth day that the impulse of the heart has diminished to a remarkable extent, and this may happen gradually, but we have observed it within twelve or eighteen hours — that is, in a patient whose heart was beating naturally yesterday its impulse is hardly perceptible to-day. Generally, however, we find that the vivacity of the heart's action is progressively and gradually lessened, and that the change is plainly perceptible about the fourth day. Instead of the normal healthy beat of the heart, there is a sluggish, laboured, and heavy motion. The diminution or cessation of its impulse is first observable at the apex, when the stroke of the heart is either not to be felt or scarcely perceptible. As the disease goes on, you will have to make pressure in the direction of the base of the heart or in the region of the xiphoid cartilage, in order to be sensible of its action at all. It will be generally found on close investigation that this cessation of impulse commences at the left side —a fact again confirmatory of the researches of Louis, that softening of the heart in fever begins in the left ventricle. Recollect, however, that there are not a few persons who, although enjoying average health, have hearts with a really feeble action, or apparently without, or with very little, impulse, and this may save you from the error of necessarily attributing to the typhous weakening or softening phenomena which may be simply natural or constitutional. Bear in mind also that feebleness of the sound and impulse may be caused by an emphysematous state of the lung, which has the effect, as it were, of burying the heart deep in the thorax.

Now, remember what I said to you about the advantage of the test of comparison, not so much of one patient with another as of the state of the same patient at different periods. If you find the heart's impulse lessened or gone, and know that it was present on the day or two previously, you have evidence that the change in the impulse is owing to the influence of the fever. Also, if you perceive the loss of impulse to be progressive—that is, that it becomes daily feebler and less perceptible—you may set this down as the result of the typhous weakening of the heart. Under such circumstances, on giving stimulants and nutrients, you may be suprised at finding the impulse greatly restored ; yet this effect, I must observe, is commonly transitory in its nature, for it is only when the disease has run through its stages and has been safely passed that you can look with any certainty for a permanent restoration of the vigour of the heart. The restoration, however temporary, of the impulse under the use of stimulants goes so far to indicate that its weakness was one of the secondary conditions of the essential disease, and as fully subject to the law of periodicity as the petechial eruption, the discoloration of the skin, or any of the other local secondary phenomena of fever.

I have told you that the loss of impulse is generally first observed at the left side of the heart, but you will meet with cases where it commences over the right cavities. But whether the signs first appear here or on the opposite side, when both cavities are engaged the impulse becomes undiscernible from the languor of the contractile power of the entire heart. If, say on the fourth day of fever, the impulse begins to languish and grows progressively weaker each day, you need entertain no doubt of its typhous character.

In these cases of diminution and at last extinction of perceptible impulse we have often observed a modification of the impulse that is interesting. It marks a feeble action of the ventricles in which the contraction is, as it were, not sudden but progressive. Instead of the suddenly occurring, promptly ceasing, and well defined beat of the heart, the impulse has a beat of a vermicular character, as if all the contractile muscles of the ventricle did not act at the same moment. In cases where the feeble impulse is visible you can sometimes satisfy yourself of this vermicular action by the eye, and, as you might expect, there is a certain prolongation of the first sound at the apex approaching bellows murmur.

Now, under such circumstances the heart is about to be, or has been, greatly weakened, and accordingly you may find this physical sign in the earlier periods, when the process of softening is on the advance, or again at a later period, when the organ is recovering. I think it is an important indication that actual softening has occurred, and that the feebleness of the impulse and sounds implied something more than failure of nervous power of the organ. It may be present, especially as a sign of recovery, for one or two days, and this is seen in cases of slow convalescence from a state of extreme prostration.

In estimating the amount of failure of the impulse I must give you some cautions before you conclude that there is no impulse. While the patient lies on his back it may happen that the mere application of the hand below the mamma will lead you to believe that impulse has ceased, yet you are not at once to conclude that this is so. You must make pressure downwards with the hand, and if still you do not get impulse you are to apply the tips of your fingers to the intercostal space firmly, and you may then feel the action. Nor are you to declare that there is no perceptible impulse until you examine the patient, turning him well on the left side and applying the hand as before. If this fails to detect the stroke you may believe that the most extreme weakness of the organ exists.

The loss of impulse is generally progressive, though sometimes rapid. You will find it at first difficult to distinguish between weakness combined with a process of softening, and simple debility without organic change. But this is of no great practical importance, at least so far as immediate action goes; it illustrates the great principle in clinical medicine, of which you have seen so many examples, that where differential diagnosis is difficult or impossible, it is often unnecessary as a guide to immediate practice. The process, like other secondary affections in fever, begins silently, without preceding signs of excitement, except perhaps rapidity of action.

There is nothing more interesting than to observe from day to day the retrocession of the local malady and the restoration of the organ to health. In general the return of the impulse is attended with that of the sounds, though we have seen exceptions to this. Thus the sounds may return before the impulse, while we have had cases in which eight days elapsed after its return before the sounds were re-established.

Let me again impress on you that the value of the lessening or the want of impulse of the heart in fever as an indication of depression, without softening, depends on the observation of a good impulse during the earlier period of the case, as this will prove that the feebleness or want of impulse was not the natural condition.

Now, as to the character of the sounds—looking at the circumstances connected with the impulse, and at the pathological state of the heart, you will be able to predicate the results of auscultation. As the impulse is lessened, it may be to extinction, so it is as to the sounds. The change appearing first, at least in the great majority of cases, in the arterial side of the heart, the sound of contraction of the left ventricle becomes feebler and feebler, while that of the right, though it may be lessened, continues. The second sound becomes relatively, though not positively, augmented, and this may be taken as showing the first phase of the lesion.

Next we may have a similar state of things as to the right ventricle, and then it commonly happens that we find the heart acting with but a single sound, and that sound the second. In a few extreme cases all systolic and diastolic sounds cease, and we have the strange condition of a heart acting, yet so feebly that it has neither impulse nor sounds—even in this state the pulse may continue perceptible.

But there are variations of these signs in different cases, all, however, showing a depressed and probably a softened state of the organ. Both ventricles may be engaged, causing diminution of their sounds, while the second is also lessened. Neither sound is extinguished, but both are greatly and apparently equably reduced. In this case, when the pulse is rapid—say 130 or 140 in the minute—the resemblance of the sounds to those of the heart of the fœtus in utero is singular. So similar are they that I believe if an observer was blindfolded, brought to the bedside, and made to use the stethoscope, he would think he was examining the abdomen of a merely pregnant woman, and not the thorax of a male subject in typhus fever.

Were we to speculate on the causes of the lessening of the second sound, we might ask, Does it depend on the condition of the heart itself, or on that of diminished resiliency of the aorta and pulmonary artery—a secondary effect of the fever? But it is unnecessary in the present state of our knowledge to discuss such points. It is enough to know that this condition is one, though an exceptional one, of the signs of debility of the heart in fever.

Now, touching the sounds of the heart, you may take it as a general rule that the diminution of impulse and the feebleness of the sounds advance *pari passu*. Yet this is not invariably the case, and I must tell you that you are not always to infer the loss of impulse from the disappearance of the heart's sounds. It is certain that in fever we may have a good impulse, apparently a healthy one, although the cardiac sounds may be very obscure. On the other hand, the sounds of the heart may be found natural and satisfactory while there still exists a decided loss of impulse. Generally, however, the two groups of phenomena are found to go together, the one being indicative of the other.

We may, for the sake of perspicuity, consider the phenomena of the sounds of the heart in fever under three forms. In the first there is a departure from the normal proportion—as to force, clearness, and persistence—which the first sound should bear towards the second. In the second we have the diminution of both first and second sounds. You will perceive that in the first form the inequality arises from weakened action at one side of the heart, while the other remains unaffected. Here both are partially enfeebled. In the third form the sounds at both sides cease to be discernible even to the keenest ear. This last change involves a condition in which successful treatment is rare, and it may supervene on one or other of the former two changes already described. Either of the first two may terminate in the last, or total cessation of both sounds of the heart.

Now, all these signs—including those which go to make up the third group of phenomena detailed—seem to indicate that the vital power, and frequently the organic structure of the heart, are profoundly affected.

It is, however, to the characters of the first sound and to the impulse that your attention in practice is chiefly to be turned. During the whole range of an investigation into these phenomena in fever, which has extended over a long series of years, neither I myself nor the gifted students who have laboured with me could ever say that we met with a single case of fever in which the peculiar phenomena of cardiac debility began with diminution or cessation of the second sound of the heart. Whatever may be the cause which produces the second sound, one thing is clear—that it has much less relation to the vital character and condition of the heart than has the first sound.

I have mentioned that where the sounds of the heart become altered in the course of a fever the change begins in the left ventricle and travels towards the right side of the heart; the systolic sound first becomes diminished towards the left, and afterwards towards the right. In cases of recovery the phenomena follow the inverse course, as we might naturally expect. We find the returning first sound audible, first over the right, and then over the left ventricle.

LECTURE XVII.

THE HEART IN FEVER, *continued—Post-mortem* appearances in extreme typhous softening —This affection not followed by chronic disease of the heart—Periods of invasion and of retrocession—Diagnosis of actual softening depends on (1) the character of the fever, and (2) the persistence of physical signs of failure of the heart— Simultaneous lessening of both sounds (fœtal heart)—Its bearing on the treatment by stimulants—SLOWNESS of pulse in convalescence from typhous softening—An- alogy to fatty degeneration of heart with slow pulse—In latter case the phenome- non, however, is constant—Occasional reversal of the order in which the signs of typhous softening show themselves—*Prognosis* more favourable with depressed than with excited heart—Former condition is more amenable to treatment—Report on an epidemic of typhus at Stockholm in 1841, by Professor Huss—CARDIAC MUR- MURS in fever, especially in advanced stages of typhoid and relapsing fever, are generally *basic* and *systolic*, functional in character, and occasionally accompanied by venous murmurs in the neck—Difficulty of distinguishing the first and second sounds of the heart in certain cases of disease: (1) *chronic bronchitis*, with weak and irregular heart and congested liver ; (2) late stages of some forms of fever— Example of the latter—*Diagnosis drawn from a want of accordance in the symptoms.*

BEFORE we proceed to consider some of the remaining secondary conditions of fever it will be right to return, in this lecture at least, to its influence on the heart, not so much as a question of pathological anatomy, but as having an important bearing on the two great objects of medical science, the cure and the prevention of disease.

We have studied some of the signs of typhous affection of the heart —a state commonly one of depressed vital energy, attended with a softened condition varying in its amount and extent, and following the laws of the secondary organic and functional affections in fever. Many of you have had an opportunity of studying this condition during life and after death. It may be described as a change in the muscular structure, which is certainly not inflammatory. There is but little, if any, change in the volume of the organ, which latter is often more or less livid, as you may see in other structures in fever. Serum is sometimes found effused into the pericardium, but beyond this there is no affection of the external covering, the endocardium, or valves. The structure of the heart, most often of the left ventricle, becomes homogeneous, and in it to the naked eye the muscular fibre can hardly be detected. It is of a dark colour, and has some resem- blance to the cortical structure of the kidneys. It seems infiltrated with an adhesive secretion, and is softened and friable, breaking down under a slight pressure. This change may be more or less general, though it commonly predominates in the left ventricle, where it may occur in patches from a quarter to an eighth of an inch in breadth and an eighth in depth. So great is the softening in extreme cases that where both ventricles are almost equally engaged, on grasping the great vessels and turning up the apex of the heart, we find the whole organ to fall over the hand like the cap of a large mushroom.

That this is a special and secondary local disease in fever there can be no doubt. I have spoken of its variations in intensity, extent, and time of retrocession. Like other secondary diseases, its frequency varies according to the epidemic character, for though it has for many years been observed in our wards and studied in connection with the necessity for and employment of stimulation, yet it was certainly more frequent before the epidemic of 1847 than it has been since that time. It was not a very prominent symptom in the famine fever of 1847 and 1848, and its subsequent rarity, as compared with what was observed in the decade following 1837, may have been connected with the general disappearance of fever in Ireland for some years after the famine fever. Like the other secondary affections, too, it often exhibits retrocession without consequent disorganization. In fact, there is no example of reactive irritation or inflammation, such as we see in the lungs or intestines, having ever occurred in the heart. Out of many hundreds of cases observed since 1837 to the present time, we have had no example of chronic organic disease of the heart traceable to the typhous affection.

The period of invasion of this manifestation appears to be between the fourth and sixth day of the fever, and its retrocession takes place at varying times between the tenth and the fifteenth day. The physical signs of weakness may be said to continue for about eight days.

The diagnosis of actual softening, as distinguished from simple debility, will depend on the character of the fever and the time during which the physical signs of failure of the heart have been present. Experience, again, shows that the progressive diminution of the impulse and sounds of the heart, which may proceed to their extinction, is sufficiently often connected with the actual softening to justify the diagnosis of this lesion.

The energy of both sounds may be simultaneously lessened, and where this takes place to a certain degree they resemble those of the fœtal heart. This, we have thought, in some instances showed an irregular and anomalous case, in which the stimulating treatment, although manifestly indicated, was not so successful as in the ordinary case of diminution or obliteration of the first sound while the second remained.

A remarkable character of the pulse—one to which allusion has already been made—during convalescence, in cases of unquestionable softening of the heart, which had been treated by free stimulation, is the progressive diminution of its rate even below the normal standard. In these cases, when convalescence is already advanced, when the heart's impulse has been restored and its sounds have again become audible, the pulse, having fallen to 72, on the next day will be found to beat but 60 times a minute. This lowering of rate may go on for several days afterwards, until at length the pulse will have fallen perhaps to 48, 40, or even 36, when once more it rises in a similarly gradual way to the natural standard of health, at which it finally remains. The return to the natural standard, however, though progressive, is effected in a shorter time than was the gradual fall in the first instance. It is difficult to assign a cause for this peculiarity of pulse, but a similar slowness of the pulse undoubtedly exists in many cases of fatty degeneration of the heart.

It is very difficult to account for this slowness of pulse supervening when convalescence is all but established, not only as to the general symptoms, but as to the heart itself, which exhibits a return of its natural vigour. In the fatty degeneration of the heart the pulse, which we have found as low as 28 in the minute, is more or less permanently slow. The rate may rise to 36, but the power of attaining the natural standard seems lost. You will remember, however, that in this condition the muscular structure is permanently damaged, while the typhous affection is under the law of periodicity.

I must tell you that although in the majority of cases the typhous change is marked in the first instance by the failure of impulse, and of the ventricular sound—these signs being most developed at the left side of the heart—you may meet cases in which they vary in their seat and order of occurrence. I have impressed upon you that fever is an essential condition. Yet when you study it in a number of cases, even during the same epidemic, though you may find among them a generic resemblance, they present infinite varieties in the local symptoms and signs—varieties as to seat, intensity, the occurrence, amount, nature, time, and complication of the secondary affections. Hence you may expect to meet with departures from the usual succession of phenomena as to the functional as well as the organic changes of the heart. The former may be ephemeral, the latter variable as to their retrocession. Signs of excitement may alternate with those of depression, and the order of phenomena as regards the first and second

9

sounds of the heart may (though this is rare) be reversed. This great principle remains, that the disturbances of the heart in fever, even when it shows excitement, are very rarely indicative of inflammation, while the nature of the morbid change is truly "something the reverse of inflammation."

Turning to prognosis, it is clearly to be more favourable in the case of depression than in that of excitement of the heart, and looking at the frequency of softening, you arrive at the conclusion—which seems a strange one—that the existence of such a change in one of the most important organs of the body may lead to a better prognosis than under opposite circumstances. The reason of this, however, is obvious. In the case of the typhous softening we can safely and advantageously employ stimulants, which are comparatively ineffective, and often inadmissible where the heart is excited. The condition of depression of the heart is certainly more frequent in the well-marked maculated fever than in the typhoid form. It begins, at all events, earlier, and the signs of progressive softening and recovery are much better defined. Still it would be wrong to say that in the typhoid cases the examination of the heart is not of great importance. When we shall speak of treatment and of the use of stimulants, you will find that in the advanced stages of typhoid a very great amount of stimulation is often borne with the best results.

Before passing from the subject of the state of the heart in fever, I wish to draw attention to a very interesting report upon an epidemic of fever which occurred in a corps of *gens d'armes* stationed at Stockholm in the winter of 1841. The observations made in this report by Professor Huss are very confirmatory of our researches at the Meath Hospital. The disease in this outbreak had most, if not all, the characters of our typhus.

The skin was maculated, with the usual accompanying symptoms of prostration, delirium, stupor, and secondary affections of the pulmonary and gastro-intestinal systems. During the earlier periods of the fever, varying from five to nine days, the sounds of the heart, particularly the first, became enfeebled. In the more advanced stages of the abdominal cases, the first sound would become similar to the second, and grow feebler until the second alone was to be heard. In convalescence the first sound was again heard faintly; then it became similar to the second, and the action of the heart was restored with the inverse series of phenomena.

In this epidemic wine does not seem to have been used by Professor Huss, but he gave tonics, such as the mineral acids, and nervine stimulants—musk, camphor, and so on ; and in the employment of these remedies he acted on precisely the same principle that we adopt in the use of wine—that is to say, he was guided by the enfeebling of the first sound and impulse of the heart, and by the other signs of a depressed vital condition.

There is one other point on which I have not touched—the existence and nature of cardiac murmurs in the advanced stages of fever. These are more frequently met with in the enteric or typhoid fever and in the relapsing forms of the disease than in maculated typhus, although even in the last-named they have been observed in the early stages of convalescence. Generally speaking they occur at the base of the heart, and are always systolic. In a few cases, however, they seem to be developed towards the apex, or they may occur in both situations at once. They are by no means so frequent or so prominent as in convalescence from rheumatic fever, in which we have observed them throughout the course of both the thoracic and the abdominal aorta. We need not here inquire whether they are anæmic or spanæmic; it is enough to know that they are not organic, and that they indicate the use of iron and a restorative treatment. In a few cases, but by no means in all, they are accompanied by venous murmurs in the neck.

I was observing just now, in the ward, at the bedside of the boy who had the pulmonary lesion (I will not call it pneumonia), with a low typhoid fever (he is under the care of Mr. Daly), how well his case illustrates the advantage of clinical study. If you take up works upon disease of the heart, you find that it is assumed by almost every writer that the first and second sounds of the heart are to be easily distinguished from each other. There are some persons who, if you were to say to them, in any given case, "I have had considerable difficulty in saying which was the first and which the second sound of the heart," would set you down as very deficient indeed, and as one who had not been properly taught. But the fact is, gentlemen, that there are many cases in which at first it is very difficult indeed to say which is the first and which the second sound of the heart. Occasionally the most experienced man will require repeated observation before he can make up his mind.

It has repeatedly happened to me that, after thinking I had settled the point, I was again thrown into doubt on moving the stethoscope an inch or two.

I mention this to show you how diffident we should be in our opinions upon these subjects, how slow we should be to condemn men because they do not come up to the mark laid down in books.

The truth, in fact, is, that they may go beyond it—that they are wiser than the authors of such books.

There are two cases in which it is often extremely difficult to say which is the first and which the second sound of the heart. One of these is that triple combination of local disease which is so common, especially in private practice, where the patient has chronic bronchitis, a weak and irregular heart, and congestion and enlargement of the liver. But there is another element very commonly to be found in connection with this combination, and that is the gouty element; so that you may have a gouty man with chronic bronchitis, with a weak and irregular heart, and with an enlarged liver. In such a case it is sometimes extremely difficult to say which is the first and which the second sound. They are closely similar; and the action is so irregular, so uncertain, that you may often apply the stethoscope for minutes together most carefully and yet not be able to make up your mind. This is one case. Well, take another—such as that of the boy above stairs.

This boy presents some very curious phenomena; and illustrates difficulties which you would not anticipate, if you depended merely upon the text-books for a diagnosis of disease of the heart. It is difficult to say whether the murmur which he has belongs to the first or to the second sound. But there is a greater and a still more important difficulty in this case—namely, to determine whether this is an organic or an anæmic murmur—and I am not ashamed to say that my own mind is not made up on the subject. It would be very easy to adopt one theory or the other, and to argue upon it; but I know thoroughly the difficulties of the subject; and I think, at this moment, it would be hardly possible to say whether this boy has disease of the valves of his heart or not. There is one consideration connected with the case which is drawn, not from physical examination at all, but from the general history of the patient, and it is this, that while organic murmurs are rare—very rare in the form of disease which he has had—inorganic murmurs are comparatively common in it.

This is a very strong point. We are here under this difficulty—a difficulty which you may meet with every day in private practice —that we are called on to give an opinion when the data that should guide us in that opinion are deficient. We want to know the previous history of this boy. If, instead of being in hospital, he were a private patient under your care, or if you had been the attendant on his family for years together, were familiar with him and intimate with the state of his heart, you would be able to say, first, if he ever had carditis; next, whether, before his late attack, he had cardiac murmur or not. But we know nothing of all this; and the only fact we have to go on is the observation of Mr. Daly that when the boy was first examined this murmur was not there at all. I myself have no doubt as to the correctness of this observation of Mr. Daly, and believe that whether the murmur be organic or inorganic, it has been developed since the patient came into the house. Can we distinguish by acoustic signs alone, gentlemen—and this is a point which bears on the subject of fever in a most important manner—the inorganic from the organic murmur? The answer to this question is simply that, in the present state of our knowledge, there are many cases in which we cannot do so; that there is no special acoustic character by which we can distinguish one of these phenomena from the other. This looks like a depreciating statement, as far as our skill in diagnosis is concerned; but the cause of diagnosis would be much more injured by attributing to it powers which it does not possess than by confessing its deficiencies. The diagnosis in the case in question is to be drawn from other sources—generally speaking, from circumstances connected with the condition of the patient, the absence of the signs of inflammation, and a variety of other points.

As regards cardiac murmur in fever, the observation has been frequently made that valvular murmur, when the patient is made to sit up, does not disappear; but we have found in this hospital that, in many cases in which a murmur was observed after fever, it was ascertained that, in an upright position, the abnormal sound disappeared, or, if it did not cease altogether, it became much less intense; so that the disappearance of the murmur in the upright position is in favour of its inorganic nature, while its persistence or aggravation points to an organic origin. So far so well. But, you will ask, is this rule absolute? This is a question which must be answered in the negative; for you will meet with anæmic murmurs which are not influenced by position; and I believe there are, on the other hand, organic murmurs which are influenced by position. There are, doubtless, some organic murmurs in which, when the heart is made to act rapidly, the murmur either disappears or becomes lost in the other cardiac sounds, so that you cannot distinguish it.

My own impression about the patient whose case we are at present studying is that the murmur is inorganic. I trust it is; but I would not say so positively, because the sound, although strongly marked— although approaching very closely indeed to the inorganic murmur— is similar to a kind of murmur which we in this hospital have met with in cases where the heart has been weakened. It is a true muscular murmur—a sound produced simply by the non-synchronous contraction of the muscular fibres—when they act vermicularly, as it were. The murmur in our patient possesses more of this character than of that of the true valvular murmur. There is another point connected with it which is of importance. If this murmur was valvular, it would imply a great deal of disease; a rough, almost rasping *bruit* in the situation of the aortic valve, implies generally a great amount of disease, commonly chronic; and, under these circumstances, you might expect that the patient would show other signs of disease of the heart. So that we here have a diagnosis drawn, as I often observed to you before, from that important source—the want of accordance of the symptoms. Supposing the murmur here to be organic, we should expect to find with this amount of valvular disease signs of dilatation of the left ventricle, or of the whole heart. And yet even when this boy had one of his lungs almost entirely obstructed—a condition which often acts in developing latent cardiac disease—the symptoms of cardiac suffering were not at all remarkable. So that there is here, to a great degree, this want of accordance in the symptoms—a condition which is against the opinion of the murmur being organic, and in favour of its being functional. A mistake, gentlemen, was often made in connection with auscultation generally— I am happy to say that it is but seldom made now—that of supposing that every disease had its special acoustic sign. Consequently the attention of students and physicians was directed to the study of physical signs from a purely mechanical point of view—to the observation merely of their acoustic characters.

There can be no doubt that it is of the greatest importance to study carefully everything connected with a diseased organ—both its physical and its vital phenomena; but what you have to learn specially is not so much how to detect or recognize a particular sign, as to know how to reason upon it when you have discovered it. It is here that the clinical student of practical experience has the greatest superiority over the mere reader. His mind is trained to reason upon the phenomena which he observes. Here we have a group of phenomena; and if we did not give ourselves the trouble to turn every possible point of the case over in our minds, we should come to an imperfect and erroneous conclusion about it.

Bear this in mind always, that there is no absolutely pathognomonic physical sign of any disease whatsoever. This cannot be too strongly stated; and I believe that we might go further, and say that there is no combination of mere physical signs which, excluding the history and vital symptoms, can be justly considered as pathognomonic; at all events, if there be such a combination, it is one of extreme rarity. We hear of certain murmurs being pathognomonic of this and of that disease of the heart—friction sounds being pathognomonic of pleurisy —crepitating râles, of pneumonia—amphoric sounds, of effusion of air and fluid into the pleura. All this is wrong; it is based upon error; and you must expunge it altogether from your minds, if you wish to be good physicians and faithful observers of disease.

LECTURE XVIII.

SECONDARY INTESTINAL COMPLICATIONS OF FEVER—General and introductory remarks— A generic resemblance between the various forms of fever—Secondary abdominal complications are more frequently observed in typhoid fever, but do not exist as its necessary anatomical character—Dothinenteritis was largely prevalent in the typhus epidemic of 1826-28—Fever must be observed independently in each epidemic and in every country—Typhoid fever almost without characteristic symptoms—Illustrative case; extensive intestinal ulcerations found after death— Vital symptoms of intestinal complications: (1) thirst, (2) swelling of belly, (3) diarrhœa, (4) ileo-cœcal tenderness, (5) increased action of abdominal aorta (6) rigidity of abdominal muscles—Three forms of abdominal swelling: (1) early and moderate tympany, (2) doughy condition, (3) slight ascites—Increased action of abdominal aorta—Case of, in perforation of the stomach—Analogous local arterial excitement in (1) whitlow, (2) rheumatism—Diagnosis from aneurism—Intestinal complications seem to interfere largely with action of the law of periodicity—Early alleviation of local irritation checks deposit, and so prevents future mischief—Hence relief of symptoms by early depletion as practised by Broussais, who misinterpreted the matter, and was led to look upon the general fever as but symptomatic of a local lesion.

GENTLEMEN, I hope that none of you will misunderstand me and suppose that I do not recognize the differences between the various forms of fever, about which so much has been written in latter times by excellent observers. That a case of fever answering to the description of the pythogenic fever of Dr. Murchison—the typhoid of Sir William Jenner and Dr. Hudson—runs a different course from a maculated typhus or a relapsing synocha, is to be admitted. All these forms vary, whether in isolated cases or in the multiplied examples which occur in epidemics. As a rule they differ as to their apparent exciting causes, their local complications, their mortality, their attendant phenomena, and their consequent effects on the economy. That follicular disease of the intestines is commonly met with in typhoid as compared with typhus may be admitted, as well as the rule that the laws of periodicity in the former are not so well marked as in the latter. But what I want you to perceive is that there is between them a great generic resemblance. The greater your intimacy with fever—the more it is observed upon a large scale, the less attention you will pay in your diagnosis, prognosis, and treatment to the question whether the disease belongs to this or to that category. This is true at all events as to the typhus and typhoid fever. Much has been written to prove that dothinenteritis may be taken as the anatomical character of the latter disease, and some go so far as to deny the occurrence of ulceration of the intestine in maculated typhus. Yet no man who has observed this fever in an Irish hospital will subscribe to such a doctrine. Dothinenteritis is, or has been, a common occurrence in the last-named form of the disease, its frequency and amount varying in different epidemics. In such a case are there two diseases, different in identity, existing together in the system? and what becomes of the alleged differences, when the management of the case is considered?

The theatre of a hospital is not the place for a systematic course of lectures. We can be here better employed, and the teacher's business is to say, like Mark Antony, "that which he knows," and to prove it by demonstration, referring to cases with which his hearers are familiar.

When we consider fever in relation to pathological anatomy, symptoms, exciting causes, and treatment, we find it a complex and ever-varying condition, with certain generic resemblances in the relations between it and the secondary affections which impress on it particular and varying characters; but to lay down rules by which each type of fever can be proved to have a separate identity is to go too far. I have told you that no two epidemics are exactly alike either as regards their essential symptoms or local complications. The results of the most careful and extended researches will enable us to lay down principles —as to pathology, prognosis, and treatment—applicable when the disease occurs in different countries and climates and affects different races of men.

I have said that this is not the place to go into the history of every observed form of fever, and into the various controversial questions that have arisen regarding them. Study the excellent works of Dr. Murchison, Dr. Hudson, Sir William Jenner, and Dr. Stewart, and use your own judgment as to how far your experience bears on the great questions therein discussed. In the mean time let us continue to study the local complications, after which we shall be in a position to deal with the question of the treatment, if not the prevention, of the disease.

It will not be necessary after these observations to take up your time by going over the beaten ground of the pathological anatomy of the

digestive tube in fever You will meet with descriptions of the tume-
factions and ulcerations of the glands in every modern work on the
subject. Let us rather take a general view of the symptoms attendant
on fever with reference to the digestive system, and as we have studied
the various conditions of the lungs and heart under the influence of
the disease, let us now consider its secondary abdominal complications.

What I have to say on this subject must be held to apply to the
several varieties of fever. Although the symptoms now to be studied
are not equally developed in all these varieties, yet when I speak of
" local lesion " I intend my remarks to apply to fevers of every kind.
We have spoken of the alleged anatomical distinction between
typhus and typhoid—the one being free from intestinal disease, the
other always presenting it. Now, it would be more philosophical,
to say that no form of fever has any special anatomical change ; that
where such does take place it is of a secondary character ; and that
when it arises in the digestive system, it is more frequently observed
in one form of fever than in another. Such a proposition might be
accepted.

The frequency of dothinenteritis as regards fever is, or has been,
greater on the Continent than in this country. The typhoid is more
common abroad than the true maculated typhus. Hence in proportion
as true typhus is epidemic, we find fewer instances of the secondary
intestinal lesion, which becomes more frequent when typhoid fever
extensively prevails. But the local disease is not necessarily characteristic of any peculiar type of epidemic. In the outbreak of 1826-28
(if ever there was a true typhus epidemic it was then) in a very
large number of cases the secondary local disease of the intestine, considered to belong to the typhoid form, was present. In fact, there
was an observable tendency towards an extreme amount of disease of
the digestive organs. It was in this epidemic that the yellow fever
appeared, with peculiar symptoms of very severe gastro-intestinal
disturbance. I cannot too earnestly impress on you all that, as regards fever and its treatment, you are not to trust implicitly to the
statements of other observers, no matter how eminent they may be,
in forming your judgment as to the cases *at the time* under your charge
Recollect that all such statements are to be accepted only as bearing
on outbreaks of fever as observed in different places and at different
times ; for both the locality and the period of an outbreak are considerations which must be taken into account.

It was a grave medical error on the part of Broussais and his disciples to declare the constancy of gastro-enteritis over the world from
observing fever in France. The same remark applies to theories as

to symptoms and treatment—doctrines formed and adopted without reference to the period and place of observation and the prevailing epidemic character. You may admit the disease of the digestive organs to be met with less frequently in typhus than in typhoid, but if you were to conclude that in typhoid fever intestinal lesion was a special and constant result, or that it was not met with in typhus, you would be wrong. Recollect what I have already told you as to the variable and inconstant characters of the local affections in fever. Cases of typhoid fever will come under observation wherein there is an absence of any direct symptom, or of any change whatever in the anatomical structure. This is an important fact, and a single case of the kind is of great value and interest.

Again, we may have typhoid fever with intestinal lesion, but without any direct symptom beyond mere loss of appetite, and *malaise*—nay, even these symptoms may be absent. I will detail for you a remarkable instance of this. The disease ran a course of forty-three days without break or alteration. There were at first some slight respiratory symptoms, but subsequently the case seemed to be one of a purely nervous character. Towards the termination, symptoms of engorgement of the air passages and of weakness of the heart appeared. At no stage of the disease was there any swelling of the belly or tenderness there. There was no throbbing of the abdominal aorta, no rigidity of the recti muscles, no diarrhœa; the evacuations were all through healthy in character. In fact, so far as the belly was concerned, not a single symptom could be detected from beginning to end. I put the state of the tongue out of the question, as in fever it is no evidence of disease of the digestive system. Not only was there a complete absence of any direct symptom of intestinal disease in this perfectly marked case of typhoid, but also the patient took his food well and it seemed to perfectly agree with him. On dissection the lower third of the ileum showed a sheet of suppurating ulcers, with extensive destruction of the mucous membrane.

The junior members of the class will learn from this case that in fever the symptoms of the secondary disease of the intestines may be singularly obscure, especially as compared with those in the lungs, heart, or brain, and when they do occur they do not give any reliable measure of the extent of disease. When the brain is affected, the nervous symptoms of pain, delirium, subsultus, coma, and so on, generally reveal the disease. The disease of the lung, and especially of the heart in its softened condition, though partaking to a certain degree of the (so to speak) silence of the secondary affections, is ascertainable by physical examination—which in the lung discovers râle and dulness, and in the heart diminution or extinction of sound and impulse.

Even the vital symptoms of these forms of disease often reveal the mischief. You may find dyspnœa, lividity, rapidity and feebleness of pulse, and so on ; but in the case of the digestive system matters are different. I think we owe to Broussais the knowledge of the fact that in fever inflammation and ulceration of the bowels may almost be described as a painless disease, the symptoms affording no reliable evidence as to the nature and extent of the local mischief. There may be thirst, some tympany, or moderate diarrhœa, and on dissection you may find ulceration, even having gone on to perforation—yet the symptoms of thirst, tympany, and diarrhœa will be insufficient to enable you to declare the amount of local disease.

The most important vital symptoms, which all vary in their amount and intensity, are thirst, swelling of the belly, diarrhœa, and tenderness of the ileo-cæcal region, and often of the epigastrium. Pain is rarely complained of. The abdominal muscles may be more or less rigid, and there is sometimes increased pulsation of the abdominal aorta.

Three forms of abdominal swelling may be noted. You may find an early but moderate tympany affecting apparently the small rather than the large intestines. Again, especially in advanced cases, you may have a doughy-like condition of the belly yielding little or no tympanitic sound, and conveying to the hand a sensation as if the integuments were thickened and agglutinated to the organs beneath. I think I have observed another kind of swelling, caused by a slight liquid effusion into the peritoneum. This can be detected by the feeling of fluctuation when the patient is placed upright. Generally, however, the abdominal swelling is principally tympanitic, while in some advanced cases the belly becomes collapsed.

About the middle period of the disease you may often find diarrhœa with or without morbid stools. The tenderness on pressure differs from that of peritonitis in not being at all so well marked. This tenderness may be general, although most commonly it is best perceived in the ileo-cæcal and epigastric regions. I would caution you, however, against using any but the gentlest pressure in seeking for this symptom ; the great rule in all examinations is to avoid giving the patient any cause of complaint or the least inconvenience.

You are also to look for increased action of the abdominal aorta— an interesting symptom, of which the analogue may be seen in the increased action of the radial artery in whitlow. I have observed that in this local manifestation of fever the pulsation of the vessel is often more equable than in ordinary nervous throbbing of the aorta. It disappears with the subsidence of the disease, and I have seen it do so after an application of leeches and poultices to the belly.

In cases where its existence is doubtful we sometimes find a marked disproportion between the beat of the radial and femoral arteries. This is a very interesting subject, and the symptom in question led us some years ago to the diagnosis of rupture of the intestinal tube. A middle-aged man, who for more than a year had suffered from abdominal pains attributed to dyspepsia, fell down in the street, and was brought into our wards in a state of collapse. The surface was cold, and the pulse at the wrist had ceased. The belly was moderately full, but painless to pressure.

These symptoms, connected with the previous abdominal pains, had all the characters of hemorrhage into the peritoneum from rupture of an aneurism. But we came to the conclusion that the case was one of perforation of the intestine from this circumstance—that while the pulse had ceased at the wrist, it was distinct and jerking in the groin. The freedom from pain on pressure seemed to favour the diagnosis of rupture of an aneurism, but you must remember that the patient was in a state of extreme collapse.

On dissection, the diagnosis of perforation of the digestive tube proved to have been correct. The solution of continuity was not, as we had supposed, in the small intestine, but in the great curvature of the stomach. The accident seemed to have occurred immediately after the man had taken a full meal, the ingesta having escaped almost wholly into the peritoneal cavity. The serous membrane presented a diffused red tinge, seen principally in the hypogastric region, apparently a very early stage of peritonitis, and as such sufficient to account for the increased local arterial action.

While I am on this subject I may mention that in certain cases of chronic aortic patency, with the usual arterial throb, in which the patient experiences an attack of rheumatic arthritis, say of the wrist, the force and vehemence of the corresponding radial artery become so exaggerated as to make it difficult to convey an adequate impression of it. It may be compared to the blow of a steel hammer on an anvil—so greatly exaggerated by the local irritation is the ordinary increased impulse of the vessel. According as each joint becomes attacked under the influence of metastasis, the violent pulsation is found in the corresponding artery. I have known this temporarily intensified impulse, when its seat was the abdominal aorta, to lead to the wrong diagnosis of aneurism, the signs of which disappeared with the subsidence of the intestinal disorder.

The diagnosis is to be drawn from the history of the case, as a violently acting abdominal aneurism is not developed in a short period of time without previous symptoms. The combination of abdominal aneurism with permanent patency of the aortic valves is rare indeed, and the existence even of a large aneurism has little if any influence on the action of the vessel above and below it. Constitutional disturbance resulting from the local irritation also aids the diagnosis, for there is nothing more remarkable than the long preservation of the general health in a case even of large abdominal aneurism.

In enteric fever you may often find a rigid state of the muscles of the belly. It seems principally to affect the recti muscles and, I think, preponderates at the right side. It may vary from day to day, and apparently corresponds with the phases of the local malady. How far this condition is related to the signs of gurgling in the ileo-cæcal region may be questioned. But this latter sign, unless when plainly localized, is not of great value.

As to the state of the tongue, you cannot in a case of fever place much, if any, dependence on it as a measure of intestinal secondary disease; you are to look on it as an index less of the local than of the essential malady. The morbidly clean, bright red, and glazed tongue may change and assume a natural appearance under strong stimulation.

Looking at the secondary disease of the intestine and its liability to reactive inflammation, I think it probable that it interferes more with the periodic laws of fever than do the respiratory affections, and many cases of protracted fever may be thus looked on as examples of an essential combined with a symptomatic condition—the first causing the special deposit, and the second resulting from the reactive irritation which may terminate in ulceration, or suppuration, and thus suspend the action of the law of periodicity. Hence the sooner we can detect and alleviate the local irritation the less will be the deposit, and the less also will be the interference with the periodic laws. The amount of deposit in essential disease, as we see in variola, seems to be influenced by that of the cutaneous vascularity and irritation. By early local depletion we can greatly diminish the degree of pustulation and its virulence. In fact, its occurrence in particular situations, say the face, can be all but suspended.

Now, this point was never considered by the school of Broussais, or they misinterpreted the matter. A patient had fever, and the application of leeches to the belly was followed by great relief of symptoms, and soon by the subsidence of the fever. Here, they said, is a proof that the fever was only symptomatic of the gastro-enteritis, and so the idea of essentiality must be given up. No, say the more careful observers; the relief in this case is from the diminution of a secondary reactive irritation interfering with the law of periodicity, which was again permitted to act on the removal or modification of that irritation.

You cannot sufficiently study in fever the relations between its secondary and its essential conditions, or the influence which the latter have on the former when a process of reactive local inflammation is set up, giving rise to symptomatic irritation, and interfering with the periodic laws. In some cases of enteric fever these laws are permitted to act, and an abortive attempt at recovery takes place. In those described by Dr. Cheyne in the "Dublin Hospital Reports" the general characters of fever subsided, the pulse fell, and appetite returned; but after a time symptoms of intestinal disease became developed, and the patient sank after the false crisis with extensive disease of the mucous membrane. It was suggested by Dr. Todd that in such cases a state of pyæmia was induced by the absorption of pus from the intestinal ulcers; but the symptoms in the second stage of Dr. Cheyne's cases were more likely due to irritation of the intestine, which interfered with the retrocession of the secondary disease and prevented crisis. No doubt in abdominal typhus you may find the mesenteric glands filled with pus, but in fever, as in variola, there seems to exist a power of disposing of purulent secretion in vast quantities, which if retained would act as a poison.

LECTURE XIX.

Intestinal Complications of Fever, *continued*—They resemble all the other secondary affections of fever in their general characteristics and relations to the primary essential malady—More frequent in typhoid, but occurring in typhus also, as, for example, in the epidemic of 1826-27—Pathological appearances observed in the intestinal tract in that fever—Yet these appearances were not necessarily found after death even where severe abdominal symptoms existed in life—Eruption of rose spots in fever.

WHEN we review the lesions of the abdominal organs in fever, we find that in their relation to the essential malady they are subject to the same general laws which govern the other secondary affections. They are—and it cannot be repeated too often—not the cause, but the result of the essential disease, whether that exists in the form of bad typhus or of enteric fever. They are various in their amount and intensity, and this so remarkably that even when looked on as secondary affections they fail to furnish an anatomical expression for the malady. The vital symptoms of the local affection are rarely prominent, so that the attention of the physician may never be called to them by the patient. This is more especially the case in proportion as the fever partakes of the characters of typhus rather than of typhoid.

But we cannot predicate in any given case or in any epidemic under what conditions or in what degrees the local affection may present itself, how far it will modify the general symptoms, or what other seats of secondary lesion the case may exhibit.

In the great epidemic of 1826 and 1827 the disease, as I have told you, was clearly a typhus fever, with every character of the affection. It was highly contagious, with abundant and well-marked petechial eruption and prominent secondary affections of both the respiratory and digestive systems. The tumefaction and ulcerations of the ileum were found well marked in numerous cases, so that if those who advocate the doctrine that such a lesion does not occur in typhus had been here at the time, and had made dissections in this hospital, they would never have defended this opinion. Let me again impress upon you that the very occurrence, or amount, or intensity of this or that secondary affection in fever varies according to the epidemic. In this fever we had all the anatomical characters of the intestinal disease—the tumefaction of the mucous glands, their vascularity and ulceration; the filling of the mesenteric lymphatics with pus, and its deposit in the mesenteric glands; sloughing of the glands of the intestines, and so on. You must be careful not to infer the symptoms and the anatomical results of disease from the observations of a single epidemic.

Discard altogether the idea which has been put forward by many persons who make too fine distinctions in medicine that this disease, of which I have given you now a rough sketch, is, or has in itself, any great value as an anatomical distinction between different kinds of fever. This is a favourite doctrine of those writers who hold that there is an essential difference—a complete difference—between the typhus fever of these countries and the fever of the Continent. The real state of the case is that, although this complication is more frequently met with on the Continent than it is here, it is not infrequently met with here also. It is also true that, although it belongs more to the non-petechial cases than to the petechial, yet it may occur in the latter and it may be absent in the former.

The tendency to this affection varies greatly with the epidemic character of the disease. In one year we may have extremely well-marked petechial typhus without the slightest appearance of ulcer-

ation or disease of the mucous membrane of the intestine—and if one
who advocated the doctrines I spoke of came to this county and made
his dissections during that period, he would probably find abundant
cases to establish his doctrine. But it might happen that if he returned after a few years he would find occasion to change his opinion,
for he would then see a fever in all its external characters the same
that he had seen before—a fever with true petechiæ and all the
characters of essentiality—but, further, a fever with the intestine
extensively ulcerated. It is incorrect, then, to say typhus fever may
not be attended with this anatomical change in the intestine; this I
wish strongly to impress upon you. The occurrence of it is, so far as
we know, accidental; at all events, it is not a necessary consequence
either of the non-petechial or of the petechial fever; but in some
epidemics we may have petechial fever with it. And, again, even in
the same epidemic we may have cases with the whole intestinal tract
perfectly free from disease, and also cases in which it exhibits the
affection extensively.

Now, in illustration of this I will read the particulars of some
dissections of fever which were observed in the epidemic of 1826 and
1827. I have stated that this was a very singular epidemic, and one
which, apparently, is unknown to the Continental writers. It was a
very extensive and prevalent outbreak; it infected many hundreds of
thousands of persons in this country. I think there were something
like 3000 beds for fever open in Dublin, and I am quite sure that if
there had been 10,000 beds, they would have been all filled. There
were in this hospital alone 300 beds, so that we had a very good opportunity of observing it. It was a true typhus fever, a maculated
fever—this I wish to impress strongly upon you—and yet in a very
large number of cases indeed there was follicular disease of the intestine. Now, such is the state of prejudice on this subject on the Continent and elsewhere, that when you mention such a simple fact as
that we had in this country an epidemic of typhus fever—of maculated
fever with ulceration of the intestine—a large number of the best
informed Continental pathologists will shrug their shoulders and
politely express a doubt as to the fact that you have told them.

But in order to show the great variety presented by the secondary
intestinal affections in one epidemic, I will briefly describe the pathological conditions observed.

The most usual appearances were extensive ulcerations in the lower
third of the ileum. These ulcers were either isolated and circular—
as large as a sixpence, with raised edges and very deep—or running
all around the intestinal tube. There was also great enlargement of

the lymphatics of the mesentery—the vessels containing purulent fluid, and the mesenteric glands themselves in a state of suppuration and destroyed. These were the common anatomical changes as far as the abdomen was concerned. There were also, in a large number of cases, typhous affections of the bronchial system. The bronchial and the intestinal tracts were the two points on which the force of the secondary affections of the disease seemed to be thrown. But in this very epidemic other cases occurred in which ulcers of the intestine were not found, and yet the disease was fatal, and fatal with abdominal symptoms. This was seen in those terrible cases of yellow fever which I shall presently describe. So that here we find a general tendency to secondary abdominal affections, but a variation in their nature ; and if this be true, what becomes of the special anatomical character of the fever?

You will not forget that with regard to the symptoms of disease of the mucous membrane and glands in fever, and especially in that form called typhoid, enteric, or pythogenic fever, or abdominal typhus, though these symptoms are more often present, yet the absence of one or many of them is not uncommon. Much attention has been paid by various observers to the eruption of rose spots, supposed to be peculiar to typhoid fever. Although we do not know anything of the rationale of this symptom, its frequency must be admitted. But, as regards its appearance, the condition of inconstancy must also be admitted, nor is its existence to be taken alone as a clear distinction between fever with, and fever without, the intestinal affection. Like all the other local symptoms of continued fever, it is not constant in its occurrence, its amount, its successive appearances, its relation to the stage of the disease, its complication with other cutaneous eruptions—measly eruptions or petechiæ, or its connection with symptoms of progression or renewal of the abdominal lesion. In the course of a protracted fever three or more distinct eruptions of rose spots may take place and you may observe the latter ones even when the constitutional state and local symptoms of fever have nearly if not altogether subsided.

10

LECTURE XX.

INTESTINAL COMPLICATIONS OF FEVER, *continued*—Division into *three* categories, with reference to the vital symptoms : I. These symptoms are absent, although the *silent* disease may be great in amount; II. Local symptoms are evident; III. Symptoms and pathological changes are both well marked—Further description of the epidemic of 1826-27—Sudden access of intense abdominal pain, followed by icterus and gangrene—Fatality of this complication—Splenic(?) abscess occurring in the first case of recovery, and discharging through the lung—Resemblance of this form of fever to the yellow fever of the tropics—Dr. Lawrence's observations—Dr. Graves' observations.

WITH reference to the vital symptoms, we divide cases of fever with abdominal secondary complication into three categories.

In the first it may be said that the local disease is silent—although, as in a case I detailed to you, its amount be great, no direct local symptoms exist, and the patient does not draw your attention to it. This may occur in petechial or in non-petechial fevers, or, to use another expression, in typhus or in typhoid. The amount of the so-called characteristic affection varies in different cases and different epidemics from a very few small ulcers to extensive disease and destruction of tissue.

In the second category there are evident local symptoms, such as early tympany, tenderness on pressure, arterial throbbing, diarrhœa, and rigidity of the recti muscles. These symptoms may occur in both forms of the disease, but are more common in non-petechial than in petechial fevers.

In the third category we place those cases observed in the epidemic of 1826–27, in which the abdominal complication widely differed in the violence of the symptoms and in the pathological changes from anything we had seen before or have seen since.

In this third class abdominal complication is attended with manifest and violent symptoms, the nature of the affection in many respects differing from the ordinary dothinenteritis in typhoid, and even as it occasionally occurs in typhus.

In the epidemic of 1826 and 1827, as I have said, the secondary affections were often marked by a great activity and severity. I have spoken to you before of this epidemic, but it is a remarkable circumstance that while the follicular disease of the intestine was extremely frequent throughout its course, yet in the particular group of cases of which I am now about to speak it was absent.

In the course of this epidemic the following extraordinary circumstance occurred: Patients who had precisely the symptoms of the general fever—whose symptoms presented nothing to draw particular attention to them more than to others—would be suddenly seized about the seventh day with extraordinary abdominal spasms—the spasms so severe that they could be likened only to the worst cases of painters' colic. In some cases the pain was so great as to make the patient scream out, and, just like the spasms in painters' colic, there was great relief given to the patient by making strong pressure upon the abdomen. In the course of a very short space of time—I believe within an hour or less—it was observed that the patient's face began to turn yellow. A jaundiced tint rapidly spread over the whole body, so that on the day on which the patient was attacked he was universally jaundiced. The kind of jaundice was curious too. It never amounted to the extreme degree of yellowness seen in true jaundice. The patient was very yellow certainly, but he had not that intense yellowness which you see in cases of mechanical obstruction of the gall ducts, or of cancer of the liver, and so on.

The horrible spasms continued for several hours. The patient then began to vomit black matter—matter at first like coffee grounds, but afterwards quite black. In a few instances he passed the same matter from his bowels, but in most cases the bowels were constipated. Then began another class of symptoms. The tip of the nose grew cold; it became pale, livid, purple. The same appearance was presented by the toes. A gangrene—true gangrene—of the nares and of the toes preceded death. In some cases death took place with the whole of these symptoms within six hours from the invasion of the attack of spasms; in others the patients lived for twenty-four or thirty-six hours. I believe few lived for more than thirty-six hours.

This disease attacked the finest and best developed men; young men from twenty-five to thirty years of age were very commonly struck down. The first sixteen of these cases died; not one was saved. The outbreak excited the greatest possible consternation; it was thought that the yellow fever was about to break out in these countries.

The *post-mortem* appearances in these patients were the same in all, and they were different—remarkably different—from those in other patients who died in this epidemic, but without these symptoms. In these cases we did not find follicular ulcers of the intestine. It is a very curious fact that the so-called anatomical character of typhoid according to many writers, was not here. What did we find? We found in the first place that the peritoneum was not inflamed, notwithstanding the dreadful pain. It had just the appearance that we see in many cases of bad fever—a certain lividity of colour. In every dissection we found intussusceptions to the most extraordinary extent, invaginations of the intestines in every direction upwards and downwards ; in some patients as many as six were observed. In all of them there was an enormously enlarged spleen, in a condition of extreme softening, so that in some patients it was difficult to take this viscus out of the body without rupturing it. In none, however, did it appear that actual rupture of the spleen had occurred during life. In none did we find any inflammation of the liver, and with respect to the mucous membrane of the stomach and of the intestines, all that can be said was that there was extreme lividity and softening in different portions of the intestine. Now I mention this fact particularly, to show that in an epidemic of our typhus fever where there is a tendency to abdominal symptoms we may have essentially different anatomical results.

I have told you that in none of these cases was the liver inflamed, and the close similarity of the anatomical appearances with those observed in the yellow fever in the Southern States of North America is very remarkable. An American physician, Dr. Lawrence, has published a series of dissections in cases of yellow fever, which exactly correspond to the *post-mortem* appearances in the outbreak I have described. I believe that inflammation of the liver is rarely observed in the yellow fever of tropical climates; and this is also true of the fever we experienced here in 1827.

But while dwelling on this subject, I may mention that the seventeenth patient was the first to recover. I do not say that his recovery was owing to the treatment adopted. It is more likely that it was due to the decreasing violence of the morbific cause; for in every great and extraordinary epidemic the first cases, generally speaking, are the most violent, and it is probable that the result of this seventeenth case was owing mainly to the fact that the intensity of the disease was on the decline. Afterwards others recovered, and the disease lost a great deal of its violent character.

One patient made a good recovery even after having lost the left ala nasi and one of her toes; but in the case just spoken of the following circumstances occurred—and it is interesting to note them in connection with the question of yellow fever generally. The patient was treated on this plan : He was allowed wine with extreme liberality. Sixteen leeches were applied to the epigastrium. He also used mercury and opium freely and after a time left the hospital to all appearances perfectly well. In the course of about two weeks he expressed a great desire to be readmitted into the hospital, stating that he was very ill.

On readmission he looked miserable. His respiration was very quick; he had a dry cough and a rapid, small pulse, with severe sweating at night; and he presented all the appearances of a person in acute phthisis. Upon a careful examination, however, we were surprised to find that there were little or no stethoscopic signs of disease of the lung. The chest everywhere sounded well, and there was hardly any râle to be found; a little sibilant râle here and there might be discovered. I may mention to such of you as have not studied the subject of acute tubercle following fever, that in almost all instances of this affection there are intense signs of pulmonary irritation. In the present case the absence of these signs led us, after a day or two, to doubt that the patient was getting tubercle, as we had at first supposed. I repeatedly examined him with extreme care over the whole chest. One morning I found nothing; next day, upon entering the ward, I saw the patient sitting up in a state of orthopnœa with a large vessel beside him completely filled with pus. There were, I am sure, three pints of purulent matter in the vessel. Upon examination I found an extraordinary change. While his chest had been quite clear the day before, the entire of the left side posteriorly was now absolutely dull; there was no resonance of the voice or tubular breathing on this side.

The patient gradually recovered, and the whole progress of the case indicated that an abscess had formed and had opened through the left lung. Whether it was a case of actual communication between an abdominal abscess and the lung, with escape of the pus into the latter; or whether it was one of those extraordinary cases of vicarious action of the lung relieving the abscess, is a matter we cannot tell, for the patient recovered and lived afterwards for many years in perfect health.

For a long time I was in the habit of looking at this case as an exceptional one in the epidemic, in which, you may remember, we did not find any example of acute hepatitis. I have since come to the conclusion that the case was, in all probability, abscess of the spleen. You will recollect that enlargement and softening of the spleen were constantly present, and this may be held to have prepared the organ for suppuration after convalesence from the fever.

Recollecting also that the sudden flow of pus took place through the left lung, it seems most probable that splenic abscess formed, which perforated the diaphragm, crossed the pleura by means of adhesions, and was finally discharged into the lung. It is possible that when the patient came into hospital the second time the spleen was a mere sac of purulent matter, and hence its condition would more easily have escaped detection from the fluid character of its contents. A case has been placed on record of abscess of the spleen in fever in which, although perforation into the lung did not take place, such an accident would have occurred had the patient survived a few days longer; for the part of the diaphragm in contiguity to the abscess was found nearly penetrated.

It is possible that this diseased condition of the spleen began to be developed during the acute stage of the fever; and taking into account the peculiar character of the epidemic, distinguished as it was by extreme activity of all the organic processes, it is most likely that the spleen passed from the softening into the suppurative condition during the patient's convalescence. Dr. Hudson, in speaking of the vomiting which so often occurs in relapsing fever, mentions a remarkable case reported by Dr. Law. In the course of less than two days the patient passed from a slightly jaundiced hue into deep jaundice, with delirium, lethargy, coma, and death. The liver and spleen were found much enlarged and congested, and so softened that they seemed as if they had been soaked in blood. May we not suppose that, if life had been prolonged, such a condition of these viscera would have ended in suppuration and the formation of abscess?

The case which I have described above was the only one in which suppuration of a large viscus came under our notice in convalescence from this fever, but it is an interesting fact that a very few years subsequent to this epidemic the occurrence of hepatic abscess was frequently noticed in this hospital, and, indeed, in most of the hospitals in Dublin. This you will see from a report, by Dr. Graves and myself, in the fifth volume of the "Dublin Hospital Reports."

With regard to the identity of these extraordinary cases of fever with the yellow fever of tropical climates, you will remember that I spoke of the dissections made by Dr. Lawrence, of America, and the close correspondence of his results with ours. Without entering at length into the question, which is fully discussed by Dr. Graves in his twenty-first lecture, I will merely say that in my own opinion the view taken by him is correct—namely, that the diseases differ only in degree. Certain it is that the most prominent symptoms of the tropical yellow fever were present in the outbreak which occurred here—black vomiting, epigastric tenderness, jaundice, and enlargement of the spleen.

LECTURE XXI.

INTESTINAL COMPLICATIONS OF FEVER, *continued*—Organic changes—Perforation of intestine—Of common occurrence in 1826-29 : (1) Generally rapidly followed by symptoms of peritonitis ; (2) but may be unattended by local symptoms in progressive cases, or again may induce only limited peritonitis (adhesions) ; (3) Symptoms of perforation may be veiled by the co-existence of intense irritation in another cavity of the body—Illustrative case—Time of occurrence of perforation as observed in *six* cases—Diagnosis of internal solutions of continuity is based on sudden development, without apparent exciting cause, of new, local, violent, and often rapidly fatal symptoms—Cases to which this rule of diagnosis is applicable—In effusion into a serous sac the degree of resulting inflammation is determined chiefly by the quality of the effused fluid—Examples—Influence of an irruption of pus in producing serous inflammation contrasted with that of an irruption of blood—Physiological difference between pus corpuscle and white blood cell—The formation of conservative adhesions seems to be rarer in peritonitis than in pleuritis—Case of hepatic abscess in which adhesions occurred and recovery followed (diagnosis from abdominal aneurism).

WE have to-day to study another of the results of abdominal complication in fever, where the ulcerative process in the mucous glands of the intestine goes on to perforation of the tube, generally resulting in effusion of its contents into the peritoneal sac. You are not, however, to suppose that this ulceration in all cases is the result of an attack of fever—it may arise under other circumstances.

Still the follicular ulceration in fever is more likely to induce perforation than other forms of this affection. You all know how common ulceration of the mucous membranes is in phthisis with diarrhœa, yet how very rarely do we meet with perforation in this case ?

I have spoken of the epidemic of 1826 and 1829 as being remarkable for the activity of the secondary organic changes. At the close of this epidemic we had several cases of perforation of the intestine in our wards, though before and since that time this accident has been rarely observed. You will see reports of these cases in the fifth volume of the "Dublin Hospital Reports"

Thus, in a large proportion of the cases observed by Dr. Graves and myself, the symptoms were those of a sudden and violent attack of peritonitis, which proved rapidly fatal, so that there was little difficulty as to the diagnosis.

But, as in other internal solutions of continuity, there may be latency as regards the accident. Perforation by no means implies escape of the contents of the tube into the peritoneal sac, and little or no local symptoms may attend the progressive ulceration—as in the case I mentioned to you.[1] In this way several perforations may occur without general peritonitis.

In other cases the inflammation of the serous membrane seems to be limited to the seat of the lesion, where the contiguous folds of the intestine become agglutinated by adhesion, which thus prevents the escape of the fæcal matter and the production of sudden and general peritonitis.

But there is a third class of cases, in which the latency of even an extensive amount of peritonitis attending the perforation, seems to be owing to the co-existence of intense irritation in another cavity of the body. A young woman was admitted with fever and severe secondary bronchial affection. In the course of five days she had some epigastric pain, which was removed by leeching. The belly became somewhat tympanitic, and the condition of the lungs got worse. The fever ran on, and in about nine days symptoms and signs of pneumonia appeared in the left lung, with tenderness of the epigastrium, for which she was again leeched over this region and also on the left side. Tartar emetic was ordered, and in a few days the pneumonia seemed to subside, but recurred. The skin then became cool, and we had hopes of her recovery; but the thoracic symptoms returned with violence, and she died after an illness of about three weeks' duration.

This was a case of tubercular fever combined with dothinenteritis. The substance of the lung was of a bright vermilion colour, perfectly stuffed with recent miliary and granular tubercles, and with intense redness of the bronchial membrane. Some puriform fluid was found in the peritoneum, and the small intestines were generally glued together by soft exudation, which, on being removed, allowed us to see no less than four perforations capable of admitting a quill in the lower portion of the ileum. Many of the follicular glands were enlarged, and—in the lower portion of the gut—ulcerated in different degrees, so that in some the bottom of the ulcer was the muscular, while in others it was merely the serous, coat. In the arch of the colon were two small ulcerations. No fæcal matter appeared to have escaped through the perforations.

This case shows how the symptoms of a severe affection in one cavity may be masked by the existence of violent irritation in another. You may see something of the same kind in delirium tremens from excess, which may be complicated with a group of local irritations of

---

[1] Page 138.

the heart, lungs, stomach, and brain, no one of which diseases presents the usual prominent local symptoms.

It is interesting to inquire respecting the period of the fever at which the perforation and consequent fatal peritonitis take place, for by this we may learn something as to the rapidity of intestinal ulcerations. You are to remember that our cases occurred at the time when the epidemic was dying out, and we may hold that the activity of the organic process for which it was so remarkable was on the decline.

In our first case—that of a man aged 36—the symptoms resembled those of ileus: great pain, violent spasms of the abdominal muscles, and tympanites. These set in on the seventh day; great aggravation of pain took place on the eighth, and he died on the thirteenth day. A perforating ulcer capable of admitting the finger was found about three inches above the ileo-cæcal valve; the mucous membrane above and below the valve was intensely red and softened; the bladder was inflamed—inability to pass water, which yielded to treatment, having been amongst the early symptoms.

In the second case—that of a man aged 32—violent pain followed a severe debauch. It returned in the course of two days, having been at first relieved by purgatives. On the return of the pain, though the belly was swelled, it was not very tender on pressure. The pulse was full and the bowels obstinately costive. In consultation with the late Dr. Beauchamp, bleeding, purgatives, and injections were ordered, the pulse continuing full and strong. During the night excruciating pain came on, with green vomiting, and the man died next morning.

A perforation was found in the last twelve inches of the ileum, corresponding with a follicular ulceration. Many similar but non-perforating ulcerations were found.

In the case of tuberculous fever which I have just now related it is impossible to fix the time of the perforation, but you will remember that there was no escape of feculent matter into the peritoneum. It would seem that a mere perforation not followed by this occurrence is, like the ulceration of the mucous membrane, a silent process as far as relates to pain.

In another case of perforation the accident seemed to occur on the fifth day. The patient had headache, for which he took two doses of epsom salts, by each of which he was briskly purged. On the fifth day violent pain, prostration, and vomiting came on. He was at once admitted with fæcal vomiting, collapse and pain, and tenderness of the abdomen. He died on the sixth day, *all pain and tenderness of the abdomen having dissappeared for many hours before death.* The usual appearances of perforating ulcer, general peritonitis, and disease of the mucous glands of the ileum were found.

In our fifth case, which was a mild enteric fever with epigastric tenderness, the countenance became anxious on the thirteenth day, the tongue glazed and dry, and the patient, a man aged 21, complained of pain in the belly. Soon afterwards hemorrhage from the bowels showed itself, and the abdominal pain became intense. Next day he had all the symptoms of severe peritonitis, and he died the following morning. The peritoneal cavity was filled with sero-purulent matter. About two inches from the ileo-cæcal valve an open perforation was found, and the mucous glands in its vicinity were in various stages of ulceration.

The last case I shall notice was that of a man aged 46, who a year previously had contracted ague. The paroxysms were stopped by bark, but thirst, anorexia, soreness in the epigastrium, and yellow slimy dejections continued. Twelve days before admission he was attacked by shivering, followed by vomiting and severe pain about the umbilical region. A bilious diarrhœa succeeded, which lasted for ten days; then it ceased, and the pain became suddenly intense, with retention of urine. The belly swelled, and the pain and tenderness were general. He sank on the third day after admission.

The peritoneal cavity being opened, a rush of fœtid air took place, the sac being found to contain much yellow fluid mixed with fæcal matter and lymph : a thin false membrane covered the peritoneum of the liver and the abdominal parietes. The small intestines were livid and covered with coagulable lymph.

One more example of perforation without effusion of the contents of the tube, and consequent fatal peritonitis, has been observed in our wards. Here the perforation appeared to be closed by merely the serous membrane of the contiguous fold of intestine, *which was not adherent,* and which showed only a slight patch of lividity. Do not forget this, as it illustrates the importance in these cases of seeking to lessen the peristaltic action of the intestine. When I speak of treatment we shall return to this subject.

The diagnosis of internal solutions of continuity is based upon the occurrence of sudden, perfectly new, local, violent, and in many cases rapidly fatal symptoms, all this often happening without manifest exciting cause. The violence of the symptoms seems to depend on changes in the mechanical state of organs, on the production of acute local inflammatory action, and on internal losses of blood, causing syncope with or without convulsions. Here the *embolic* pathology confirms principles already in use so far as the solids are concerned, and extends their application to the fluids; for there is in one sense a solution of continuity, not indeed of the tissues of the suffering organ, but in the current of the fluids which supply it.

The same general rules of diagnosis apply to many different cases, such as rupture of the heart or of an internal aneurism ; perforation of the pulmonary serous membrane from the lung ; opening of an empyema into the lung, causing expectoration of pus and pneumothorax ; perforating ulcer of any portion of the digestive tube; rupture of the urinary bladder, uterus, or gall-bladder; the opening of an abscess of the liver into the peritoneum, pleura, or pericardium : and rupture of a vessel in the brain.

The cases of peritonitis from perforation we have been considering are examples of an acute local inflammatory action, the result of a solution of continuity.

Now, as regards the diagnosis from sudden inflammation of the perforated organ, much depends on the quality of the fluid which escapes into the sac. The effusion of the contents of the intestinal tube, urinary bladder, or gall bladder, is commonly attended with new and violent inflammation ; while more bland fluids, such as blood or the contents of an hydatid sac, do not produce these violent effects. The sudden effusion of purulent matter, on the other hand, is often followed by intense inflammation of a serous sac—as we see in phthisis with pulmonary fistula, and in hepatic abscess opening into the peritoneum.

Of this latter accident we had a remarkable example in our wards many years ago. It occurred in 1828, when abscess of the liver was observed in many instances. The early symptoms of hepatic irritation were rather obscure, but three weeks before admission the patient had sweatings and nocturnal perspirations. The right side was dilated, but the intercostal spaces were well marked. There were all the signs of hepatic tumour. In the course of a fortnight the swelling increased, and as the symptoms indicated abscess, although there was no fluctuation, Dr. Graves' operation was performed. In the course of a week a fluctuating tumour appeared between the median line at the epigastrium and the lower end of the wound. The patient was greatly prostrated. A lancet was pushed from the wound into the tumour, when in place of the expected matter there was an effusion of dark bile. No jaundice existed at the time. The circumscribed tumour subsided, but the fulness of the side remained. In the course of four hours the patient had two very copious motions, consisting of purulent matter tinged with bilious and fluid fæces. It was plain that the abscess had opened into the intestine. Next morning the improvement was remarkable; the swelling had much diminished, and in a few days had altogether subsided. The patient improved so much as to take exercise, but continued to be affected with an obstinate diarrhœa.

In little more than three weeks from the subsidence of the tumour a small hard swelling appeared in the epigastrium: it rapidly increased and became fluctuating. The diarrhœa continued. Thirteen days having elapsed, he was suddenly seized with excruciating pain in the epigastrium. It was so severe as to produce an almost convulsive state. He now had the usual symptoms of perforation and of peritonitis, with this exception, that the disease, after its first violence was spent, ran a course of eight days before death took place.

We found the peritoneum filled with fluid, intermixed with large masses of gelatinous exudation, which in some places showed a commencing organization. This exudation was laminated, and its interior was traversed by bloodvessels of a deep blue colour. An abscess, the size of an orange, communicating with the peritoneal sac by an opening capable of admitting a quill, was found in the left lobe of the liver. In the right lobe was a cavity lined with a dense membrane, and communicating with the duodenum by an opening which admitted the finger with ease. This accounted for the consequent diarrhœa on the subsidence of the first tumour.

In another case, in which a vast hepatic abscess existed, the operation of puncture was immediately followed by dreadful pain in the lower part of the belly, and a sensation as if matter was escaping into the peritoneum. In a few hours the patient, a woman, showed every symptom of acute peritonitis. There were vomiting and screaming, the pulse 140, small and wiry; and the knees drawn up. These symptoms all subsided in a few days under the opium treatment, but she sank exhausted in nearly a month from the operation. Universal adhesion was found, and the abscess contained nearly four pints of purulent matter.

The influence of an eruption of purulent matter in exciting serous inflammation, so far as we have observed it, differs very much from the effects of hemorrhage into a serous sac. I have seen a case in which, from a rent at the origin of the aorta, a gush of blood into the pericardium took place on three separate occasions. After death no evidences of pericarditis were discernible. In a second instance, where an aneurism of the abdominal aorta opened into the pleura on three occasions, with a considerable interval between the first and second and between the second and third hemorrhages, no trace of pleuritis could be discovered.

This character of the blood is in direct contrast to the irritative effect of a purulent fluid on a serous membrane, and goes far to show that there must be some essential physiological difference between pus and the white corpuscles of the blood. Here, as in many other points, physiological conclusions are to be tested by the facts of pathology, and no matter how similar the white blood corpuscle and the pus cell may appear under the microscope, we must believe that the vital characters of the two are different.

Since perforation of the peritoneum occurs more frequently than perforation of the pleura, it is interesting to consider whether adhesive inflammation is a less frequent occurrence in the former than in the latter lesion—at least when *we speak of cases where the irritation is prolonged from the underlying tissues to the serous surface*. That this seems to be the case in chronic disease there can be little doubt. In the ordinary tuberculous disease of the lung, partial adhesions of the pleura are almost constant, and consequently empyema and pneumothorax are very exceptional. We know little of perforation in acute suppurative disease of the lung, and it is certain that in chronic ulcerations of the intestine, as in phthisical diarrhœa, it is very rare. Adhesion may be absent in hepatic abscess—as is seen in India, where the abscess may come forward so as to cause discoloration of the integument and yet the peritoneum be not adherent over it. This comparative insusceptibility of the peritoneum to the adhesive process is mentioned by Mr. Annesley.

That adhesion of the serous membrane in cases of fever with ulcerated intestine is rare seems certain when we consider the frequency of the complication and the number of recoveries in cases where perforation has never occurred. Yet this accident, like every other complication in fever, varies in frequency with the epidemic constitution.

Still, were you to hold that adhesion and local inflammation of the peritoneum never attended cases of underlying suppuration, you would be wrong. At the time of the prevalence of hepatic abscess in this hospital the disease was often observed as a primary and idiopathic affection, and we had a case in which the signs of adhesive inflammation assisted in the diagnosis.

The patient, a young and strong man, after exposure to cold and damp from sleeping on the grass, was next day attacked with intolerable pain in the loins. He had fever of an inflammatory type. After some days the pain in the back ceased, and a tumour with excentric and strong pulsation made its appearance in the right hypochondrium. The pulse became more rapid, and copious sweatings set in.

The case was considered to be one of· aneurism of the hepatic or of the abdominal aorta. We came, however, to a different conclusion, and looked on it as one of acute hepatic abscess, for the following reasons:—

1st. The history of the case and the time of life of the patient.

2d. The existence of fever, at first of an inflammatory and then of a hectic type. Such a condition, so far as we are aware, is unknown in aneurism.

3d. The pulsation was indeed excentric, and so far like that of aneurism. Yet we knew that a pulsation communicated to a sac filled with fluid and *lying upon an artery* acquires this character. This fact, therefore, did not exclude the possibility of hepatic abscess.

4th. That when the hand was laid on the tumour *a deep inspiration enabled us to feel well-marked friction.* This was very important, as aneurism of the abdominal aorta has little, if any, influence in causing adhesion of the peritoneum, though aneurism of the thoracic may be attended with local pleuritis and adhesion.

In a few days the contents of a large abscess were discharged per anum, and the patient recovered.

We have seen that the ordinary chronic ulceration of the intestine in phthisis rarely spreads to the serous membrane. The comparative insusceptibility of the peritoneum to adhesive inflammation in acute secondary disease of the intestine increases the obscurity of the diagnosis of this lesion in fever.

Dr. Beatty[1] details cases of inflammation in ovarian and splenic tumours, in which the *frottement* of peritonitis was plainly felt. He also quotes Dr. Bright, and then remarks : "It would appear that this method of diagnosis of disease of a serous membrane is applicable only in those situations where one at least of the opposed surfaces is adherent to a solid existing body. I am not aware that such phenomena as have been mentioned can be perceived in inflammation of the peritoneum under ordinary circumstances, where the soft, pliable walls of the abdomen are in contact with the mass of the intestines."

---

[1] Contributions to Medicine and Midwifery, p. 298.

LECTURE XXII.

SECONDARY NERVOUS OR CEREBRO-SPINAL COMPLICATIONS OF FEVER—when they predominate, prognosis is unfavourable—Of all secondary typhous affections they are least connected with organic change—Probable reason : mucous membranes and skin undergo anatomical change more readily than serous membranes—Cerebral inflammation rarely observed in fever—Purpuric fever of 1867 an exception—Absence of organic change in typhous cerebral derangement does not lessen its importance as regards prognosis and treatment—Inadmissibility of routine treatment either antiphlogistic or by stimulation, in fever—Results obtained by Louis as to relation between head symptoms and pathological change in fever—Actual cerebritis, when it does occur in fever, is a *tertiary* phenomenon—Dr. Hudson's cases—Study of analogies is of importance in essential diseases ; thus relief of headache in early stage of some cases of smallpox by leeching is analogous to good results of moderate depletion in early stages of some cases of fever—Further examples of the effect of lessening vascular supply in controlling development of smallpox eruption—Analogy in case of secondary affections of fever—Nervous symptoms arise from *three* conditions : (1) influence of fever-poison, (2) uræmia, (3) specific secondary inflammation, probably erysipelatous in character.

WE are to-day to study the nervous or cerebro-spinal symptoms of fever. I believe it may be held, that, of the various symptoms indicative of suffering of organs in fever, these are the most remarkable; and, when developed to a certain point, the grounds of a worse prognosis than any others. And yet, so far as investigation has gone, they are less often connected with organic change than those belonging to the digestive, respiratory, or circulatory systems.

Is there any reason for this ? Not that the question should materially influence our practice. Yet, looking at the results of dissection in fever, it may be held that the surfaces of relation—the mucous membranes and skin—undergo anatomical change far more frequently than the serous membranes. Of the three great cavities of the body the cerebro-spinal is the least liable to secondary anatomical change ; an interesting fact when we reflect on the number of violent and extraordinary nervous affections—epilepsy, chorea, tetanus, hydrophobia, mania, and others—on all of which anatomy sheds but a negative light.

The first thing to be laid down is that, as regards fever in this country, or rather as it has hitherto occurred in this country, inflammation, either of the substance of the brain or of its serous covering, is rarely observed. The researches of Louis show how little cerebral symptoms in fever are to be relied on as indicative of the presence of inflammation. Dr. Murchison[1] says that he has repeatedly known the most severe cerebral symptoms during life without abnormal vascularity of the membranes after death, and, further, that he has met with only two instances where the appearances would justify the opinion that inflammation had occurred in typhus. In another place, in speaking of the diagnosis between cerebritis and the delirium of fever, he adduces the existence of the eruption in the latter disease.

But you will be ready to admit that the cerebral symptoms in fever, in regard to their connection with organic change, are under the same law as those of the digestive and pulmonary systems, and that they share with these the characters of inconstancy in occurrence, in amount, and in their connection with organic change. This inconstancy you will see influenced by the epidemic character and in isolated cases; and whether the symptoms are or are not associated with organic change, they also show a subjection to the law of periodicity.

I can add my testimony to that of Dr. Murchison as to the rarity of cerebritis in fever; indeed I never saw an example of it in the dead body before or after 1867, when the epidemic (if it may be so called) of the purpuric fever with cerebro-spinal symptoms furnished many cases to our wards. This was an example, as it were, of an epidemic within an epidemic—like the occurrence of the yellow fever of which I have already spoken. Arachnitis as a secondary affection of the brain and spinal cord was then common enough, so that the name of cerebro-spinal fever could be justified, *if the existence of organic change of the nervous centres is to be made the ground of nosological distinction.*

It is, then, to be admitted that, so far as the actual state of our knowledge of the affections of the three great cavities in fever is a guide, those of the brain are the least connected with anatomical change. It is possible that at some future day chemical or microscopical research will succeed in discerning anatomical change corresponding with the manifold nervous conditions of fever. As yet, however, this has not been done. On the other hand, if you were to conclude that nervous symptoms are of less importance because we cannot connect them with ascertained organic states, you would fall into great error—as regards treatment and prognosis they are of the greatest importance, for they reveal a state of deranged function which may be, and often is, fatal, although there is neither inflammation, nor deposit, nor any known constant or distinctive anatomical change.

The assumption of inflammation of the brain in the presence of

---

[1] Continued Fevers of Great Britain. Second edition, p. 260.

violent nervous symptoms in fever constitutes one of the greatest dangers to which young physicians are exposed, when they come to deal with the most formidable complication of the disease ; aye, and old physicians, too, whose clinical education has been imperfect. I have known of the application of leeches to the head in an advanced case of cerebral fever with delirium ferox to be followed by sudden sinking and death. I have told you how an eminent apothecary in this city, the late excellent Mr. Packenham, while he was an appren‐ tice in one of the first establishments in Dublin, would be commonly sent to remove the leeches from the temples on the death of the patient. The doctrines of the anatomical school—a school which denied essentialities, and with which all diseases were symptomatic of a local irritation—naturally led to a routine practice. The more violent the local symptoms, the more intense the inflammation was held to be, and in consequence the more vigorously and continuously the antiphlogistic treatment was pursued. I once saw in Paris a caricature in which a patient was stretched in bed *in articulo mortis* surrounded by three physicians. His countenance was hippocratic, and it was plain that the hour of deliverance from the disease by death was at hand. The principal figure among the attendant physi‐ cians, intended for Broussais, exclaims, " Encore des sangsues. "

But the doctrines of Broussais, of Bouillaud, of Clutterbuck, and of Armstrong are now matters of history, thanks to the researches of Louis and of Andral into the pathological anatomy of fever— " that disease" (to use the words of Louis) " called gastro‐enteritis" —and thanks to the influence of the writings of the fathers of British medicine—of Sydenham, Haygarth, Fothergill, and Heberden—and on the Continent of John Peter Frank. Truth, though for a time obscured, conquers in the end. The teaching of these great men has triumphed over the innovations of the so‐called physiological medicine. A more accurate observation, a truer interpretation of phenomena, a greater respect for the recorded experience of such men as those I have mentioned, have resumed their sway over the medical mind, and every day the routine application of the antiphlogistic or the stimulant treatment is less and less seen. It is right, however, to observe that the disuse of the routine antiphlogistic treatment is not altogether to be attributed to more modern research.

When studying fever, you will find that what applies to one symptom applies more or less to all. Thus, when we study the relation between organic change and delirium, we may safely adopt the same conclusion with regard to all the nervous symptoms, such as coma, convulsions, and so on. Louis, in his work *Recherches sur la*

11

Gastro-Entérite (page 155), compares the results of twelve dissections in cases of fever where delirium was absent, or only passing and slight, with those of twelve other dissections where this symptom was most violent and persistent. In a former lecture I have given the results of his observations, but I may be pardoned for reproducing them here in a tabular form.

DELIRIUM ABSENT.	Cases	DELIRIUM PRESENT AND VIOLENT.	Cases
Redness of cortical substance of the brain	4	Slight reddening of cortical substance	5
		Slight softening of brain . . .	1
Inflammation of optic thalamus .	1	Livid venous injection of mem-	
Slight softening of brain . . .	1	branes of the brain . . .	1
Brain anatomically healthy . .	6	Brain perfectly healthy . . .	5
	12		12

Now, looking at these tables, it is impossible to avoid seeing that there is no constant relation between the anatomical changes of the brain and the symptoms. In the general progress of fever, as I have told you, the nervous symptoms may be considered of the greatest importance, and in the present state of our knowledge we must refer them to the effects of the poison of fever. Whether that poison acts directly and in the first instance on the nervous centres, or indirectly on them through the medium of the blood, is a question which may still be asked. They are, at all events, in their early stages to be looked on more as functional than as organic symptoms. But, in the nervous as in the pulmonary and abdominal symptoms, we find inconstancy and irregularity in the visible alteration of the organ. It would in any case, however, be an error to assert that there are no cases of secondary nervous engagement, in which local antiphlogistic treatment is to be used. We might as well say that there are no cases in which cupping of the chest, or the application of leeches to the ileo-cæcal region, was useful.

That actual cerebritis does occasionally occur in fever is certain. It is very probable that it is a tertiary phenomenon in the case—the steps being, first, fever; then, deposit; and, lastly, reactive inflammation. I do not apply the observations I now make to the cerebrospinal or purpuric fever, although when cerebritis does occur in fever it seems to depend on an epidemic tendency. You will see in Dr. Hudson's work[1] an account of three cases in which true inflammation of the brain and its membranes was proved on *post-mortem* examination to have occurred in the course of fever. In one case head symptoms

---

[1] Lectures on the Study of Fever. Second edition, p. 252.

of a very severe nature became developed about the eleventh day of maculated typhus. Four days later the patient died. On examination the dura mater was found sensibly thickened, the subarachnoid fluid considerably increased in quantity, and the vessels of the brain and its membranes much congested. The cerebellum and medulla oblongata were to some extent softened. The second patient from the time of his admission lay in a state of increasing stupor, with ptosis of one eye, strabismus, retention of urine, and finally dysphagia. Here there was intense venous congestion of the cerebellum and upper part of the cord and a circumscribed collection of yellowish-green pus lay included beween the arachnoid and the under surface of the cerebellum. The arachnoid itself bore traces of inflammation. In a third case similar appearances were observed.

Dr. Hudson also quotes some cases of a like kind which were communicated to the Pathological Society by Sir Dominic Corrigan. "While," says Dr. Hudson, "you must endeavour, on the one hand, to avoid the mistake of ascribing the nervous derangements caused by the toxic action of the fever poison to cerebral inflammation, you must, on the other, avoid the opposite error of ignoring the existence of true inflammation, when this is indicated by the groups of symptoms enumerated above, whether it occurs in the form of acute congestion of the brain, as in some epidemics of typhus, of epidemic cerebrospinal arachnitis, of arachnitis, or as the effect of previous injury, or of reactive irritation and inflammation, set up in the advanced period of typhoid fever."

In the investigation of disease, especially in that of fevers, the study of analogies is of great importance; and looking at the liability of essential affections to induce secondary local conditions, we may expect the brain also to be subject to this liability, the result being a neurotic or functional condition followed or not by anatomical change. Why it is that the latter result seems so rare we have as yet no means of determining. It may indeed, unless reactive irritation occurs, be overlooked in examinations after death. It is not easy to distinguish the toxic influence of fever from the signs of primary or of reactive inflammation. Yet, although it be admitted that the nervous symptoms are generally functional, the relief afforded in certain cases by a few leeches, the cold affusion, and the use of ice to the head, indicates a condition which—if not actual meningitis—is related to or may possibly be a precursor of it. And it may be asked whether the secondary effect of fever may be locally modified or arrested by a lessening of the blood supply. I have published a case of variola which illustrates the arrest of local development of the pustules.

A young and healthy woman was admitted with severe fever of a sthenic type. She was about three days ill, and complained of intense headache, far more violent than that met with in the early periods of ordinary fever. The face was flushed and turgid. Looking on the case as exceptional, we applied leeches freely to the temples. This was followed by relief of pain; the redness of the face disappeared, as did the fulness. Next day smallpox vesicles appeared, on the breast and arms, and there was soon a plentiful crop of pustules running into confluence over the entire body, *with the exception of the face,* where but one or two small and aborted pustules formed.

We have found, too, in variola, that where the appearance of the vesicles on the face was attended with heat and vascularity, the application of leeches rendered the after-pustulation so much more benign that this mode, together with the use of light poultices, has been found most efficacious in preventing the subsequent pitting of the face, and we have therefore commonly employed it.

In a remarkable case of severe confluent smallpox the patient had been an inmate of the surgical ward for a chronic affection of the knee, for which the joint was strapped with mercurial plaster. Of this I was not aware till the stage of decrustation arrived, when the strips of plaster which had tightly bound the knee fell off, and this singular appearance was seen. The face and body generally presented black, thick, and fetid crusts, but the knee for a space of seven inches was of a pearly whiteness, without a trace of pustulation, and contrasting strangely with the condition of the skin above and below the joint. Here the pressure by the straps had lessened the vascular supply.

Now, regarding the eruption of smallpox as a secondary and local manifestation of that disease, as there is no doubt it is, we see it, in the instances just quoted, controlled by local depletion or lessening of the blood supply. The similar relation between the nervous symptoms in fever and the local treatment I have referred to is at once interesting and suggestive.

We may hold in practice that the nervous symptoms in fever arise from the following conditions:—

a. The influence of the poison of fever.

b. The occurrence of the uræmic condition.

c. The occurrence of an inflammation, probably of an erysipelatous and also of a specific nature, analogous to that in the other secondary affections of fever.

Of these the first two may be considered as functional or neurotic, and, remembering the quality of inconstancy as to the period of appearance of the secondary symptoms in fever, we find that any, or any combination, of these may occur at various stages of the disease.

LECTURE XXIII.

NERVOUS COMPLICATIONS OF FEVER, *continued—Cerebro-spinal fever*—Phenomena of fever inconstant and variable, except, perhaps, the phenomenon of increased temperature—*Type* of fever also varies in different epidemics—Two examples: (1) *yellow fever* of 1826-27, (2) *malignant purpuric*, or *cerebro-spinal fever* of 1867—Dr. E. W. Collins' report on latter—There exists a "constitutional element" in the disease, so that the cerebro-spinal arachnitis can hardly be held to be a primary, idiopathic affection—Evidences of essentiality from presence of other phenomena in connection with the skin, etc.—Reports to the *Medical Society of the King and Queen's College of Physicians in Ireland* on the epidemic of 1867—Inconstancy and variability of the symptoms in the outbreak—Dr. H. Kennedy's views—Symptoms of the disease—Petechiæ—Early setting in of putrefraction—*Retraction of head:* sometimes persistent after disappearance of other local and general symptoms, and sometimes persistent after death—Recapitulation: Points to be considered in connection with epidemic of 1867: (1) yellow fever of 1826-27, (2) cerebro-spinal arachnitis of 1846 (Dr. Mayne), (3) coincidence of cases of malignant measles in 1867, and (4) hæmorrhagic and purpuric smallpox in epidemic of 1871-72.

I HAVE on many occasions sought to impress on you that fever is a condition which, though possessing a generic character, exhibits infinite varieties in most of its aspects, whether it be looked on in its sporadic cases or as occurring in great epidemics. There is no point of view in which any of its phenomena can be regarded as constant, except perhaps that of increased temperature. The epidemic of one period is found to differ from that of another, whether we look at its commencement or decline, its intensity or mortality, or the influence of remedies. And this quality of variability applies to the sporadic cases also, whether considered individually or collectively. The disease varies in its contagiousness in different epidemics as the condition of receptivity in healthy bodies varies, and this state of receptivity is different according to the period. It is changeable as to its degree of intensity, the number and nature of its complications, and the vital phenomena of the secondary affections, their progress and their influence on the disease as to its danger and its periodic laws, and all this whether local symptoms are merely functional or reveal organic change.

This will prepare you for the occurrence at irregular intervals of time of groups of unusual cases having on the one hand a generic resemblance, yet varying as to their local manifestations, and this is what we mean by the term of *epidemics within epidemics.*

Now, the variation from the type of the general and coexisting epidemic may be seen in both the essential and the local characters. We have had two most remarkable examples of this in Dublin. One of these was the yellow fever of which I have already spoken, characterized by violent and sudden abdominal spasms, followed rapidly by jaundice and mortification of the nose and toes; and the other the disease which has so many names—the cerebro-spinal fever, the malignant purpuric fever, epidemic cerebro-spinal meningitis, *febris nigra,* etc.

Now, I recommend all of you to carefully study the report on this disease by Dr. Collins in the *Dublin Quarterly Journal,*[1] which may be taken as a model of what a scientific and faithful medical report should be. This variety of fever appears first to have attracted attention in America early in this century. Dr. Collins shows that the first account of the cerebro-spinal fever is that of an epidemic which prevailed in Geneva in 1805. The disease showed itself in various places in Europe and in America. Then it continued in America, and in 1837 it became a wide-spread epidemic, occurring in Germany, England, Ireland, and Denmark, and appearing at many ports in Spain, North Africa, and Italy. In the *British and Foreign Medico-Chirurgical Review,*[2] you will find an excellent *résumé* of the reports of the American, German, and British physicians. This article is written in that philosophical spirit which has so long distinguished the periodical just mentioned. The name in use in America for this disease was *the spotted fever.* Discussions arose about the nature of the disease, some holding it to be an essential fever related to typhus, if not typhus itself; others, a true cerebro-spinal meningitis. But it is plain that the relation between the nervous symptoms—and also the state of the brain and spinal cord—and the general symptoms was not fully understood. The great fact of the secondary lesions in fever varying in amount, prominence, seat, result, time of appearance, was not yet appreciated, while the doctrine of the anatomical school, that fever was symptomatic of a local irritation, made men look upon the structural change as the cause of all the symptoms, while it was truly the effect, though when it occurred it produced special phenomena of a striking kind. It is true that Dr. Gordon found the marks of cerebro-spinal inflammation within five hours from the occurrence

[1] Vol. xlvi. August, 1868, p. 170.   [2] Vol. xlii. p. 389, and vol. xliii. p. 1 32

of the first symptoms of the constitutional malady, though the special signs of cerebro-spinal irritation were wanting, and Levy has recorded another case of singular rapidity of morbid action. Arguing from these cases and from another in which extensive exudation in the meninges was found after thirty hours of illness, Dr. Collins, while admitting a constitutional element in the disease, holds that, since the products of inflammation became developed in so short a period of time, the inflammation itself from which they sprang cannot be considered other than primary and as forming *along with the constitutional element* the pathological essence of the disease.

Now, the admission of the constitutional element is to give up the doctrine of primary cerebro-spinal meningitis; for what is this but fever, with secondary nervous symptoms and organic states?

"Congestions," writes Dr. Collins;[1] "plastic, purulent, sero-purulent, or serous exudations; sometimes even alterations of the nervous substance itself, of ever-varying extent, singly or together, bear their testimony to the nature of these inflammatory processes. But these inflammatory changes, constant though they be, are not the only, nor are they always the most important, features of the disease. Behind them all, as in other affections, modifying and at times predominating, lies another, a constitutional element, which gives to the disease so many of its varied and most appalling characters. This constitutional element, the importance of which cannot be over-estimated, is remarkably exemplified in those malignant and rapidly fatal cases of *meningite foudroyante*, so called, which occurred within the past two years throughout this island. The lesions here found, in many instances, have been only varying degrees of congestion of the pia mater, and similar experience is not wanting from the records of other epidemics, so that some French writers have even given to this form of the malady the title of *forme congestionelle*."

Now, this term "*meningite foudroyante*" is improper. It conveys a false idea of the whole disease, leading to the belief that all its symptoms, the rapidity of its progress, and its fatal results are only measures of the intensity of a primary local inflammation. But that the "constitutional state" of Dr. Collins is of the nature of fever generating local disease—as scarlatina commonly generates sore throat; measles, bronchial irritation; and typhus and typhoid, pulmonary and abdominal diseases—is obvious when the relation between the local and constitutional state is considered. Its amount is variable, and does not necessarily correspond to the violence of the symptoms. In some of the most rapid cases there is nothing observable but

[1] Loc. cit. p. 201.

congestion of the pia mater, and the degree of meningeal inflammation
has been found, as in the secondary affections of fever, to vary according to locality and time—in other words, according to the local
epidemic.

To show that the cerebro-spinal arachnitis can hardly be considered
a primary idiopathic affection in this disease, the coexistence of other
local affections is to be noticed. Thus, great swelling of the eyelids
and conjunctivitis, with deep-seated injury of the eye ; deafness, often
without, but occasionally with, purulent discharge; aphthæ; swelling
of the parotid, submaxillary, and cervical glands, with or without
consequent suppuration, have been described. Epistaxis, meteorism,
diarrhœa, enlargement of the spleen, broncho-pneumonia, and occasionally pericarditis, have been noticed by various observers in different localities and at different periods.

Yet there are other evidences of its analogies to essential disease—
the occurrence of herpes; of a dusky discoloration of the skin, as in
typhus; of extraordinary petechial spots running occasionally into
vast ecchymoses, so as to evoke the designation of black death, and
the occurrence of a condition of the joints similar to that described
long since by the late Dr. MacDowel. This at first simulates rheumatic arthritis, but soon shows the signs of purulent deposit. All this
confirms the view which was long ago taken in this hospital, and more
lately set forth by Stillé, that this disease is a combination of an essen
tial specific condition, analogous to fever, with an important local and
consequent lesion of the nervous centres. The variations of phenomena, both essential and local, though these present a generic resemblance, the differences of results of *post-mortem* examination—all are
plainly referable to the laws of essential epidemic disease occurring
at various times and in various parts of the world.

That the remarkable local affection, which gave a name to the epidemic we are considering, agrees in its general characters with the
secondary lesions of other varieties of fever, is evident from the truly
able and practical paper by Dr. Gordon in the forty-third volume of the
Dublin Quarterly Journal; and also from the records of two successive meetings of the Medical Society of the King and Queen's College
of Physicians in 1867. At these meetings not less than twenty-seven
observers of the disease in Ireland during the epidemic of 1866 and
1867 recorded their experience of it. I do not know of any greater
illustration of the healthy state of medical opinion in Ireland than
that afforded on this remarkable occasion. Most of those who gave
reports of cases and the results of their experience were physicians

to some of the Dublin hospitals, while reports were also read by some military surgeons then quartered in Ireland.

The occurrence of the nervous symptoms and the condition of the nervous centres had received great attention from most of the observers. I may state that these meetings were more for the purpose of recording individual experience than for discussion, of which there was very little ; and when among the reporters were men of such mark as Drs. Hudson, Gordon, Lyons, Hayden, Law, Banks, Henry Kennedy, and Moore, you can understand the great importance of the occasion.

Now, I claim no originality for the views I have submitted as to the primary or the secondary nature of the cerebro-spinal disease. Gentlemen, there is nothing more deplorable than the contests among our brethren respecting priority in observation and doctrine. I have spoken of this in my lecture on medical ethics, and have shown you that when several observers are working for the same object and at the same time—similar views will occur to many of them simultaneously. This applies to all investigations. It is of the first importance that the truth should be made known, but by whom it was first suggested matters little indeed.

If you study the cases brought forward at the College of Physicians, you will find that the character of inconstancy attended the symptoms of meningitis, and also the structural alteration. In one of the very worst cases which I saw with Dr. Lyons death took place in little more than twenty-four hours. The patient was a fine young man, an officer in a cavalry regiment. There was no retraction of the head. Dr. Lyons recorded two other fatal cases in which the peculiar cerebro-spinal symptoms were absent. In the 52d Regiment five cases were reported by Mr. Haverty. The third case proved fatal in sixteen hours after admission. There was no pain in the head, no retraction ; nothing unusual was found in the brain, but at its base an increased quantity of serum, which was of a dark colour. In a case which occurred in this hospital with recovery, there was no retraction of the head. The patient had slight converging strabismus and dilated pupils. In a case by Dr. MacSwiney no lesion of the brain or spinal cord was discovered, and Dr. Kennedy stated that many similar instances had been met with by others, in which, as in Dr. MacSwiney's case, there were no symptoms of arachnitis and no lesion of the nervous centres found after death. Dr. Banks, also, said that in many fatal cases in this epidemic no signs of cerebro-spinal meningitis were discovered after death.

Dr. Kennedy remarks on this subject as follows: "Taking, then, all the facts at present known, and more particularly the one that our typhus fever has, within these two years (he spoke in 1867), been frequently complicated by spinal arachnitis, into consideration, it appears to me that no other conclusion can be arrived at than that the late terrible disease which has visited us is a specific fever, and that the spinal arachnitis is but a complication, which may or may not be present."

It is needless to insist on the importance of all this, as showing (what might have been predicated) that the disease in its essence was not primary inflammation of the cerebro-spinal meninges. We have seen fatal cases in which it might have been said that there were never any symptoms of inflammation of the nervous centres, while, on the other hand, every shade or degree of such symptoms have been met with. We had one case here in which convulsions continued through the whole illness; and the state of the brain and spinal marrow varied from the condition of freedom from disease in some instances to one in which the base of the brain and spinal cord were bathed in pus.

This variability in the amount of the local disease is thus strictly analogous to what we observe in the secondary intestinal lesions of typhoid.

It appears, then, that a form of cerebro-spinal disease with meningeal inflammation has been observed to commonly but not universally attend this singular malady in America and in Europe. It has been revealed by pain in the head, rachialgia, opisthotonos, trismus, and occasionally convulsions. Yet it throws no light on the constitutional state to which it appears secondary. It is variable in its occurrence, inconstant in its amount, and incompetent to account for the general malady. In short, it has all the characteristics of a secondary rather than of a primary local malady. It is often associated with other forms of local visceral disease.

There is nothing more appalling than the appearance of many patients in this affection—the dark petechial spots soon become confluent, and vast black ecchymoses form. In a patient whom I saw with Dr. Croly a few petechial spots appeared on the neck on the first day of illness. Next morning these had become black, and increased in size so rapidly that they seemed to grow under the eye of the observer. At eleven o'clock the spots were extremely large, and in the course of two hours the entire right arm and half of the right side of the chest had become continuously black, with large patches over the rest of the body. Soon after this a fit of convulsions came on, and the patient died at half-past two. The duration of the illness was about thirty hours.

Another case is given by Dr. Croly in which the disease set in with vomiting, followed by severe diarrhœa. On the second day blue spots, soon becoming black, appeared on the sufferer's legs, and shortly before death on her arms and face. She died in convulsions with forcible retraction of the head. The duration of illness was twenty-eight hours.

In some instances, where this terrible disease had run a rapid course, putrefaction appeared to have set in at a very early period after, or even before, death. I was called to see a patient in whom the symptoms had first developed themselves but twenty-eight hours before. He had just died as I entered the room, and I shall not soon forget the overpowering stench of putrescence which rose from the still warm body. The ordinary medical attendant assured me that the stench had been observed some time previously to death.

Two interesting facts in connection with a remarkable symptom of this disease—I allude to the retraction of the head—deserve to be mentioned here. The first is the occasional long continuance of the rigidity after all constitutional and local symptoms have disappeared. I saw a boy in whom the retraction was so great that he could lie only on his belly, and in this position he remained for several weeks, during which time his general health was excellent; he took much nourishment and gained flesh. In another case the retraction did not appear until just at the subsidence of the constitutional condition. It increased with the patient's convalescence until at last, when all febrile condition had ceased, it became so extreme that his head was bent backwards almost at a right angle with his body. This extraordinary retraction subsided with remarkable rapidity, and had quite vanished within 48 hours.

The second point is the occasional persistence of the rigidity after death. It has been supposed that the muscles which have been thus contracted during life are not liable to the *rigor mortis*, but in a remarkable case published by Dr. Gordon in his *Report on Cases of Fever with Cerebro-spinal Meningitis*[1] all the constitutional and local symptoms of the disease were present, opisthotonos being extreme, and continuing after death. On the fifth day of the disease the patient, a girl aged 15, lay on her abdomen, and refused to allow herself to be moved on the back, or on either side. Her spine presented a most wonderful and uniform curve, concave backwards; her head was also curved backwards on the spine of the neck. Dr. Gordon had not seen

[1] Dublin Quarterly Journal, vol. xl. p. 412.

so much opisthotonos in the worst cases of tetanus. She had no pain
or tenderness on pressure on any point of the spine. She died on the
ninth day of her illness, and after death the body presented a very
frightful appearance. It was still prominently arched forward. It
was of a dusky blue colour, with a copious eruption of black spots, of
various sizes, from that of a small pea to a crownpiece; some small and
circular, others large and irregular in form.

Now, in reviewing the results of our experience in this hospital, together with the published reports of the disease in Ireland, Germany,
and America, we must, I think, agree with all the best observers that
to look upon the affection as simple and idiopathic cerebro-spinal
meningitis would be erroneous. It is quite true that the frequency of
actual disease of the cerebro-spinal centres is a most striking peculiarity, yet that this condition should be placed in the category of local
affections secondary to an essential malady is more than probable.
Like this class of diseases generally, even where it shows itself early
in the case, the cerebro-spinal complication does not seem to take the
initiative. We have had examples here in which the symptoms of the
local malady failed to appear until after the seventh or even the ninth
day, although the other characters of the disease were strongly marked.

I have already spoken to you of the character of inconstancy in
amount which it has in common with other secondary lesions, and not
only in amount but in intensity. Like them, too, it may occasionally
be absent. Nor can we attribute the remaining phenomena of the
disease—the enormous ecchymoses, the rapidly increasing and dark
petechiæ, the gangrene of the skin, and the tendency to general putrescence—to the occurrence of a primary cerebro-spinal inflammation.

In connection with the extraordinary epidemic in Ireland of which
I have been speaking, the following circumstances are worthy of re-
membrance :—

First. The occurrence of the cases of so-called yellow fever, described by Dr. Graves, in the epidemic of 1826 to 1830, in
which there was blackening and mortification of the feet and
the nose, with jaundice, black vomit, and splenic enlargement.

Secondly. The outbreak of cerebro-spinal arachnitis in Dublin and
its neighbourhood in 1846, an account of which is given by
Dr. Mayne in the *Dublin Quarterly Journal,* vol. ii. p. 95. The
collapse stage in the worst cases he describes as closely resembling cholera. This stage was ushered in by violent pain in the
abdomen, rapidly followed by vomiting, and not infrequently
by purging. The extremities then became cold and bluish, and
the pulse a mere thread. There was no cutaneous eruption or
hemorrhage.

Although Dr. Mayne does not deal with these cases as examples of essential disease, but rather looks upon them as primary inflammation, yet analogy and the history of the *febris nigra* make it highly probable that the cerebro-spinal inflammation was not a primary affection in the strict sense of the word. In the collapse cases noticed by him, after the lapse of a few hours, reaction, more or less perfect, ensued; the surface became hot, the pulse full and frequent (from 120 to 140); the stomach often continued irritable, whilst an intolerable thirst tormented the sufferer.

Thirdly. The coincidence of cases of malignant measles with the recent epidemic of cerebro-spinal fever—a fact noticed by Dr. Gordon, and of which I have recorded a remarkable example in the *Transactions of the Medical Society of the College of Physicians.*

And, *fourthly.* The extraordinary prevalence of purpuric and hemorrhagic smallpox in the late terrible epidemic in Dublin.

I think that when you reflect on what has been now said, and on these latter remarkable facts, the doctrine of a cerebro-spinal meningitis independent of the general causes of essential disease, whatever these may be, cannot be entertained.

LECTURE XXIV.

NERVOUS COMPLICATIONS OF FEVER, *continued*—*Hysteria*—Occurrence of hysteria, especially at an early stage, of unfavourable import—View that hysteria is always symptomatic of uterine excitement is quite erroneous—Nymphomania only a local and accidental manifestation—Hysteria is observed in males as well as in females in fever—Case of erotic symptoms in typhoid fever occurring in a young girl, reported by Dr. A. W. Foot—In early stage of fever hysteria generally is the precursor of severe nervous symptoms—Its appearance may lead to serious complications later in the disease—Illustrative cases—Hysterical symptoms are sometimes connected with actual or organic disease, *especially in acute affections*—Dr. Cheyne's observation: *Hysteria a ground for a good prognosis in every disease, fever alone excepted*—Outbreak of hysteria, affecting the abdomen, in female fever ward of Meath Hospital—Anomalous symptoms in advanced stages of fever often due to hysterical state—Case of typhous hysteria in the male followed by cerebritis.

ONE of the nervous conditions in fever still remains to be considered. I refer to hysteria, the occurrence of which, especially in the early periods of fever, should always excite apprehension as to the result. I have often told you that you are to reject the common notion that hysteria is always symptomatic of uterine irritation, and that the occurrence of hysteria in a woman was owing to ungratified desires. I would advise you not to enter practice, whether your patients be in the humbler ranks of life or in the more refined walks of society, with this gross, degrading, and ignorant idea.

We cannot doubt that in certain cases of hysteria there is evidence of excitement of the genital system, but this result of the general disease is only one—it may be—of a series of local excitements. The hysteric condition may affect the brain, and you may have intense pain, coma, mania, and convulsions. If the lung be affected, dyspnœa, cough, expectoration, even hæmoptysis, may be observed. Hysteric palpitation and syncope occur when the disease falls on the heart, vo-miting when it affects the stomach, paralysis when the bladder is engaged, and so on. It is easy to understand that if the disease fastens itself upon the uterus and the genital system, symptoms of nympho-mania may be produced.

In fact, in cases of hysteria with excitement of the genital system it has merely happened, and accidentally, that upon that system the brunt of the disease has fallen, while, if any other organ had been affected, there would have been no symptoms of nymphomania; but mania, convulsions, palpitation, cough—the *tussis ferina*—or uncontrollable vomiting might have been present, according to circumstances.

Indeed, the occurrence of hysteric symptoms in fever in the male as in the female is almost conclusive that it is a special nervous affec-tion, the origin of which is unknown—an affection which may engage every great organ in the body, which is not symptomatic of irritation of any one of them, and whose seat is in the nerves of animal and organic life.

Let me again impress upon you that the old and still too common view of hysteria is to be rejected as one based on ignorance of the female constitution and of medicine. You will hear it advocated only by men of gross and prurient ideas. It is true, that, when the genital system happens to be engaged in the hysteric state, there is a liability to nymphomania, and you may hear expressions and witness actions in the purest females that may surprise you ; but remember that these are but the symptoms of a secondary local manifestation of a general malady. Hysteria, as its name implies, was held to be symptomatic of irritation of the uterus, just as fever was considered as symptomatic of cerebritis or muco-enteritis.

It is true that in fever we have not yet observed any erotic symptoms in the male subject, but in the young female they are occasionally met with. A case of this kind recently occurred in these wards under the care of Dr. Foot. A young woman was admitted on the eighth day of an enteric fever. Her pulse was 100 and temperature 99.5°. She was talking and gesticulating in such an erotic manner that the nurse suggested her separation from the other patients. She laughed incessantly, and exhibited all the symptoms and action of violent excitement of the genital system. This continued all that day and night. Next morning the pulse was 114 and the temperature 101.3°. The head, hands, and feet were very cold and livid. The heart's action was weak. This patient was a blonde, with very light hair and blue eyes. She hid her face from the physician, then jerked it round, took a look at the class, and hid it again. She took a double meaning out of every question put to her. In reply to ordinary questions as to headache, etc., she said, with a knowing laugh, "I know you all well. I won't let you; you won't succeed. I know what you're about." In words such as these she addressed both the physician and the class in general. It was impossible to get an answer from her. Her manner and conversation were jocular, immodest, and disrespectfully familiar.

She was ordered 30 grains of chloral at once, and immediately went to sleep. After the effects of the chloral had passed off she was ordered 30 grains of bromide of potassium every third hour. Next morning she was a different person—timid, respectful, gentle—and she did not recollect a word of what she had said the day before. This fact was further ascertained through the nurse to be true, as shame might have led her to feign forgetfulness to the students. On this day, the 10th of her illness, several rose spots appeared for the first time on her chest. She subsequently went through a well-marked enteric fever, on the 28th day of which her temperature permanently fell, having ranged during her illness between 104.8° and 97.2°. As there was constant and characteristic diarrhœa, and as the lungs became the seat of congestion at one period, the case afforded an example of secondary complication of the three great cavities of the body.

The patient's manner subsequent to the hysterical attack was most decorous. She did not appear to possess a *particle* of what is called the "hysterical temperament." So far from seeking for or seeming to like any attention, she was so distant and indifferent to the pupils as sometimes to appear impolite. She bore an excellent character prior to admission, and her parents intended to have nursed her at home, but got alarmed "when she got out of her mind," and brought her to the hospital.

Many a time I have known of a deep wound inflicted on the delicacy of the purest girl by the expression of these—I may call them brutal —views on the part of the attendant—views which show that he is at once ignorant of the physiology and of the pathology of the female

constitution, and of the moral nature of that sex, which is the deposi-
tary of all that is pure and delicate and moral in this life. That man
is unworthy of confidence or of the name of a ph ysician who thus
drags his profession into the mire.

In the early periods of fever hysterical symptoms generally usher
in a great severity of many of the nervous conditions of the disease,
while their later occurrence gives rise to singular and often embarrass-
ing complications even after the fever has run its course.

This is illustrated by the case in the wards. The girl had recovered
from fever, when she was agitated at seeing one of her friends brought
sick into the ward, and soon fell into her present condition. She lies
in a prostrate and stupid state, though answering questions rationally.
She complains of pain at the top of her head. The breathing is
natural, but at times hurried and croupy. Any attempt to examine
the throat brings on the most violent spasms, attended by hysterical
singultus. Now, has this patient irritation of the brain or of the
larynx? It is most probable she has neither, but you must remember
that she has recently had a continued fever, and so we must act as if
she were threatened with cerebral or laryngeal irritation, although of
course in a very tentative way.

A case which left a deep impression on my mind occurred with us
some years ago. It shows how actual organic change may be masked
by the hysterical complication. A young woman was an inmate of
this hospital for many months, presenting a succession of the most
violent and various local symptoms of hysteria. In fact, almost every
organ of her body was in turn attacked. She had long-continued
and incessant vomiting. For many weeks she took no food, although
with little if any emaciation. She had hemiplegia, palpitation, rapidity of pulse, constipation, tympany, and retention of urine, and these
symptoms succeeded one another or were present in various combinations. But the most prominent symptom was a spasmodic and
unceasing cough, so loud as to be heard through the house; indeed, I
have often heard it at the gate of the hospital. This was attended by
frequent attacks of stridor—so severe as to threaten life—and these
would alternate with convulsions, or some other symptom. During
the latter the stridor would completely disappear. Many months
passed by, during which this girl left and was readmitted into hospital
on several occasions. Soon after her last admission she showed for
the first time symptoms of fever, which eventuated in an attack of
general though modified smallpox. During the continuance of this
attack all the hysterical symptoms completely subsided. Some weeks
elapsed, during which she continued well, when the *tussis ferina* and

the fits of stridor returned exactly as before. We looked on it simply as a renewal of the old condition, and, as many and various remedies had been tried before, the case was regarded as one which might be left to nature. In a few days she died, asphyxiated. On dissection, to our surprise, we found a great amount of inflammation and deep ulceration of the larynx, with total destruction of its ventricles.

I do not think highly of that man's mind or heart to whom the death of a poor patient with recent, unrecognized, and probably remediable disease is a matter of indifference. Did the ulcerative disease coexist with the hysteria? It is not likely that it did, for the latter was of long continuance, while this laryngeal ulceration was obviously acute. Were its symptoms occasionally suspended during the convulsive paroxysms? Did the variolous disease, by its derivation, cause a lull in the laryngeal condition, or did the hyperæsthetic state of the larynx predispose it to organic change consequent on the exanthem? Unhappily we cannot solve these questions now, but there is one lesson to be learned from this sad case, and it is this: that, in dealing with hysterical patients, we must not fall into the common mistake of considering their local symptoms as in all cases unconnected with organic disease.

We are not, then, to neglect local symptoms, and to consider them as merely neurotic in the hysterical condition. That they may be, and commonly are so, is certain, especially in cases of chronic disease. But in an acute disease like fever the occurrence of hysteria should make us especially cautious in our prognosis as to coming nervous symptoms. The late Dr. Cheyne, of this city, used to say that the hysterical complication was a ground of a good prognosis in every disease, fever alone excepted, and this observation may apply to all forms of essential and of symptomatic fever.

Some time ago we had a remarkable manifestation of the hysterical state in fever. A young woman who was all but convalescent, and who had nearly passed through her disease before admission, was suddenly attacked with violent pain in the belly, which was swollen and tympanitic, with extreme hyperæsthesia on pressure. But the corresponding symptoms of peritonitis were absent. There were loud and constant screaming and all the other evidences of a violent hysterical attack. In the course of two or three days five other patients in the same ward became successively and similarly affected, and you can well imagine the scene presented by six women in the same ward and for several days and nights in this state. It seemed as if they were possessed, and labouring under the most violent form of demoniacal mania. There was nothing remarkable in the character of the fever

12

at the time. Some of them had simple continued and others typhus fever. Convalescence followed in all the cases, though in two of them, and in one especially, symptoms of enteric inflammation supervened, and were met by the usual treatment.

These facts show how even in a fever ward hysteria will spread by contiguity.

The most common form of the combination of the hysterical state with fever is met with generally in an advanced stage of the disease, when the patient shows signs of the hysterical state by complaining of anomalous symptoms, the alleged severity of which is in no way in accordance with the constitutional condition. She becomes unreasonable, capricious, and complaining. She watches for sympathy, refuses sustenance, and may be detected in feigning symptoms. Retention of urine is common, so as to require catheterism—an operation which should be, if possible, performed by a female attendant.

But it is in cases where the nervous symptoms which properly belong to fever are preceded by a well marked hysterical state that head symptoms of a severe kind may be anticipated. In one of the most severe cases of typhus fever with cerebral symptoms that I have seen, the patient, a middle-aged man, of excellent physical development and the most splendid intellectual attainments, exhibited perfectly formed hysterical symptoms for thirty-six hours after sickening of fever. Symptoms of violent head-affection then set in, which were treated by local depletion. The case terminated favourably.

PART II.

TREATMENT OF FEVER.

LECTURE XXV.

INTRODUCTORY REMARKS—Principles on which the treatment of fever is to be based—True meaning of the word *empiric*. Historical retrospect—The Symptomological, the Anatomical, the Rational or Eclectic Schools—*Essence* of fever cannot be determined by pathological anatomy—*Etiology* of fever is indefinite.

BEFORE entering on the treatment of fever it may be well to consider the principles on which it is to be based, and which the best physicians from the earliest times have followed. Though the application of these principles has varied according to the prevalence of this or that theory of disease, still, when we look at the recorded experience of practical men, we shall find that there has been in the main an agreement as to questions of prognosis and of treatment. Notwithstanding all that has been done in the morbid anatomy of fever, including the results of the microscope and of chemical research, I believe that our predecessors were, as a rule, as good physicians in fever as we are ourselves. Indeed, it may be held that in the highest quality of the medical mind, the almost intuitive perception of what is right to do under existing circumstances, they were—notwithstanding all our boasted advance in pathology—our equals, if not our superiors. The older British physicians—Sydenham, Haygarth, Heberden, Fordyce, and Fothergill in England; Gregory, Cullen, and Alison in Scotland; and Harvey, Cheyne, and Graves in Ireland—were all great physicians, whose practice was based on a study of the history and symptoms rather than the organic changes. These true lights of medicine were eclectics, and so were not wedded to any exclusive doctrine or practice. As I have said before, they were more symptomatologists than morbid anatomists—that is, their practice was founded rather on the general vital conditions than on the supposed state of any particular system. They looked on a case of fever as a whole, and dealt with it as a whole. They did not, like Paracelsus, advise their followers to burn the writings of Hippocrates, Galen, and Avicenna; or, like Broussais and some more modern professors, impugn the morality or the intellectual powers of the great men who preceded them.

The class of physicians to which I allude did not assume any distinguishing name. They were all imbued with the modesty of science, and did not affect to be the apostles of any new doctrine. They were, however, agreed on some great points, of which that of essentiality of disease was the chief one. This view of fever is well expressed by Fordyce, whom I have long since quoted in speaking of fever. "Fever," he says, "is a disease which affects the whole system; it affects the head, trunk, and extremities; it affects the circulation, absorption, and the nervous system; it affects the body and it affects the mind: it is therefore a disease of the whole system in the fullest sense of the term. It does not, however, affect the various parts of the system uniformly and equally, but, on the contrary, sometimes one part is more affected than another."

All the great observers whom I have enumerated believed—and acted on that belief—that our knowledge of the nature of fever is of a negative character, and though the earlier of them did not fully apprehend the history of the organic secondary lesions, yet it can be inferred from their writings and their practice that they looked on them less as the cause than the consequence of fever. To all intents and purposes, then, they recognized what we now call the secondary affections of fever, and met them as they arose, always keeping in view the previous and associated constitutional state so commonly marked by prostration of nervous energy. They recognized the laws of periodicity. In a word, their principles of management of fever were based on "observation rendered fruitful by study;" the recorded experience of the past was to them a light in the wilderness, not a matter to be ridiculed or sneered at; and so, though unassisted by the scalpel, the microscope, or chemical research, they worked out the true principles of treatment by studying the living rather than the dead. Their treatment has been called *empiricism*, as if this term was necessarily one of reproach.

I address myself now to the junior members of this class. I wish to impress upon them that those who so use the term display ignorance alike of its meaning and of its derivation. The class of men of whom I speak practised empirically—that is, they *practised from observation and experience.* Their empiricism was an enlightened empiricism, based on a just appreciation of facts as regards the living, rather than of those concerning either *post-mortem* changes or therapeutic influences. In truth, the term empiric has been applied to one who is truly not an empiric—to one who, ignorant of the natural history

of disease and of the influence of his so-called remedies on the health
or life of his patient, practises recklessly and for his own profit, not for
the benefit of the sick. To such a class the old-fashioned word "quack"
applies, rather than that of "empiric." You may ask me: Are we all
to be empirics? I answer: Yes, in the true sense of the word, for the
benefit of our patients, not ignorantly or for our own advantage. The
great men whose names I have mentioned were empirics of this kind.
They had learned from long experience that the adoption of certain
modes of treatment, differing according to circumstances, would be
attended with beneficial results, although even the most gifted of them
could not tell why it was that such effects were produced.

All they professed to know was that such was the fact, and the line
of treatment was adopted simply because it was proved to be useful.
This was pure empiricism; but who will refuse to say that the practice
of it was not only justifiable but commendable? In fact, in the
present state of medical knowledge we must all be more or less
empirical in our practice. The gentleman who has the case of dumb
ague under his charge in the wards prescribed cinchona, and therefore
is an empiric; for he cannot explain, any more than I can myself,
why the remedy is useful in such cases. He knows only that cinchona exerts a specific remedial effect on the disease, and so he employs
it empirically, yet conscientiously and wisely.

The symptomological school of physicians in their treatment of
fever invariably looked to the general condition of the patient first,
and afterwards to the state of his local organs. And so these men,
acting mainly by the light of their own genius, sagacity, and experience, adopted the same principles of treatment which we advocate
here, and which are now endorsed by the best men in Europe, aided
as they are by all the appliances of modern science. These old physicians, to use the impressive words of Dr. Graves, "fed fever" liberally,
yet judiciously, with nutriment, with wine, with tonics, and with diffusible stimulants.

We now come to a school of practitioners who adopted a diametrically opposite plan of treatment in fever, who looked less to the patient's general condition and more to the secondary and local affections
of the disease under which he was suffering. They discovered, or
thought they discovered, *cerebritis, gastritis, hepatitis, pneumonia,* and
so on, according as symptoms arose indicative of engagement of the
brain, the intestinal or the respiratory system; and they asserted
that those physicians who dared to treat such symptoms of local inflammation by the administration of food, wine, and bark were nothing
short of privileged assassins, to be denounced as legalized murderers.

Shortly after my election to this hospital, at a time when the fever wards were under the charge of Dr. Graves, a gentleman fresh from the schools of Paris, an ardent believer in the so-called physiological doctrines of Broussais, called on me to say that he could no longer continue to attend in the fever wards. I asked his reasons for this determination. He said, "I cannot longer witness such wholesale murder. I every day see Dr. Graves, in manifest cases of *gastro entérite*, administering wine, brandy, and nutritive food, when the tongue is red and all the symptoms of enteric inflammation are present." "But," I said, "when you speak of 'wholesale murder' have you seen any cases in which this practice had fatal results?" "No," he replied; "that's the extraordinary thing; but I suppose your Irish constitutions are peculiar. Yet I cannot bear to see it any more; I must go away." And so this fettered *doctrinaire* lost the clinical teaching of the "great Dublin practitioner," as Graves was called by Trousseau many years later.

This second school of physicians we may fairly designate "The Anatomical School," who denied essentialism and mistook the effect for the cause, and whose simple treatment was starvation and local depletion. I may here observe that the practitioners of this class used to style themselves "The Physiological School," but their *physiology* was very bad indeed. They based their theory and practice in fever on morbid anatomy rather than on pathology. They sought to explain all the symptoms of the disease, local and general, by referring them to the sympathies of a part of the digestive system when under inflammation; while they failed to recognize that this inflammation was not the first link in the chain of morbid phenomena, but was reactive and secondary in its nature.

We now come to the Rational School, though its disciples have not assumed any such distinctive name. It might be termed "The Pathological School," for pathology signifies only the physiology of disease. It is this school, shadowed out by the old English writers, still more developed by John Peter Frank, its views and doctrines long taught by Graves, which has been now followed by most right-thinking men at home and abroad. It is in this school that so many of our countrymen have been educated, who in various parts of the world have so nobly upheld the repute of British and Irish medicine. It may be termed "The Eclectic School," for it adopts whatever is true in the teaching of the past, and rejects whatever is mischievous, erroneous, and bad. It admits the essentiality of fever—that strange but general condition which—it cannot be too often repeated—differs from any other condition of the living body, varying in form, in intensity,

duration, and secondary complications, subject to the laws of periodicity, and in which the rules of diagnosis of local diseases applicable
in other cases must be modified.

Now, if we inquire to which of the preceding schools, the symptomological or the anatomical, the present rational or eclectic system
more nearly approaches, you will find that it is far more closely
related to the first than to the second. In the present healthier state
of medical opinion, the general condition of the patient in fever is
looked on as of more importance than the local affections. *"The whole
is more than the part"* is the golden principle to be recognized in the
treatment of all essential diseases. You are not to adopt any exclusive theory from the condition of one part, and you are never to permit the occurrence of a local affection to sway you overmuch in your
management of the general disease, if from your knowledge of the epidemic character and the actual condition of the patient, you determine that a decisive mode of treatment is necessary—for example, the
use of food and stimulants. You are not to be stopped from giving
them because some local affection might seem to prohibit their use,
for I believe in ninety-nine out of a hundred cases you may override
this seeming objection with safety and advantage.

The anatomical school, as I have shown you, fell into the great error
of regarding the local diseases in fever not only as primary but as
necessary affections. You are to hold a diametrically opposite
opinion; it is in the higher knowledge of the laws affecting the local
diseases in fever—its consequence, not its cause—that the rational
and eclectic school has its chief merit. We of that school know well
that, although these local diseases are so common that their occurrence is the rule rather than the exception, yet they vary according
to many circumstances. Some of these are utterly unknown to us,
while of those the existence of which seems probable—such as climate
and epidemic influence—the *modus operandi* is hidden from us.

I have shown you that the so-called anatomical or physiological
school explained the various symptoms in fever on the principle of
organic sympathies, but they cannot be thus accounted for. Fever
may exist without the presence of any notable anatomical change. A
single case of this kind would overturn the entire theory, and I believe
that the more you see of fever the more readily will you admit,
especially in typhus, that the severity and the mortality of the disease
are directly in proportion to the toxic effect of the poison and the
freedom from anatomical change.

I have brought before you examples of the cessation of fever coincident with structural change. The general principle which comes

into view on looking at the most wide-spread epidemic affections is, that their victims do not die of local organic disease; or, to put it in other words, that the destructiveness of these affections is in the inverse ratio to the amount of anatomical change produced by them. If this be so, it furnishes a crushing argument against the anatomical theory of fever, and recommends to our minds the paramount importance of considering the vital rather than the organic state.

One more important consideration I beg to recommend to you. The anatomical school held that between the local affections in fever and idiopathic inflammation there was no difference, but we hold fast to the opinion that, though similar in physical signs and in anatomical character—at least to a great degree—to primary disease, they are widely distinct in their vital characters. Although to the eye, even when armed by the microscope, the character of these secondary changes may be precisely similar to those of idiopathic lesions, yet similarity of physical aspect by no means implies identity of vital character. Consider two cases of iritis apparently the same: you have an opportunity of examining the structures after death; will you then find an anatomical difference between the two? Or if you do, will this explain the fact that in one case simple antiphlogistic measures would suffice to subdue the disease, while in the others a specific treatment is necessary?

Gentlemen, you will perceive the vast importance of recognizing the vital characters which are extended to the products of disease, and this applies to all physiology.

In Goethe's drama of Faust the Devil possesses himself of the professor's gown, and sitting in his chair is consulted by some of the students as to their objects of study. He decries anatomy as a means for clearing up the problem of life. I have often thought that the words of the great German poet and philosopher, which I have previously quoted, are strangely applicable to the question of the vital character of disease, which is something varied, although hidden, not to be seen, measured, weighed, or analyzed.

Before passing now to speak of the treatment of fever in detail, I would remind you that we cannot by pathological anatomy determine the essence of fever. We may even go further and say that no *post-mortem* or *ante-mortem* investigation has discovered what is its cause, why this condition presents itself in so many forms—some of them sufficiently distinct and, as it were, concrete, others more or less indefinable—one form passing into another, varying at different times in history, apparent exciting cause, epidemic character, degree of contagiousness, mortality, and the amount and nature of the secondary changes. It may be that destitution has been often attended with relapsing fever, that decomposing human exuviæ may induce typhoid or enteric fever, that typhus springs from overcrowding; yet I would exhort you to avoid all exclusive doctrines as to fever, whether you deal with its exciting causes, its classification, its pathology, or its results.

As far as we can judge, the relation between the particular form of fever and its apparent exciting cause is by no means constant. Destitution is followed by every form of fever. The presumed exciting causes of typhoid—such as impure water, defective drainage, putrid emanations—will be followed by typhus in one case and by typhoid in another. While saying this, I believe it to be sufficiently made out that typhus is more immediately connected with overcrowding than typhoid, and that the latter form of fever is more related to the defective sanitary conditions I have just specified. But all this has little to do with treatment, the great principles of which are constant, while their application varies in the individual case or in the special epidemic.

LECTURE XXVI.

No specific line of treatment—Respect to be had (1) to the essential disease, (2) to its local and secondary effects—Failure of specifics in early stage of fevers—Want of success in the endeavour to found a science of therapeutics on experimental physiology or pathology—Effects of the action of the law of periodicity wrongly attributed to the adoption of therapeutical measures—Sustenance by *food* and *stimulants*—Two sources of danger to the fever patient; (1) primary effects of the fever poison in causing depression, (2) supervention of secondary local disease—Views of Dr. Graves on the subject of giving food in fever.

IN our study of the treatment of fever we shall best consider the question first in regard to the essential element of the disease, and next in reference to its local and secondary effects. You will meet with a certain number of cases in which your attention will be compelled more especially to the constitutional state, and this throughout the whole course of the malady; while even in the most prominent local complications you are not, in your treatment and prognosis, to overlook the essential condition. Let us apply ourselves to the first of these questions.

Is fever, independent of local complications, a condition which can be cut short, or can its duration be materially abridged? In other words, is there any known specific treatment for any kind of continued fever?—has any means been discovered of cutting the process of fever short, or of anticipating the time when, by the law of periodicity, the peculiar condition of organic life which we call fever will cease, and the system be again governed by its natural laws?

Now, I believe that no direct or specific treatment which would have these effects has been as yet discovered. When I was a younger man, some idea that a fever might be cut short, particularly if it were dealt with in its earlier periods, influenced most, or at least many, practitioners. Each physician had, according to the teaching he had received or to the theories he had formed—less from experience than from *à priori* reasoning—his own favourite and routine method of proceeding. Some employed emetics to effect the object in view; others, diaphoretics; many used purgation, blood-letting, or even the exhibition of mercury, while each appealed to examples of recovery after such proceedings in justification of them.

I believe that all these courses of proceeding were not only futile, but harmful—futile in this, that they did not arrest the fever, and harmful because their effect too often was, in ordinary words, *to spoil the case:* that is to say, to interfere with the pathological laws which govern disease as physiological laws govern health. Among these laws that of periodicity is chiefly to be mentioned. There were other bad effects. Copious sweating or venesection produced debility. Purgatives predisposed, as we have seen, to dangerous disease of the digestive tube, while the use of mercury, especially in rheumatic fever, clearly increased the cachectic and anæmic condition in convalescence. Some of the worst cases of recovery from rheumatic fever which I witnessed were those in which the system had been saturated with mercury in the early stages of the disease.

The error involved in the adoption of any of these practices was that of not recognizing the natural history of fever. These men acted vigorously in the first period of the disease, and thereby commonly tended to exhaust the system, not knowing what the duration of the case might be, when all the powers of nature would be called on to induce a favourable result. You, gentlemen, have not had an opportunity of becoming practically acquainted with what I am about to tell you. It often happened that, after the employment of some of these measures, a remarkable lull in the symptoms followed; the febrile state was greatly ameliorated and sometimes almost disappeared, the patient expressed relief, and everything seemed to justify the course which had been adopted. But the "snake was scotched, not killed," and in a short time the disease showed itself again, running its course unaffected—except for evil—by what had been done.

I have spoken of rheumatic fever. See the number of specifics that have been proposed for its treatment—mercury, opium, bark, iron, alkalies, acids, and so on. I will say nothing of the system of Bouillaud—the bleeding *coup sur coup.* The very number and variety of the so-called specifics for the disease leads to a conviction of their little value as remedies. But it would be well were their effects only negative, for experience shows that they are too often injurious by their interference with the ordinary and normal laws of the disease. As I have just said, rheumatic fever was commonly treated by mercurialization, with the result that convalescence was in almost every case protracted and uncertain.

In truth, gentlemen, that part of medicine which involves therapeutics has always been—and we may say, is still—in the most unsatisfactory condition. There is no part of medical science in which the principles of right reasoning have been so largely and so continuously neglected or outraged; and though in our own time experimental physiology or pathology has been had recourse to as a basis for a rational therapeutical science, yet how very far are we from any satisfactory conclusion on the matter? This is to be accounted for from various reasons. Experiments have been made on animals, and the results have been held to apply to man, not only in his normal but in his diseased condition. For example, to determine whether a mercurial is ever efficacious in bilious derangement, calomel is given to a dog, in whose gall-bladder an open fistula has been made; and the question of its fitness in *man, when in disease,* is tested by the quantity of bile which flows from a canula in the gall-bladder of *a healthy dog.*

But it is in relation to our immediate subject, and especially to the periodicity of disease, that the most fruitful source of error in modern therapeutics exists. The essential disease, as well as its secondary effect, is subject to periodic law. Both spontaneously subside, and when that subsidence follows on the exhibition of this or that remedy, a therapeutic fact is held to be discovered. Yet this subsidence may be in no way connected with the effect of the remedy. It probably would have occurred without it; it may have been delayed or otherwise interfered with by the action of the medicine itself; nay, further, the subsidence of the essential or of the local part of the disease will occur even after the use of many and different remedies. The false reasoning which has been held to apply to one applies equally to all, and so the therapeutic experiments lead to erroneous conclusions.

I have shown you that the study of the diseased or healthy organism reveals more of the effects than of the essence of disease. Hence you must be cautious in adopting any therapeutical system based

upon visible organic change. In the study of therapeutics we should
depend principally upon experiment and induction in disease as observed in man.   Professor Acland has observed that if but a few well-
instructed men were to take up any one remedy, and continue to
record the character and history of the case, and the results of the
particular agent, making as it were their hospitals medical observa-
tories, we should in time have such a mass of facts— the results of unbiassed observation—as would enable us to draw safe conclusions.

The therapeutist of the present day has great advantages over his
predecessors, particularly in the assistance which is now given by
chemical and microscopical research.   But he must also possess assistance of other kinds.   He must know the principles of accurate
reasoning, he must deal with vital phenomena, of which our knowledge is so deficient that we have to study their modifications experimentally, as yet without any direct reference to structure or to vital
chemistry.

The laws of periodic action must be considered, and—as he pro-
ceeds—he must inquire whether the simplest local, as well as the
most complex general, affection is not more or less subject to some of
these wonderful laws.   He must study the question how far medical
interference is capable of extinguishing morbid action, of merely post-
poning it, or, lastly, of deranging a process which was to end in its
removal.   He must well understand how certainty in medicine is to
be approached only by the balance of probabilities, and he must be
thoroughly acquainted with the difficulties which are involved in those
medical statistics which result from the labours of more than one
observer.   Other circumstances will suggest themselves—such as
locality, race, habit, age, sex, and previous history.

In dealing with the treatment of fever, and looking upon the disease
in its aspect of essentiality—that is, as a condition independent of
local disease and capable, after a period, of spontaneous disappearance—the question of the use of sustenance by food or stimulants
should first engage our attention.

We have seen that there are two prominent sources of danger to
the patient in fever—one, exhaustion from the direct influence of the
fever poison in depressing the vital energy ; and the other, the frequent
development of local disease.   But we are never to forget that when
fever assumes the typoid form its duration is very uncertain.   It may
last from three to six weeks, so that if the sustenance of the patient
be not attended to he may sink from inanition.   On this point you
should read Dr. Graves' ninth lecture, in which he teaches how to feed
a patient in fever.   I remember once, when he and I were going

through the convalescent wards, he expatiated on the healthy appearance of the patients, many of whom had gone through long fevers. "This is all owing to our good feeding," he said. "Will you, when the time comes, write my epitaph, and let it be—'He fed fevers'?"

Now, this expression of one who was the representative man in medicine in Ireland has been carped at by some of those whose criticism means only fault-finding—a wide-spread class like the critic in Goldsmith's *Citizen of the World.* "The work might have been better if the artist had taken more pains." It has been supposed that Graves advocated high feeding in fever indiscriminately, but you know too much to believe this. He speaks of the danger of the starving system, and shows how the practice arose from the doctrines of those who taught that fever was only symptomatic of inflammation. He shows the effect of abstinence in producing symptoms similar to those of the worst fevers, as exemplified in the wreck of the "Alceste" and of the "Medusa." "You may," he says, "think that it is unnecessary to give food, as the patient appears to have no appetite and does not care for it. You might as well think of allowing the urine to accumulate in the bladder, because the patient feels no desire to pass it. You are called on to interfere, where the sensibility is impaired, and the natural appetite is dormant; and you are not to permit your patient to encounter the horrible consequences of inanition, because he does not ask for nutriment. I never do so. After the third or fourth day of fever, I always prescribe mild nourishment, and this is steadily and perseveringly continued through the whole course of the disease."

He continues: "An attentive consideration of the foregoing arguments has led me, in the treatment of long fevers, to adopt the advice of a country physician of great shrewdness, who advised me never to let my patients die of starvation. If I have more success than others in the treatment of fever, I think it is owing in a great degree to the adoption of this advice. I must, however, observe that great discrimination is required in the choice of food. Although you will not let your patient starve, do not fall into the opposite extreme: you must take care not to overload the stomach. When this is done, gastro-enteric irritation, tympanites, inflammation and exasperated febrile action are the consequences. I have witnessed many instances of the danger of repletion in febrile diseases. A case of this kind occurred some time ago in this hospital, in a boy who was recovering from peritonitis. In another case, in private practice, an incautious indulgence in the use of animal food was followed by a fatal result. A young lady ate some beefsteak, contrary to my orders, at an early period of convalescence from fever, relapsed almost immediately, and died of enteritis in thirty-six hours."

He then speaks of the care and judgment which are necessary in giving food, particularly in the beginning of fever. He recommends well-boiled gruel made of groats and flavoured with sugar, thin panado, and, as the fever advances, speaks of good and well-made chicken broth as one of the best of nutriments—to be employed, however, at first experimentally. He advises that "all kinds of food and nutriment should be given by day, and the patient should, if possible, be restricted to the use of fluids by night. The natural habit is to take food by day and not by night, and in sickness as well as in health we should observe the diurnal revolution of the economy." Again, the usual period of meals should be observed, and the space of time for giving chicken broth, jelly, arrowroot, and other mild articles of diet should be from eight o'clock in the morning to eight in the evening.

With respect to drinks, he considers that the patients are generally allowed to drink too much. "It may be urged that they have a strong desire for fluids; but they should not be gratified in everything they wish for. The continued swilling of even the most innocent fluids will bring on heaviness of stomach, nausea, pain, and flatulence, and predisposes to congestion and intestinal irritation." Further on he says: "You should never allow them to take a large quantity of fluid at a time; you should impress upon them the danger attendant on such a practice, and tell them that a spoonful or two, swallowed slowly, allays thirst more effectually than drinking a pint at a time." Again: "The abuse of ordinary drinks—as common water, whey, barley water, soda and seltzer waters, and effervescing draughts—is a frequent source of tympanitic swelling in fever."

I have now shown you that Dr. Graves was no advocate for the indiscriminate and too liberal employment of food in fever, and that he was fully alive to the dangers both of the want and the excess of food even in convalescence.

In addition to the prejudices with which the inflammatory doctrine imbued so many minds, with respect to the use of food in fever, a new set of arguments was raised against it, in consequence of the experiments of an American physician. I allude to the case observed by Dr. Beaumont, and so often quoted since. In this remarkable case various medicinal substances and articles of food were introduced through an external fistula into the stomach; their effects were noted, and also the conditions of temperature, vascularity, etc. The results were subsequently published in connection with the action of the stomach upon food. One of the results stated to have been thus obtained was, that the existence of the state of fever altogether suspended the process of digestion. Here was a statement which had the appearance of being founded upon strict observation. It influenced a number of young men; but did it influence those who had once been in charge of a fever hospital? Not at all; because such men knew well that, no matter what Beaumont might say about the stomach not digesting when the patient had fever, in thousands of cases patients in fever digested remarkably well, required food, and derived benefit from it. In a large number of cases of typhus fever the stomach has an excellent power of digestion; and, I believe, if we were bold enough, we should find that many articles of food usually forbidden to fever patients might be given to them with safety.

A remarkable incident was related to me which shows that the stomach in fever is capable of digesting even a rather coarse article of food. A lady who had been recently married was attacked with extremely severe petechial fever; she was covered with dark-coloured maculæ, and disease had run to about the twelfth or thirteenth day. She was attended by several eminent physicians. Her case was an extremely bad one, and her life was all but despaired of. She was violently delirious. Her husband, himself a physician, had occasion to leave the house on some business. At the period of the dinner hour of the family the servants were cooking a rump of beef and cabbage, and the odour of it filled the house. In her delirium the patient called for some of the dish. Her sister, who was attending her, believing she was dying, determined to indulge her, from the feeling that it was right to accede to the request of a dying person. She proceeded to the kitchen, and, as soon as the beef was boiled, brought up a very large mess, smoking hot, to the lady's bedside, when she devoured it with great avidity. Shortly afterwards her husband came in, and was told what had happened. He became terrified, and sent for physicians in every direction. Four or five assembled; time was pressing, and all agreed that something should be at once done.

Each of these physicians had his own suggestion to offer—one recommended an immediate emetic; another, a drastic purgative; a third, a purgative injection; a fourth, a large dose of calomel; a fifth, a powerful blister. At length the late Dr. Harvey, then Physician-General and a man of the greatest practical knowledge in medicine, joined the consultation, all members of which except himself were in a state of intense excitement. At the time the stomach pump was not in fashion, but every one agreed that some great effort should be made to get the corned beef and cabbage out of the lady's stomach. Dr. Harvey was entreated to go upstairs immediately to see the patient, who was declared to be in coma. His first observation was characteristic of the man. "Some of you," he said, "help me off with my coat." He proceeded leisurely to the bedside, where he remained for some minutes, which appeared to the anxious consultants below an inordinate period of time. He came downstairs slowly, and on entering the room was again surrounded, all of them declaring their willingness to forego their individual opinions and to abide by his decision, for not a moment further was to be lost.

He was quite unmoved by the situation, and simply said, " By ——, *I'd* let her sleep it out !" and took his departure. She did sleep it out, and in the course of some hours awoke much better. Her recovery was perfect.

Now, I do not tell you this anecdote to induce you to feed your patients with salt beef and cabbage in fever, but it is very important as showing that in the advanced stage of a maculated typhus fever the stomach is capable of digesting such an article of food as salt beef, and that it proved in the particular case innocuous. Dr. Harvey was too good a physician not to understand the evils of the *nimia diligentia medicorum* in fever, and the result showed the value of his practical knowledge. The supposed coma was natural sleep—a most favourable circumstance, and he knew his art too well not to decry any interference with it.

There can be little doubt that in many cases of advanced fever a greater latitude in the use of food might be adopted with advantage. But you must remember that, in the lower ranks of life, the power of the stomach to deal with a variety of food becomes less and less. Ordinary nourishment commonly answers well where greater delicacies would be rejected or would disagree.

LECTURE XXVII.

STIMULANTS IN FEVER—Views as to the nutrient properties of stimulants are to be received with caution—*Anticipative* use of stimulants—Meaning of the term—Considerations to be taken into account in resolving upon this method of treatment: (1) prevailing epidemic character of the disease, (2) previous condition of the patient ("Sinking of vital power"—Illustrative case—Stimulation often unsuccessful in the intemperate, and in those whose brains are overworked), (3) development of symptoms of severe typhus, (4) development of *fever odour*—Contrast between typhus and typhoid as regards period at which stimulation is called for—*Condition of the heart, a guide*—Physical signs of cardiac weakening.

FOLLOWING the consideration of food in fever we shall next take up that of diffusible stimulants. Their employment we have had together a full opportunity of studying, and those of you who are practising pupils have learned to prove their value and importance in every form of fever. You have learned also to avoid routinism, and you well know that when we speak of every form of fever we do not mean every case of the disease. We have had cases in which no wine was used, in which it was sparingly employed, where it was not used until after the middle period of the fever. In many cases, too, you had to use it and other stimulants with great boldness and for many days, beginning at an early stage of the disease. Again, wine had sometimes to be omitted, though the disease still was running on ; and, lastly, its exhibition or its withdrawal had to be alternated several times in the course of the disease.

Many of you have also learned that in fever the common error of delaying the giving of stimulants to a very late period of the case is a practice fraught with mischief, attributable to the prevalence of the doctrine that fever and all its local symptoms were induced by inflammation. By this system all the good of the anticipative use of stimulants is lost.

Any unbiassed observer of fever will admit that between the condition of vital prostration and what is termed "waste of animal tissue" there is no constant relation. We cannot deny the occurrence of metamorphosis of tissue and waste of organic substance as incidental to fever; on the contrary, we believe that these phenomena are remarkably perceptible. But we must also hold that there is a prostration of vital energy—a thing *per se*, which is totally unconnected with loss of organic substance. Do not for a moment forget this—that the

13

forms of disease in which we find the greatest prostration of vital power are those wherein we discover least signs of organic mischief. A striking example of this is found in cholera, and in the various forms of continued fever.

Now, I must tell you that the views of my lamented friend Dr. Todd are to be received with caution. One thing is certain—that whether we look on wine and brandy as food or simply as stimulants, the great point is to know when and how to administer them beneficially. We have not indeed attempted to decide the question experimentally as to whether stimulants act as food by repairing the wasted tissues, for in all our cases food and stimulants were given together—our object being rather to save life than to settle an abstract physiological question; and many of you had cases of weakened heart in fever where the influence of stimulants was too rapid to be accounted for except on the principle of a direct action on the nervous system.

It is true that we have seen life prolonged for several weeks by stimulants alone. Some years ago a patient in one of the small wards had long used a fabulous amount of spirits. He lived on brandy or whiskey for a month, during which time he swallowed nothing else, and cost the hospital a good deal more than his life was probably worth.

If Dr. Todd's views were to be carried out in every case of disease, essential or otherwise; if, in short, we were to administer stimulants on the *routine* principle—regarding them as nutrient substances, calculated to supply the waste of animal tissue, and as it were rebuilding the organic structure, we should find ourselves lamentably disappointed. The adoption of such a system found very few supporters among experienced physicians.

But let us do justice to Dr. Todd's memory. As practical men, in the present state of our knowledge, we have little to do with questions of physiology, and to him belongs the merit of showing that the use of alcohol may be resorted to or at least borne in states of disease where it was held to be dangerous. He has still further shown the error of the anatomical school, which referred everything in acute disease to inflammation; and though he may have fallen into a routine practice, we should be slow in holding him answerable for the errors of some of his followers.

Even in many essential diseases you will find that stimulants are contra-indicated or badly borne. I do not say that in such, an opposite mode of treatment will succeed, but there are many cases of essential disease—of puerperal fever, pyæmia, malignant scarlatina, small-pox, and others—in which, though the vital strength is fearfully prostrated, for some reason which we cannot explain stimulants are too often powerless for good. There can be no doubt that the efficacy of stimulation is closely connected with the prevailing epidemic character of disease, and thus it was observed in our late visitation of small-pox that wine and brandy were often productive of good effects. But still the proposition is true that stimulants in the class of diseases I have mentioned are not followed by the same happy and almost heroic effects which we so often witness in typhus fever.

We may dwell upon the question of the use of stimulants in fever as regards, first, the anticipative treatment, and next the treatment urgently called for by the circumstances of the case. By the term *anticipative treatment* you are to understand the administration of stim-ulants at an early stage of fever, when, although there may be no very pressing vital symptoms calling for their use, the sagacity of the physician enables him to foretell the occurrence of great prostra-tion of vital energy. Under such circumstances he gives stimulants *by anticipation.*

In comparing the relative value of these two modes of proceeding, I am of opinion that the anticipative method is that which will tend most to the saving of human life. In adopting this line of practice the physician does not wait until the patient has been labouring for many days under the exhausting influence of the disease. He does not withhold the needful aid until the 10th or 12th day, when the prostration of vital energy has assumed a formidable aspect, when the prompt use of stimulants is suggested by common sense, and when often, unfortunately, the system is incapable of responding to the remedy. For you will learn that where the powers of life have re-mained long without support, a downward process may commence from which no effort can rescue the sufferer.

In the anticipative treatment we follow the old maxim, "venienti occurrite morbo," and he who knows when to adopt it has gained a high place in practical medicine.

In determining on the employment or the contrary of the anticipa-tive treatment, the following considerations must be present to you

First, the epidemic character or habit of the disease; secondly, the previous condition of the patient.

What we have to guard against is a sudden sinking of the vital energy, shown by special conditions of the nervous and the circula-tory systems. I have told you, that, with respect to these and the other systems in fever where the strength has been unsupported, the down-ward tendency goes on until a point is reached from which there is no revival. In these cases there is between the heart and the nervous centres a great sympathy, and the condition of the one—which is revealed by manifest physical signs, and with which you are all now familiar—gives you a clear conception of the state of the brain and the spinal marrow.

This failure of the heart, like the other secondary affections, is under the law of periodicity, yet I believe it may occur in chronic cases, but with this difference—that having become established it continues until the end. A gentleman of energetic and industrious habits, who lived well and took his bottle of wine daily, and who never showed any disease of the heart, became subject to attacks of ordinary gout. He was persuaded to undergo a protracted course of hydropathy, during which the candle was burned at both ends, for no wine or stimulant was allowed for more than a month. His condition was remarkable; he had no pains, no fever, the pulse was about sixty, weak but regular, and when asked to describe his symptoms he said, "I have no complaint to make, but of a strange weakness of body and mind which is quite new to me." He lived for several weeks, the failure of the heart increasing every day, while no amount of stimulation had any effect in restoring its vigour, and he died without any ascertainable cause beyond mere nervous exhaustion. The process of death was peculiarly slow.

This sinking of the vital power, not accounted for by any apparent loss of organic tissue, takes place in fever, and it is with a view of arresting its progress that we have recourse to the anticipative treatment. But there are various grounds for adopting this line of conduct; for example, if you know that in the epidemic, a great number of cases assume well-marked symptoms of prostration, say on the seventh, eighth, or ninth day, you will on the fourth or fifth anticipate their occurrence by commencing the use of stimulants. Even in the middle of the course of a fever case, or at any period of its progress, you will do right to guard against the occurrence of sudden prostration, which, when once it has set in, especially in mature age, may resist the most active stimulation.

But there are collateral circumstances to which you must look—such as the previous history of your patient, his habits of life, his previous health, in short, whether he brings into this contest with a formidable disease a constitution affected by previous illness, bad habits, or nervous exhaustion. You will also ascertain whether any ignorant attempts to cut short the fever had been made; the patient may have been bled for supposed inflammation, he may have had cathartics, mercury, tartar emetic, or powerful diaphoretics. In such cases you have solid reasons for adopting the anticipative method, though the patient may not as yet have fallen into a state of prostration.

The full administration of stimulants is generally called for when the patient has passed the age of eighteen or twenty. In children we are obliged to have recourse to stimulants, but we employ them in a modified manner; their energetic use is indicated principally in adults between the age of twenty-five and forty-five, and here we employ them at an early period, not so much to combat existing prostration, but to anticipate the depression of vital power which sooner or latter is almost certain to ensue.

In estimating the chances that the employment of stimulants will be followed by success, much will depend on the previous habits of the patient. We have long found that the greatest triumphs of the stimulating treatment were seen in patients of strictly temperate habits, who seem more capable in fever of bearing large quantities of stimulants without intoxication. In private practice we often find that stimulation cannot be carried on so boldly as in hospital; and this appears to be connected with the previous habits of the patient, not in the way of intemperance in the use of wine, but in that of over exercise of the brain. Men engaged in anxious callings, or in intense mental exertion, are bad subjects in fever, and bear the stimulating treatment imperfectly. Thus it is that professional men so frequently succumb—witness the frightful mortality among the medical men of Ireland in the famine fever. In many such cases, with symptoms of profound adynamia, stimulants are badly borne, and hence—when the disease, as too often happens, is of a malignant character—the patient makes but a poor fight, and adds to the list of victims who have fallen in the discharge of their duty.

For the first few days your patient may make little complaint. There are often remissions in which he declares himself much better; but if the symptoms of essential fever are gradually developing themselves, if petechial spots begin to appear, and particularly if the skin exhibits the dusky discoloration so characteristic of typhus, you may expect severity of symptoms. This discoloration appears, and after a time recedes, as the petechiæ come and vanish, and like them too is subject to the law of periodicity.

Another indication for the early exhibition of stimulants is the peculiar fever-odour sometimes present from a very early period. Benign fevers rarely are attended with this peculiar odour, which belongs to more malignant forms of disease.

You will observe that the symptoms I have particularized are more closely connected with typhus and with typhoid fever, and accordingly we find that early stimulation is much more frequently indicated in the former than in the latter; in other words, the free use of stimulants, when necessary, is called for at a later stage of the disease in typhoid than in typhus. It is right, however, for us to bear in mind that some of the cases requiring the most powerful stimulation have been of typhoid fever in its advanced and complicated condition.

It is in petechial typhus that the anticipative treatment is most frequently called for, and will be found to answer best. In typhoid fever the occurrence of prostration is commonly later observed, and is of more gradual development. As we have already seen, this form of fever is less manifestly under the law of periodicity than true typhus, and the character of its secondary affections is more variable.

Physicians have from the earliest times been in the habit of determining on the administration or withholding of stimulants in fever by the state of the pulse. But—at least in the early periods of fever—the pulse taken alone is not to be depended on. It may be, up to the fourth day, full, throbbing, and resisting, and this has often led to errors in practice of both commission and omission. I have shown you that even under these circumstances an examination of the heart may reveal the commencement of a change in the vital condition of that organ. It was this temporary excitement of the pulse that led to the practice of bleeding, and of employing other depleting measures, by which the vital power was expended at an early stage of the case, and the influence of the law of periodicity was interfered with.

This ephemeral state of arterial excitement led, on the other hand, to errors of omission. The apparently inflammatory condition caused apprehension—the existing state was alone attended to, and the probable future in the case disregarded. You will not fall into these errors. The secondary debility of the heart may have commenced at a time when this pseudo-inflammatory state still existed, while in fact the pulse continued full and bounding, and the temperature high.

Take this rule with you into practice—that in the treatment of fever, and at almost any period of fever, you are not to be guided by the pulse alone. It must be observed in relation to the action of the heart—remembering that a full and good pulse may coincide with a feebly acting heart—a heart under the influence of the fever poison, often as it were on its way to the state of softening. All this you see bears on the question of the anticipative treatment.

Now among the most reliable indications for the early use of this treatment are the physical signs of weakness of the heart.

A man, aged 30, was admitted on the sixth day of typhus fever.

He was the fifth of his family who within a short time had severe maculated typhus. The impulse of the heart was scarcely perceptible, and there was already a distinct preponderance of the second sound. On the next day the impulse was imperceptible, even when he lay on the left side. He was ordered twenty ounces of wine, a blister over the heart, and beef-tea. The following day the impulse could be felt, but the sounds resembled those of a fœtal heart. The wine was increased, and two glasses of brandy were also administered. On the 12th day the pulse had fallen to 80, and the sounds of the heart were greatly improved ; on the 13th day the impulse of the heart was restored, its sounds were proportionate, and the pulse had fallen to 76. The diminution of the first sound of the heart led us to the exhibition of stimulants boldly, and at an early period of the case. On the 7th day the impulse was imperceptible, while on the 8th the first sound had disappeared ; and although the other symptoms did not seem to call for active stimulation, wine was ordered in free doses from this indication alone. The symptoms of cardiac debility were observed at so early a period as the sixth day, but it is probable that the typhous affection of the heart had commenced even before admission to hospital.

So far as the heart is concerned, the following are the physical signs which seem to indicate the anticipative use of stimulants. I have put them down in their chronological order :—

(1.) Early subsidence of the first sound, observed over the left ventricle.

(2.) Diminution of the first sound over the right ventricle.

(3.) The heart acting with a single, and that the second sound.

(4.) Both sounds being audible, but their relative intensity being changed so as to represent the action of the heart of a fœtus *in utero.*

(5.) With these signs, a progressive diminution of impulse, which occasionally becomes imperceptible, even when the patient lies on the left side.

During convalescence, as we have seen, the signs of recovery of the heart are usually observed first on the right side, and afterwards over the left side.

With reference to the anticipative treatment, we have spoken principally of the results of physical examination, as indicative of the typhous weakening of the heart in the early stages of fever. I have stated, that, although in the commencement of a typhoid fever any bold exhibition of stimulants is not often called for, yet in its advanced stages we have sometimes to make free use of stimulation.

I have observed that students were occasionally under a misapprehension about the doctrines which we have long held in this hospital with respect to the condition of the heart as a guide for the use of wine. They have come to the erroneous opinion that we are to give wine only when we find the want or diminution of the first sound of the heart, and that we are not to give wine where the heart is acting well. This is a mistaken view. As to the state of the heart in connection with the effect of stimulants, we have ascertained that the efficacy of stimulants is often directly as the debility of the organ. It has also been ascertained that the power of bearing stimulants, their effect upon the nervous system, their good effects on the general condition, are directly as the weakness of the heart.

We may lay down as a rule, that there are three conditions of the heart to be looked at by the practical man in the treatment of fever.

In one, we have an excited heart—a violently excited heart all through the case; and this, although the symptoms be those of extreme adynamia, although the surface be cold, the breath cold, and the pulse so feeble that it cannot be discovered. Nay, the heart may act with great force for several days, and yet there may be no pulse at the wrist. This is one case.

In the next case, we find an exactly opposite condition, in which the systolic force of the heart is diminished. This is shown by loss of impulse, by diminution—and, in certain cases, by extinction—of the first sound of the heart, while the second remains. This is a case which calls for wine, and in which you should give it; it is a case in which, in the vast majority of instances, wine will agree with the patient.

There is a third set of cases in which the heart does not seem to be implicated at all in the course of the disease—in which, notwithstanding the existence of the most extraordinary group of symptoms affecting various organs, the heart, in the middle of the storm, seems to be in a state of calm and quiet.

If we compare these three conditions with a view to prognosis, we may arrange them in this way. The excited heart all through, with feeble pulse and with adynamia, is unquestionably the worst. There is no worse symptom in fever than an excited heart. It is especially a bad symptom when, with that excitement, we find a feeble pulse. Next will be the case of sinking of the heart; and the most favourable condition is that in which, as I said before, the heart seems to escape disease.

You are not, however, to suppose that because you have an excited heart you are not to give wine; or that, because the heart is not affected at all, you are to withhold wine if in either case the general symptoms of the patient require it. You are not to found your exhibition of wine or other stimulants upon any one thing; you are to take the general state of the patient into consideration. What we have done is to discover an intelligible practical rule which will guide you in the use of wine in certain, I think in many, cases; but you are not to suppose that because a man has a clear first sound of the heart, therefore you are not to give him wine. You are not to suppose that because the heart is safe you can do without wine. Now, in a case recently under your observation, although the heart seemed to escape, or was at most only feeble through the course of the disease, frightful adynamia existed; day after day the patient's face was Hippocratic, or almost so; the general character of the disease was that of the most terrible putrescent fever—yet his heart escaped. And here is the result. We have given that man upwards of twenty bottles of wine and twenty-four ounces of brandy, and now, on the twenty-eighth or thirtieth day of the disease, we have the satisfaction of feeling that his case may be set down as among the triumphs of medicine.

I wish also strongly to impress on you the great importance of the use of other forms of nourishment in this disease; for we must not only keep up the nervous energy of the system by wine, but we must support nature by food. There is no greater mistake in fever than that of the withholding of food.

LECTURE XXVIII.

STIMULANTS IN FEVER, *continued*—Signs in connection with the heart of the agreement of stimulants: (1) return of impulse, (2) return of first sound, (3) gradual fall in the rate of the pulse—In cases of "fœtal heart" great boldness in stimulation is needed—No certain rules as to quantity of wine and whiskey or brandy required—Examples of free use of stimulants in malignant typhus—Case of Hardcastle (typhoid fever)—Eruption of vesicles as a secondary complication—Bed-sores.

WE are to-day to consider practically the use of stimulants in fever. This is a matter difficult to be taught orally. The exhibition and the management of stimulants in fever are among those points in practice which are best learned at the bedside, so that when I am addressing the advanced students—men who themselves have already largely shared in the responsibilities of the fever wards—I do so as a fellow-student on the one hand, and a brother practitioner on the other.

Many medical men who have received little beyond a surgical education, or who have not had a case of fever on their hands before they entered into practice, and who probably have never attended in the wards of a fever hospital, on their first meeting with the disease, are timid in the use of wine in fever, and have not learned that in this disease the symptoms of inflammation are commonly fallacious. This, as I have before said, is from the nature of their medical education. Here we see the wisdom of that regulation of the University of Dublin, in accordance with which all candidates for the degree of Bachelor of Medicine must show that they have personally attended at least five cases of fever before being admitted to examination.

As experience increases, men become less timid in the use of wine, and accordingly we find that those physicians who are sneeringly termed men of the old school, are often the best practitioners in fever; they have learned by experience in middle life what you have been taught in your student days, and they know, by their perception of the vital phenomena, when to give or not to give stimulants, when to increase, to diminish, or to omit them.

Now it is a great thing to possess a simple rule which will guide the practitioner who has had little or no experience in this matter, in the exhibition of wine—and I believe that in the observation of the physical signs of the heart, he will obtain such assistance. You will not suppose that I advise you to be guided solely by the state of the heart, but I say that in solving the question as to the use and the management of stimulants, you are to ascertain and consider in every case the condition of the organ *plus* the general symptoms and history.

We have already studied the anticipative use of wine. Let us suppose we have a case of maculated typhus, say on the sixth or eighth day—the pulse not very weak, and at 115 or 125 in the minute; you find that the impulse is not strong, or it may be absent, unless when the patient lies on the left side—the first or ventricular sound is lessened. Under such circumstances the use of wine is called for, and there is a strong probability that it will agree. You begin with six or eight ounces of good port in the day—given in divided doses, together with proper food.

It will always be right that in such a case you should see the patient in the course of six or eight hours, to judge whether the stimulant has agreed; in a few cases even at this period of the fever the depression of the heart goes on rapidly, and if so, the stimulant will have to be increased. Should things on the next day remain without change, and should there be no signs of the stimulant having disagreed, you may continue. By-and-by it may happen that the first sound of the heart disappears, so that the organ acts with a single sound, even over both ventricles. This indicates increasing debility, and calls for a free use of the stimulant, and, in many cases, the employment of brandy, for which a good vehicle is warmed milk with a little sugar.

Now, in most cases of typhus fever in this country with favourable result, the prostration of the patient, of which the heart is commonly so good an index, begins to disappear at about the twelfth day, but you may find evidences that the wine has agreed even before that period. Of these the principal are :—

1st. The return of impulse.

2d. The commencing re-establishment of the first sound.

3d. The gradual coming down of the rate of the pulse.

Of these, the second and the third are the most important, for the return of impulse is sometimes the commencement of an excited state of the heart—always an unfavourable symptom in fever. When the first sound is restored in its normal manner, the process is gradual, being commonly first perceived over the right ventricle, and when completed it has its natural character.

But with regard to prognosis, the best indication of the agreement of stimulants is the lessened rate of the pulse; even a slight diminution, say of two or three beats in the minute, is of great importance. If at your next visit the diminution of rate goes on, it is a great encouragement to a good prognosis. Remember how often we have seen a good result when the only favourable point in the case was that the pulse became slower and slower while stimulants were being freely used. Still, to say that the falling of the pulse under stimulants is a certain ground for a good prognosis would not be justifiable, as we shall see presently.

In cases of extreme nervous prostration and debility of the heart, as shown by the fœtal character of the sounds—or in some instances by the extinction of all sound, while the pulse continues—great boldness may be used in the administration of stimulants. It is true that in examples of the "fœtal" heart the ventricular sound continues. Yet we have found that the lessening of the second sound is an important sign of generally deficient vital energy, and the necessity of free stimulation. Of this I offer no explanation, but of the fact I am certain.

It is very difficult to lay down rules as to the quantity of wine or other stimulants that may be required by circumstances, and you have seen cases in which the patients took a quantity of stimulants, which in the state of health would have produced intoxication. We have commonly given from 16 to 24 ounces of wine with half a pint of brandy in the day; and in many cases we might have given more, and with advantage.

In a severe case of maculated typhus with extinction of the first sound over both ventricles from the seventh day, 96 ounces of wine with five ounces of brandy were exhibited. The coming down of the pulse was remarkable.

Thus on the 7th day it was at 124
"	8th	"	120
"	11th	"	116
"	12th	"	96
"	13th	"	80
"	15th	"	76

On this last day the skin was cool, the impulse perceptible, and the sounds proportionate.

This case also showed that peculiar character of pulse which we have observed in many examples of the debilitated heart in fever treated by free stimulation, the pulse having been restored to its natural rate, and convalscence all but established. It continued to fall even as low as 32 in the minute, when it rose progressively to its natural standard.

Thus in this case the pulse was—

17th day	.	.	.	.	.	60
18th "	.	.	.	.	.	50
22d "	.	.	.	.	.	32
25th "	.	.	.	.	.	60

The convalescence was perfect on the 18th day.

This case was a model example of typhus, in which recovery was not interfered with by any secondary lesion. The falling of the pulse so far below the natural standard is not constant, but I have always looked on it as showing that the heart had been greatly weakened, with or without muscular softening.

I have told you that no rule can be laid down as to the actual quantity of stimulants to be exhibited. Every case has its own peculiarities even in the same epidemic. You will have differences in the necessity for stimulation, differences in the degree of vital prostration, in local complication, and in all the physical signs of the heart as to their nature, combination, mode of subsidence, and behaviour under treatment. As a general rule the freer the case is from manifest local complication, *apart from the vital depression of the heart,* the bolder may you be in stimulation. But you are not to allow the local complications—except that of active irritation of the brain—to deter you; and even in certain cerebral cases, where circumstances call for it, you may use stimulants tentatively.

Two cases of most malignant typhus occurred to me some years ago. Both the patients were medical men; one was a young man of a non-excitable and phlegmatic temperament. In this case the use of stimulants was commenced at about the eighth day, and ran on for more than a week. The symptoms were extreme prostration, continued—though not profound—coma, weakness of circulation, coldness of breath, enormous vibices, a general purpling of the skin, and paralysis of the bladder. A worse case so far as the essential disease was concerned could hardly be conceived. Fortunately the power of swallowing was unaffected, and you are not to despair of any case of fever as long as deglutition remains. During ten days the stimulants given were so varied and in such large quantity that his friends refused to continue them, thinking it would be a dreadful thing that the patient should leave the world in a state of intoxication. We could not persuade them that we knew better, and we had to send one of the class of this hospital to mount guard over the case, and to administer the wine and brandy perforce. By the twenty-first day, when the disease subsided, he had taken at least two dozen of wine, including port, Madeira, and champagne, with six large bottles of brandy. The recovery was perfect and without any accident, and the gentleman has since enjoyed many years of the best health.

In the second case I did not see the patient until the twelfth day. He was a man of high mental culture and activity of mind and body. He had been attended by a physician of the anatomical and antiphlogistic school. In place of food he had got mercury, and in place of wine, tartar emetic. A glass of claret had been permitted on the day before we saw him. There was no disturbance of the brain, but he was covered with a petechial eruption approaching to purpura. The surface was cold, and the pulse almost imperceptible. From the middle of the calf of each leg downwards, and over both feet, the surface was black, the skin hanging in loose wrinkles, giving an appearance as if the patient had on a pair of black socks. We expected mortification of the legs and feet, but, within twenty-four hours from the commencement of the stimulating treatment, the circulation was fully re-established, the blackness had disappeared, the feet had become warm, and the fulness of the limbs had returned. I need not tell you that stimulants were used boldly. In the first eight hours sixteen

ounces of brandy were given. The patient made an excellent recovery, and is still in the best health.

In both these cases the patients had been of very temperate habits.
The disease was a most severe but uncomplicated typhus, the nervous
system not excited, and the stimulants agreed throughout. Both
cases were thus well adapted for the bold and continued use of the
stimulant treatment.

Gentlemen, there is at present in our wards a patient whose ·case I
would commend to your most attentive study. I refer to the young
man Hardcastle, in whom the general symptoms of fever are presented
in their most aggravated and appalling form. This patient is a native
of England, and had been but a short time in Dublin. His case is
full of instruction.

I have mentioned that he is not a native of Ireland because it is
probable that this circumstance has acted in modifying the symptoms
of his disease. Had this patient been attacked with fever in his
native place, he probably would have shown the symptoms of ordinary typhoid fever, and the case would have been a comparatively
mild one. But at all events, this much we may believe, that different
countries present endemic, sporadic, and even epidemic fevers, with
characters in some degree peculiar to themselves; and we are not yet
able to explain why fever in one country differs so much from fever
in another—why maculated typhus should be so common in Ireland,
and comparatively rare in England—or why the fever in Paris should
so commonly present a particular local lesion. Many causes doubt
less act; and I suppose among others, such as climate, diet, soil, and
so on, the race and temperament are to be reckoned.

I have suggested that if various families of mankind have a physiological stamp, they probably have also their pathological peculiarities.
However this may be, it becomes a curious subject of inquiry, to determine what are the modifications of the symptoms of the fever in
Ireland or in any other country, when the patient is not a native of
the country, and especially if he has not been long resident in it. The
most extraordinary case I ever witnessed was that of a gentleman, a
native of France, who, after a long exposure to contagion during the
famine fever, contracted maculated typhus here. He was a man of a
sanguineo-nervous temperament, and exhibited during his illness a
succession of symptoms widely different from those which we commonly see in the spotted typhus of this country. He was profusely
maculated, and the peculiarity of the case consisted in the irregular
manifestations of various local symptoms—principally engaging the
nervous system—and the inconstancy of the general condition, espe-

cially with reference to excitement or collapse. This gentleman
happily recovered, after passing through a storm of disease such as I
and his other attendant, Dr. O'Ferral, had never seen before.

Hardcastle is a young man who has been well educated, and he is
evidently above the rank of the ordinary hospital patient. His symptoms have been, from an early period of the disease, alarming in the
highest degree. You will seldom see a worse case of adynamic fever.
We may safely say, that for the last fortnight, both by day and by
night, there has been an uninterrupted struggle between medical art
and the fell disease which is upon him. During that time he has been
lying more like a decomposing corpse than a living man ; but he has
been kept from dying by the bold and constant exhibition of stimulants, by tonics, and by food.

Some of you may wonder why it is that we thus go on with the
increasing exhibition of stimulants—the untiring efforts to support
life—although for the last ten days, at least, we have been hourly expecting his death. The answer is, that we believe his disease to be
one which may subside, sooner or later, under the law of periodic
action. His recovery will then take place—not in consequence of
the action of any specific which has the power of curing fever, but
from causes the nature of which is hidden from us. We are like the
defenders of a post attacked by a powerful enemy, but yet expecting
succour, and we seek to hold the place until that succour arrives.

There are two points in this case worthy of notice. One is that
the nervous system has been so little engaged. He has had occasionally a slight delirium, and latterly some agitation and slight subsultus
tendinum ; but though he generally appears sunk in stupor, it is not
true coma, but rather the stupor of exhaustion, for, when you rouse
him, his intelligence appears to be good. Is this escape of the brain
to be looked on as favourable, or the contrary ? According to an old
and well-founded opinion, all anomalous circumstances in fever are to
be feared. You know the aphorism, "*Pulsus, vultus, et urina bona: et
æger moritur.*" This contains an important truth ; but, in typhus, the
want of nervous symptoms is in general favourable ; for of the symptoms referrible to one of the three cavities, doubtless those indicating
nervous lesion are the most formidable.

The second point to which I wish to direct your attention is, that,
although this patient presents the symptoms of typhus so decidedly,
he cannot be said to have any maculæ or petechiæ. In fact, his skin
has been unaffected ; there has been none of the so-called exanthema-
tous eruption of typhus ; and, even at this advanced period, the
existence of petechiæ is so doubtful, that I would not say that he has

them. Yet, if ever a man had the *typhus gravior*, this man has it. His surface exhales the peculiar odour of typhus, strongly marked; he is prostrated to the last degree; he has been kept alive by the most powerful stimulation; he has a feeble heart, and well-marked secondary affections of the intestinal and bronchial surfaces; his mouth is full of sordes; his tongue black, dry, and cracked; his breath fetid. The stethoscope indicates a general and severe bronchial affection, and there is a wasting diarrhœa.

I am not going to take up your time by a discussion as to the distinctive characters of typhus and typhoid fever. But it would be, I think, difficult even to the advocates of the distinction, to declare in which class this case should be placed. In this instance, as in most others, the settlement of the question is of little value; for, whether the disease be typhus or typhoid fever, the treatment should be no other than that which we have so far carried out. I may say this much, however, that the presence or absence of an early eruption having some similarity to an exanthem, or, again, the presence of petechiæ, appears to be insufficient to justify our drawing a strong line of distinction between these diseases. I would advise you to receive with more than caution the doctrine, that the early eruption in typhus is a true exanthem, and that its absence in any given case points out that the disease is not typhus, but typhoid fever.

Again, it is stated that the non-maculated fevers are often protracted and dangerous; so they are, but not so often as they are short and easily managed. And I have not seen that relief of organs in typhus, which some describe as the rule, when the eruption appears. How, then, are we to look on the eruption. Certainly not as a distinctive mark between two different diseases. Gentlemen, we know that typhus fever will run its course and destroy life, without the necessary production of any hitherto ascertained anatomical change. We know further, that in many cases local alterations are formed, but that there is the greatest inconstancy in different epidemics, and in different patients during the same epidemic, in the seat, amount, time of appearance, and results of these local changes. The cutaneous rash is plainly one of this group of secondary affections; and its absence or presence can no more be said to distinguish the disease, than the absence or presence of any other of these affections. I think we may admit that an early and florid eruption is often met with in typhus, which is well marked in other respects also; and again, that such cases generally require and bear stimulation.

To return to the case of Hardcastle. We observe that there has been as yet no tendency to the critical or periodical retrocession either of the secondary diseases or of the general affection. The fourteenth day passed by without any crisis, or without any subsidence of the disease; the eighteenth day passed by; the twenty-first day has passed by; and he is now in the twenty-fourth day of this terrible disease, kept alive by the use of wine, administered every hour, and also by the free use of hot brandy punch. He presents an appearance to-day to which I wish specially to direct your attention. You may remember that Saturday last was the twenty-first day, and it was then reported to me that the patient was getting a bed-sore. Upon examining him, we found in the ordinary situation of bed-sores a blush of redness and a slight degree of œdema; but beyond that there was nothing remarkable. There was this point, however, which I observed at the time, although it was not until to-day that I thought it of importance, namely, that there was already a solution of continuity of the skin. Now, this is remarkable, and if such a case should occur to me again it would awaken my attention. In the ordinary cases of bed-sores we seldom see a solution of continuity of the skin at an early period; we see lividity, blackness if you will; but a solution of continuity of the skin before the ordinary appearances of mortification have occurred, is extremely rare.

In this patient, on Saturday, just at the very centre of the livid patch on the skin, there was a slight solution of continuity. During the evening the nurse observed that several dark-coloured vesicles or pustules were making their appearance on various parts of his body. Mr. Parr saw these on Sunday, and he found that between the shoulders there was an eruption of livid tumours, which appeared to be something between vesicles and pustules. To-day (Tuesday) such of you as saw the patient will not soon forget the extraordinary appearance of his back. I have been attending on fever in this hospital since 1827, and I never saw anything of this kind before.

Now, it is a very remarkable circumstance, that this eruption of gangrenous vesicles or pustules should have occurred upon the twenty-first day; and this case, as far as it goes, appears to strengthen an opinion, which I have long held—that we were in error in attributing what are termed bed-sores in fever, simply to mechanical causes. The general idea is, you know, that they are simply the result of pressure long continued on a particular part of the body, from the neglect of turning the patient in bed—of pressure combined with the effects of position. Now there can be no doubt that these are predisposing causes, but whether they are the sole and entire causes is another matter; and I am almost convinced that the bed-sore in fever is often one of the group of secondary affections analogous to the ulceration,

14

or the tumefaction and ulceration, of the glands of the intestine—or to the bronchial affection which occurs in the middle stages of the disease—or to the other secondary organic diseases of fever. And if analogous to them, it should be more or less observed to be under the law of periodicity; it should appear and disappear at a certain time, or, at least, exhibit a tendency to do so. We have observed this very curious fact. There are cases in which the system seems to be in such a state that bed-sores will form from the slightest possible causes— that is to say, whenever there is any irritation or pressure, no matter how slight, a bed-sore will form in any part of the body. Some years ago we had a patient in this hospital, who, after the twelfth day, showed this tendency. She had bed-sores on the nates, and one on each shoulder. Then the tendency to the multiplication of these sores increased, and every morning two or three new ones were discovered. Wherever there was the slightest possible pressure, we found a gangrenous spot—in the fold of the arm; in the fold of the pectoral muscle; where the mamma leant upon the arm; where the head leant upon the hand in sleep; where one leg lay on the other—the mark of a black hand was stamped upon the surface. In every possible position in which anything like pressure was made, or irritation excited, there were bed-sores; and this tendency went on day after day, up to a certain day, until there were about thirty sloughs in different parts of the body. From that day—I might say from an hour of that day—no more bed-sores formed, although the constitutional symptoms had not subsided. The patient then had to go through the process of throwing off all these sloughs, of granulation of the cavities from below, and of their cicatrization. She was kept lying on her face for upwards of a month, and finally recovered.

Now what I want to draw your attention to in the case of Hardcastle is, that this extraordinary eruption of gangrenous patches on his back is not of the nature of bed-sores in the ordinary sense of the word. These patches are not produced by pressure. We find them in great abundance in the hollow of the back, where pressure is relieved by the pelvis and by the shoulders. We find them in abundance in the interscapular region; but if we wanted additional proof it is this— that we find them on the anterior portion of the thorax. They came out as vesicles. These vesicles became hard at the top, then black, and soon the mass dropped out; and this patient's back is now as if you took a sharp gouge and punched out circular portions of the flesh in a vast number of spots. Now it can hardly be doubted that this singular appearance is an example of a secondary disease affecting the surface; and it is very remarkable that it should have appeared on one of the critical days—upon the day when, in the ordinary course of fever, the disease should have subsided. It strengthens greatly the opinion, that not only is the general disease under the law of periodicity, but that the secondary alterations are so too.

As a general rule, gentlemen, in prognosis, the occurrence of any vesicular eruption whatsoever in fever is bad. We have in fever several forms of vesicular eruptions. But suppose you take a patient's hand to feel his pulse, on the eighth or tenth day of fever, when he is otherwise going on well, and you are surprised at seeing a vesicle upon his arm. Do not neglect this—do not overlook it. The mere circumstance of that solitary vesicle forming so silently, without any pain, without any notice, points out that there is mischief before you —that the case is likely to go wrong. It is a very important prognostic. Here we have on this patient an eruption of vesicles running rapidly to deep gangrenous destruction of the part, for some of the cavities formed by them are singularly deep, though circumscribed.

Now, suppose that in place of that disease attacking the skin, upon the fourteenth day, or whatever day you please, it should attack the intestine. Suppose that the typhous matter suddenly infiltrated a gland in the intestine, which should fall as suddenly to gangrene, and that there was a solution of continuity ; you will at once see the progress of the worst form of the typhous secondary disease of the intestine. You may look on this man as at this moment turned inside out. On the surface of his skin you are able to learn the history of the worst form of the typhous ulceration of the intestine. This extraordinary condition of his surface no one will say is inflammation of his skin. Apply the same view, and will you say that the disease of the intestine is inflammation of that part ? Certainly not.

Whether this man is to live, gentlemen, or to die, I believe none of us can venture to say. Of course the chances are enormously against him ; but I have said that in the treatment of fever you are never to despair so long as the patient can swallow. So long as he is able to take nourishment, or to swallow wine, no matter how dreadful or apparently hopeless the symptoms may be, you are not to desert him, but—to use the phrase of our glorious sailors—you are to fight the ship while she swims. In a disease under the mysterious law of periodicity, every hour of compelled life is a clear gain. And, over and over again, you will find that your efforts will be crowned with success. You will see a patient lying with his back icy cold ; you will see him pulseless—his lungs filled with secretion—his belly tympanitic—with dreadful diarrhœa—the lower extremities gangrenous—himself in a state of insensibility—and yet, even under these circumstances, a recovery is possible. But that recovery can be effected only by the steadfast determination of the physician not to desert his post until the vital spark has actually fled; and, if you commit an error in holding on—in hoping against hope—at all events it is an error on the right side.

LECTURE XXIX.

STIMULANTS IN FEVER, *continued*—Case of Hardcastle, continued—Treatment by food and stimulants in extreme cases—Presence of cerebral symptoms to a great extent unfavourable to the exhibition of stimulants—Necessity for daily observation of the effects of the treatment in each case—Signs of disagreement of stimulants—*Routine* practice is in every instance to be deprecated—Fallacies of the numerical system in therapeutics—History of *routinism*—Its results—Description of routinism in the treatment of fever.

WITH reference to the case of Hardcastle, with which we were occupied at our last lecture, we may hope that the symptoms have at last yielded. The great interest of this case consists in its having been an example of a fever in which the patient was scarcely maculated, yet in which the stimulating treatment had to be pursued with an activity as great or greater than that which we are called on to employ in the worst cases of spotted typhus.

On looking over my notes I find that on his admission, which was on or about the seventh day, he had a few scattered maculæ on the abdomen, of a large size, and of a leaden gray colour. He then had diarrhœa, abdominal tenderness, and ileo-cæcal gurgling; and the sounds of the heart, though weak, preserved their natural mutual relations as to force and duration. Doubtless the patient at this period might have been well described as labouring under typhoid and not typhus fever, according to the distinctions now in vogue; but on the 14th, or the 21st, or the 24th day, he would be a bold man who would declare that the case was not typhus of the worst description.

He is now at the 28th or 30th day of his illness, and we have every reason to believe that all will now go well. Since the eruption of gangrenous vesicles or pustules, which occurred on the 21st day, there have been no new appearances of this form of disease, there has been no new bed-sore, nor have the gangrenous patches spread, as might have been expected; two of them are in the form of sinuous cavities, but even these show signs of healing.

These sores were treated first, you will remember, by the simple, and afterwards by the fermenting, poultice; but as the latter gave considerable pain, the nurse returned to the simple poulticing, and now we have changed our plan, and are using stimulating dressings to the ulcerated surfaces.

In the management of these sores, whether they be the ordinary bed-sores or examples of the gangrenous pustules, both of which appear to be of the nature of the secondary affections of typhus under the law of periodicity, it sometimes happens that we have to deal with extensive sinuses. I have seen them at times of not less than six inches in length. In most cases the best treatment for them will be stimulating injections, using the vulcanized India-rubber bottle with a long and slender ivory pipe. It is generally requisite at first to wash out the sinus with tepid water, and afterwards to inject some of the metallic solutions—diluted solutions of sulphate of copper, nitrate of silver, or sulphate of zinc—and when the discharge is very fetid, you may use the decoction of bark, or solutions of chloride of lime or soda. An excellent dressing when the sore is open is the Canada balsam combined with oil, or a mixture of equal parts of castor oil and balsam of copaiba. You will derive advantage, also, from the employment of pressure by means of flat compresses of lint, and a roller when it is possible to apply it, or in other cases you may employ strapping with adhesive plaster. When the sinus is in a depending position, and matter accumulates in its lower portions, it is sometimes necessary to make a counter opening; but this operation should rather be delayed until the system has improved; the case is then to be treated as an ordinary surgical one.

Now let me draw your attention to the diligence with which the administration of wine has been pursued in this case. We began its exhibition on the 2d of November, which was the eighth day of the disease; on that and the next four days, the quantity administered was six ounces daily. The wine used all through was port, of an excellent quality. From the 6th to the 11th he had twelve ounces daily, and from the 11th to the 18th his daily allowance was twenty-four ounces. During the next three days it was reduced to eighteen ounces; and from the 21st to the 25th, to twelve ounces per diem. On the 26th and succeeding days he had ten ounces; on the 28th the quantity was reduced to eight; on the 4th of December he had but four ounces; and the wine was omitted altogether on the 5th. Besides all this, a tumbler of hot brandy-punch, containing two ounces of the best brandy, was administered whenever the patient's state seemed to require it. In this way we used about twenty-four ounces of brandy, seven bottles of porter, and 432 ounces of wine, while, in addition, bark, musk, and ammonia were freely exhibited.

Some may suppose that this quantity of wine was excessive. Such is not my opinion, nor will it be yours when you come to treat the typhus of this country in a large hospital. I am sure we might have given him with safety much more, and I doubt if we could have done with less. The result of the case confirms what I have said to you before, that in fever, no matter how terrible the group of symptoms may be, *you are not to despair so long as the patient can swallow.* Bear in mind, too, that Hardcastle has been carefully fed throughout with chicken broth, beef-tea, and jelly ; and we have now passed that period when, under the law of periodicity, his terrible disease should subside.

The principal symptoms were extraordinary prostration, coldness of the surface, and feebleness and irregularity of the heart's action; and it was not until the end of the eighth day of the exhibition of stimulants in great quantities that any favourable influence was produced on the circulation. The case strongly illustrates the advantage of persisting in the use of stimulants, although for days together no amendment seems to follow their employment.

I cannot too strongly impress upon you that even under apparently desperate circumstances life may be saved by the repeated introduction of small quantities of food and stimulants. Here we see the advantage of skilled nurse-tending. In the practice of a friend of mine a case occurred in which the power of deglutition was all but lost, the vital powers were sunken to an extreme degree, the action of the heart almost imperceptible, the eyes staring, with contracted pupils; while the symptom of lachrymation, regarded by experienced men as one of the worst in fever, was present. It was thought by all except the physician that the patient should be left to die. He, however, did not utterly despair. A large blister was applied to the occiput and nape of the neck, and a teaspoonful of brandy and beef-tea was administered every ten minutes during many hours. A slight motion of the eyelids was at last perceived. This was followed by deglutition, and after some time reaction had taken place.

Some would say that in this most severe case the recovery was to be attributed to the blistering. It is more probable that it was connected with the action of the periodic laws, favoured by the continued introduction of stimulants. In such a case the use of enemata of beef tea or of milk, containing in addition a small quantity of brandy, and also quinine, as recommended by Dr. Graves, is indicated.

As to the employment of wine in a case seen for the first time, you will remember that in fever those who have been previously of temperate habits are generally the best subjects for the stimulating treatment. In our wards great quantities of wine have produced the best effects in the peasant class. Such men are by no means habitually intemperate. They may exceed now and then on the occasion of a fair or a wake, but their habitual drinks are milk, water, or tea. It is not so with the artisan class, who indulge in ardent spirits. Here I beg of you to remember what we have seen as to the anticipative treatment, and also that having to deal with a case of fever—say, in its first week—you cannot predicate how long it will continue. This is particularly true in the typhoid form, especially when affecting the adult.

It would seem as if the frequent habit of alcoholic stimulation in health rendered the brain less capable of supporting wine under the condition of fever. At all events, you have seen that the use of stimulants where the patient had been a drunkard has by no means the same admirable result observed in men of a different habit.

The freedom from symptoms of cerebral excitement, particularly when attended by heat of the head and increased action of the cerebral arteries, is of course favourable to the use of wine.

But there is another cerebral condition which renders the use of wine in fever less often advantageous. It is met with in those whose occupation has long entailed a close and intense mental labour. Such subjects you will meet more frequently in the middle classes of society than among hospital patients, and in them we find that, while other circumstances indicate the free use of stimulants, their tranquillizing effect is not seen, and they have to be omitted or used only at intervals. This is one out of many reasons why the overworked professional man, especially if he be a physician, is so bad a subject for fever. Indeed, whenever you are called to treat a medical brother in typhus or in typhoid, you may lay your account at having a rock ahead.

In the course of a case of typhus or the more prolonged examples of severe typhoid, in which you are giving wine, you must every day be on the look-out for symptoms that the stimulant is no longer necessary or is disagreeing. Such a change is common, showing that the period has arrived when the stimulant is beginning to have the intoxicating effect which it would have were the patient not in fever. It is not easy to describe accurately this state, and you must learn it by observation. There is an undefined general excitement, some-times with heaviness and even a degree of delirium, often of a novel kind, together with loss of sleep. Symptoms not unlike many of those in the earlier stages of the case appear, while the pulse is more resisting and the patient complains of thirst and general *malaise*. Now, some of you have seen this group of symptoms in the advanced stages of fever where stimulants had been employed at first with great advantage, and you will remember the benefit which followed their disuse or diminution. This is a most important point of practice. Coincident with the use of wine or other stimulants you may have observed a gradual subsidence of the symptoms of fever, the re-establishment of the heart's action, the coming down of the pulse, the cleaning of the tongue, and an improvement in the nervous symptoms. Under these circumstances the wine may be diminished gradually.

But where there are indications that it is beginning to disagree, and that, in place of having a calming, it has a disturbing, effect on the brain and heart, *although at first the opposite state had been induced*—then the omission of the stimulant may take place at once, and the patient be supported on bland and unstimulating nourishment. You must have seen examples in our wards of the happy effects which followed the disuse of stimulants.

When, in a protracted fever in which stimulants had been clearly indicated and had manifestly agreed in full quantity, symptoms of a more general disturbance of the system supervene, you must consider whether this condition is owing to an exacerbation of the essential disease or to the influence of stimulants; in other words, whether the time has not arrived when their sanative action has given place to an opposite effect. Under such circumstances your course may be often, and safely, a tentative one. Such a course is recommended by Dr. Murchison when there is a question as to the giving of stimulants in the early stages of fever; and here likewise you may feel your way in an opposite direction and watch the effect of a certain diminution of the remedy.

Now, gentlemen, before concluding this lecture, I wish to say to the junior members of the class, and indeed to you all, that physicians are to be met with who boast that they do not give stimulants in fever, while, on the other hand, there are men in whose practice their use is a matter of routine. In either of these categories you may meet those who refer to and compare the numerical results of their practice. But these men have not learned how inconsequential are such comparisons. They have not learned how fallacious the results of the numerical system are in indicating a line of practice to be adopted *in all cases.* They have not perceived that life may be saved or lost by the adoption of this or that system—the advocates of stimulation saving those cases which required it, and their opponents those where it was injurious or unnecessary.

It is true that the observations of the numerical school have been directed to determine what treatment in a certain disease will be followed with success in the greatest out of a given number. But this is not what the practical physician wants to know. Is it not rather what is best for him to do in the case of A, B, or C ? A certain treatment may have been successful in 75 per cent. of a group of cases, but he knows that this will not justify him in adopting it exclusively in all or in any of the remaining 25 per cent.

He has learned that fever, in the general acceptation of the term, is a condition with laws of periodicity, and that, therefore, all therapeutic conclusions as regards it will have to be estimated by a reference to this characteristic; and, lastly, that fever is a varying condition, its cases—although capable of being arranged into groups —having certain similarities, but also infinite varieties, in local and essential symptoms ; in amount, period, and degree of complications ; in the influence of remedies and in the epidemic character. Therefore in its treatment, and with reference to therapeutics, each case must be considered *by itself.*

It is plain that dependence on the numerical system will encourage routinism—a line of conduct so opposed to the proper dealing with disease; for to adopt a practice deduced from the results of comparison of numbers is but to justify routinism under the show of authority.

It is hardly necessary to observe to the senior members of this class that the use of wine and other stimulants in our wards is in no way a practice of routine. Gentlemen, you have seen many cases during the last year in which wine was sparingly or not at all used in the course of the fever, simply because it was not required. Food was regularly given, while careful watching was practised, so as to detect early any sign of failure of the energy of the brain or circulation.

It will be well to look at the various illustrations of routinism in the treatment of fever which we have known in this country. The Irish physicians of the last century might be called routinists in one respect—namely, that they employed wine and tonics in most cases liberally, if not indiscriminately. Like the old English physicians, however, they were eclectics, and so did not fall into many of the errors of their successors. Their doctrine of putrescence merely implied prostration of the system—in other words, debility was the condition to be guarded against and met; and doubtless, in the whole class of adynamic and essential diseases, if they erred, the error in practice was one on the right side. Drs. Quin, Plunket, and Harvey, all used wine freely in maculated typhus. Indeed, a bottle of Madeira daily was commonly ordered by them. To a certain extent they used it anticipatively, for they did not wait for the advent of extreme prostration.

The next phase of routinism was of a different and opposite nature. The doctrines of Broussais, which taught that the essential disease was symptomatic of local inflammation, while the reverse was true, turned the minds of men into a wrong direction. The idea of inflammation was opposed to the exhibition of stimulants and tonics, and the practice of medicine was reduced to using direct or indirect depletion.

The theories of Clutterbuck and of Armstrong supplemented those of Broussais as to inflammatory action being the cause of fevers, and so that new routinism in practice was generated, of which the leading characters were starvation and evacuation. The laws of periodicity in fevers were ignored, as was also the great fact in medicine that symptoms diagnostic of local disease when the patient has not essential fever cease to be so when he has.

Thus was established the routine practice of the adoption of evacuants, of bleeding, of diaphoresis, and even of purgatives. The system was pertinaciously reduced through every outlet, while little or nothing was introduced to supply the deficiency. The disciples of Broussais by applying leeches to the abdomen and by starvation reduced the patient to a state of inanition. Those of Clutterbuck did the same by depletion of the head for imagined cerebritis, and those of Armstrong operated similarly for the reduction of a supposed inflammatory diathesis. The depleting effect of acute disease, the reduction of the volume of blood by the fever itself, the waste of tissue —were overlooked, while every new interference with the powers of nature more and more impaired the *vis medicatrix*.

We may attribute to the same cause that timidity in the use of wine in fever which is still observable in the practice of some of our brethren, especially those who during their student lives have not been brought into daily bedside contact with the disease. I remember some few years ago receiving an urgent call to see a lady in fever. I was entreated to lose no time in going, as the patient was so low, so far gone, that she had actually been ordered wine! I found the lady at about the fourteenth day of a low enteric or typhoid fever. She was extremely weak, and suffering under great mental depression and physical exhaustion, which had been present from the commencement of the attack. I recommended the immediate use of wine. "Oh," was the answer, "she has been ordered wine, and is now taking it." On inquiry it turned out that what had been ordered was light claret, the quantity being *one or two teaspoonfuls in cold water twice or thrice a day.* Now, this was the treatment of a physician whose opinion was in general not to be despised, but who had, like many of his contemporaries, been brought up not only in ignorance of the use of wine, but in a terror as to its effects on the supposed inflammatory condition of fever. My advice as to the quantity and quality of the wine was looked on as daring and innovating, but was nevertheless followed, and with full success.

Closely following on the routine local and general antiphlogistic treatment in fever was a method which seemed to spring from the adoption of the views of Abernethy as to the influence of derangement of the chylopoietic viscera in introducing disease. A patient might or might not have a continued essential fever, but the intestinal and renal secretions showed derangement. Here the treatment recommended itself by its simplicity—a mercurial pill at night, followed in the morning by doses of infusion of senna, with rhubarb and gentian and Epsom salts, the care of the attendant being mainly directed to the appearance of the tongue and the inspection of the evacuations. This practice would be continued for days, the digestive organs obstinately refusing to right themselves, notwithstanding the treatment, until the patient began to sink, and was perhaps attacked with peritonitis, the result of perforation. Let me tell you a case of this kind.

A gentleman previously healthy was attacked with symptoms of fever, and attended by two professional men long since dead, one a physician, the other a surgeon. He was treated for many days on the mercurial and purgative plan. I need not say that the fever continued, and as at last there was considerable sinking of the vital powers, a consultation was asked for by the patient's friends, and an eminent consulting physician of Dublin saw the case. He suggested that the treatment had been carried sufficiently far, and recommended chicken broth and a moderate use of wine. A light tonic, consisting of an infusion of cascarilla with a few drops of dilute muriatic acid, was also ordered.

This was in the morning, and within two hours, the consulting physician having to leave town, I was hurriedly summoned to the case, it being alleged that the patient had been poisoned by the medicine. Violent pain had supervened *just at the moment of swallow-ing the first dose of medicine.* It was easy to see that perforation and peritonitis from long-continued intestinal disease had taken place. Nothing that I could say would induce the friends to take this view of the case, and to my surprise they were backed up by the medical attendants. I even drank some of the mixture in their presence. The patient sank in the course of some hours, and it was only by my declaring that a coroner's inquest should be held that I got permission to examine the body. The ileum was extensively ulcerated, and complete perforation had occurred in no less than four places. In one, probably that which caused the effusion into the peritoneum, the opening was the size of a fourpenny piece.

The coincidence in time of swallowing the first dose and of the effusion into the peritoneum was singular. It was hardly down when the patient cried out, " I am poisoned! I am poisoned !" and re-mained in terrible pain until be was moribund.

Here was a case of enteric or typhoid fever in which the intestinal disease was doubtless aggravated by the continued catharsis for many days. In the Report of the Meath Hospital, by Dr. Graves and myself, many cases of intestinal perforation are given where at the commencement of the fever hypercatharsis had been induced by the exhibition of doses of saline purgatives. Looking at the routinism then prevalent, the case I have detailed was probably not an excep-tional one, and curiously illustrates that a knowledge of medicine is not necessarily implied in the legal qualification for practice.

But as the principles of right reasoning in medicine are better inculcated and understood, and as larger views of the pathology of fever—such as those taught by John Peter Frank, by the fathers of British medicine, and by modern writers, like Christison, Graves, Watson, Murchison, Jenner, and Tweedie—are more generally known and made use of in medical education, the older as well as the newer forms of routinism will disappear. The time is coming rapidly when routinism in its successive phases will be forgotten, and the state of fever be dealt with in a philosophical spirit.

Before concluding this lecture let me give you an extract from one of the writings of a witty medical satirist, the late Dr. Brennan, of Dublin, commonly called " The Wrestling" and sometimes " The Turpentine Doctor." It is entitled " A Receipt to Make a Fever," and is a picture of the practice of the day three-quarters of a century ago—unhappily, not yet extinct:—

Any patient, when you get him,
First of all, be sure you sweat him:
The next day you need not heed him,
But the third take care to bleed him.
When he's sweated and he's bled,
Then, of course, you'll shave his head;
Clap on five-and-twenty leeches,
Tho' the first cost a crown each is.

When to sink he does incline,
Blister legs and give him wine.
Tell his uncle or his brother
That you'd like to see another—

Yet let nobody approach
But a doctor in a coach;
For a coach does mighty wonders
In concealing doctors' blunders.

The writer then passes in satirical review the different consulting physicians of Dublin, concluding with himself:—

If they talk of Brennan's knowledge,
Say, "He is not of the College,"
Or, to joke if you incline,
Smiling mention—*Turpentine*—
And you may throw in—by dad!—
That you know he's wrestling mad.

The patient dies:—

When with drugs you well have swilled him,
Tell his friends *the fever* killed him;
All that could be done was done—
The worst you ever saw, but one:
And this is a mighty consolation
In such an awful visitation.

LECTURE XXX.

TREATMENT OF THE LOCAL SECONDARY AFFECTIONS IN FEVER—Relative importance of
these affections as regards *prognosis*—BRONCHIAL AFFECTIONS—Necessity for administration of stimulants and nourishment—Danger of exhibition of tartar emetic
—Failure of emetics—Turpentine-punch—Dry-cupping, poulticing, blistering—
Internal remedies: bark, ammonia, spirit of chloroform, turpentine—ACUTE CON-
SOLIDATION OF THE LUNG—Its *three forms*—Treatment of the first form by dry-cupping,
blisters, quinine, turpentine, and wine—Of the second form by local depletion
simultaneously with the administration of wine—Of the third form, *externally* by
iodine and blisters, *internally* by tonics and iodide of potassium.

FOLLOWING the plan which I have laid down in this course of lectures, I shall to-day direct your attention to the management of the
secondary local affections of fever.   We may classify these under four
headings, according as they involve the nervous, circulatory, pulmonary, or digestive systems.

We are we to attempt to classify these local affections with respect
to their importance as regards the parent disease and the safety of the
patient, it would be difficult to determine whether the nervous, circulatory, pulmonary, or digestive symptoms should be considered as
entitled to the first place.

In reference to *prognosis*, the predominance of cerebral symptoms
may certainly be held to be of unfavourable import, and one reason
for this is that their presence often interferes so materially with the
attempt to combat prostration by the administration of stimulants.
But, apart from this consideration, the preponderance of cerebral symptoms is more serious as always indicating—not necessarily organic
change in the nervous centres—but a functional disturbance in them
which reacts on all the other systems of the body.

If, however, we were to classify the various phenomena connected
with the different systems of the body in fever according to the
amount of their corresponding anatomical changes, we should say
that the pulmonary affections are the most liable to changes of this
description.

Thus, notwithstanding all the researches which have been insti-
tuted respecting the anatomical changes in typhus and typhoid fevers,
no one can at present venture to say what condition of brain corresponds to this or to that symptom in these diseases; no one can
accurately determine the state of the brain as regards its anatomical

changes from the observation and study of any symptom. We may recognize a condition of brain in fever in which stimulants will not be borne, and another wherein they are useful, but we may be unable to reduce either of these to an anatomical expression. As we have seen in a former lecture, there is no symptom in ordinary fever whereby we can determine the presence of actual and progressive *cerebritis* or *arachnitis*. One patient will be in a state of high delirium, with injected brain, another will have an injected brain in the absence of any such symptom.

These are important facts, most necessary to be kept in mind ; but you are not to infer from this that we are altogether powerless in the treatment of the cerebral symptoms of fever. All that has been said shows only, that, in dealing with the special condition of existence to which we give the name "fever," our pathology must not be too material in its character or tendency, and that the symptoms of merely functional suffering are infinitely varied in nature, time of appearance, intensity, and their degree of combination with organic change.

I have said that of all the secondary diseases of fever those affecting the pulmonary system are the most frequently attended by anatomical change, and among these—THE BRONCHIAL AFFECTION—for primary bronchitis it does not seem to be—most especially so.

It is remarkable how silently this affection will be developed in proportion to the severity of the fever. From superficial observation the presence of serious bronchial disease might never be suspected, but on exploring the chest morbid sounds may be heard universally in front and behind. Yet there may be no severe cough, no extreme dyspnœa, or lividity of countenance.

Frequently with this secondary disease in malignant typhus an extreme degree of weakening of the heart, with softening of that organ, will be found associated. By having regard to this complication we obtain the key to the treatment which is especially indicated in these cases—namely, the free administration of stimulants and nourishment.

Here, also, the anticipative method of treatment is often indicated, for the secondary bronchial affection with a weakened heart places the patient in a position—it may be—of the most imminent peril. The heart grows weaker, and there can be little doubt that its weakened condition is repeated in the muscular fibre of the lungs and bronchi. The bronchial tubes are loaded, mucus is copiously secreted, the muscles which assist the act of expectoration become paralyzed, and, should relief not be afforded, the almost inevitable result is asphyxia and death.

These observations are simply suggestive of the necessity of adopting a decided and active system of treatment. The more closely you investigate cases of this kind, the more convinced will you be that paralysis of the circular fibres of the expectorant muscles takes place; and here we have one—perhaps the principal—reason why the liberal administration of stimulants is found so successful under such circumstances. It may be that even after recovery from the primary disease death will ensue from purely mechanical obstruction in the lungs and air-passages. This is another reason for adopting the principle of meeting the disease early. I never saw a case of death from secondary bronchial effusion except where the disease had been overlooked at first.

Now let us advert to the general mode of treatment of this complication. Suppose you are called in to a patient, say on the fourth or fifth day of typhus. You find a râle in the large bronchial tubes, extending next day into the smaller tubes. Will you call this "bronchitis" and treat it as such? Certainly not. You have before you a patient in a certain condition as regards the respiratory functions, which condition is under the influence of the parent malady. If there be any inflammation present in such cases, it is specific, asthenic, and reactive, not to be treated by antiphlogistic means. The presence of the râle is not to induce you to bleed or to apply leeches, but what you have to trust to is active and energetic stimulant derivative treatment. Some physicians recommend in such cases the exhibition of tartar emetic. Where this course is followed the patient may sink.

Now, the inveterate habit with which men in our own time were imbued, of attributing every local symptom in fever to inflammation, led to the practice of giving mercury in this condition. But you will easily see the unfitness of such a course when time is pressing and it is absolutely necessary to modify the vital, and relieve the mechanical, state of the lung which threatens asphyxia. My friend Dr. Mackintosh, of Edinburgh, strongly advocated the use of emetics in this condition; but I do not recommend them—at least they have not been hitherto successful in our hands. You will meet cases in which they will not act at all. I have seen the most powerful emetics, of various kinds, exhibited without any vomiting whatever being produced. I have known cases in which, after milder remedies had been used, the sulphates of zinc and copper utterly failed. Or the full action of the emetic may occur, and be followed by great relief of the chest; yet in a short time the suffocative state will return, and, the sensibility of the stomach being destroyed, the patient sinks asphyxiated.

But the course of treatment under these circumstances long

followed in our wards is dry cupping, blistering, and the free exhibition of turpentine in whiskey-punch. By this course our late excellent apothecary, Mr. Parr, saved many a life when the patient was almost *in articulo mortis.* He would administer a tumbler of strong punch with two or three drachms of spirit of turpentine, and repeat the dose, if necessary, in a short time. Often has he said to me in the morning, "Sir, I had to *punch* three cases last night—they are all doing well." The effects were simply wonderful, and illustrate the principle that you are not to despair in a case of fever so long as your patient can swallow.

This reminds me of a translation by Dr. Brennan in the *Milesian Magazine:*—

> Si quid novisti rectius, istud candidus imperti.
> Si non, his utere mecum.
>
> Doctors ! if you have better drugs than mine,
> Say where they're hid ; if not, use turpentine.

In this theatre my late colleague, Dr. Graves, dwelt largely on the value of this medicine in the secondary affection of the lungs in fever, and he has been followed emphatically by Huss of Stockholm.

In the less urgent cases you are not to forget that the disease may show a sudden and violent exacerbation; and I have often heard practitioners account for the occurrence of tracheal rattle and fatal asphyxia and excuse themselves on the supposition of a sudden effusion into the chest, when, in truth, the bronchial tubes had for days been engaged, and the affection unrecognized and neglected.

I repeat that in fever, especially in typhus, with a weakened heart, the affection of the bronchial tubes may be developed insidiously and to a great extent.

With respect to external and local applications in ordinary cases of this secondary affection, I have already spoken of the use of dry-cupping. Amongst other means may be mentioned the repeated application of turpentine fomentations; of poultices consisting wholly of linseed meal, or of linseed meal and mustard in varying proportions; and of moderate-sized blisters, covered with a linseed poultice, so that the vesicating action shall be favoured by the warmth and moisture of the poultice.

Of internal remedies, the decoction of bark, with ammonia and spirit of chloroform, is most frequently indicated ; or moderate doses of turpentine may be employed with good effect. The confection of turpentine administered in peppermint water is found to be a valuable preparation. But above all it will be necessary to support our patient's

15

strength by the judicious administration of suitable nourishment, and wine or other stimulants.

ACUTE CONSOLIDATION OF THE LUNG in fever may be considered, with regard to practice, under several forms: First, that in which symptoms and signs of anything like acute or sthenic inflammation do not occur. The disease is in these cases more or less silent or latent, and recognizable chiefly by physical signs. You are to treat this affection by dry-cupping, blisters, quinine, turpentine, and wine.

But between these cases and others where a greater activity of the ordinary inflammatory symptoms is observed, indicating that a local antiphlogistic treatment may be employed with advantage, there exists an intermediate form which includes cases of almost infinite shades and varieties of character.

In cases of the secondary pneumonic affection which possess many of the characters of acute sthenic pneumonia, there may be pain in the side, great local increase of temperature, and distress of respiration. Here the application of a few leeches, or of the scarificator and cupping-glass, may be followed by immediate and marked relief to the patient. In many such instances the use of wine is not to be intermitted on account of the practice of local depletion. There is a point of great importance in practical medicine—one which I wish to impress strongly upon you—namely, that lines of treatment apparently opposite or antagonistic may, under certain circumstances, be employed simultaneously with success. Your treatment is to be influenced not by the *name* of a disease, but by the condition of your patient; and you may relieve local irritation by local blood-letting while you support the general system, and deal with the essential disease by the use of stimulants.

When describing in a former lecture those consolidations of the lung, especially of its upper lobe, in fever, which seemed to partake of the nature of a crisis, I said that it was often a matter of doubt whether the clearing of the lung was to be attributed to the remedial measures employed or to the spontaneous subsidence of the condition in obedience to the law of periodicity. However, a small blister or two may be used, and the application of the tincture of iodine externally, with the exhibition of iodide of potassium in combination with a tonic, may be of advantage.

I need not say to the students of large bedside experience that it is sometimes difficult to distinguish between a primary pneumonia with a symptomatic fever and states of the lung secondary to typhus or to typhoid. You will, also, be prepared to hear that this difficulty has been more commonly met with since the period of change of type

in disease. Still, during the last few years, several cases of primary
pneumonia have come under our notice, in which, though with less of
the general violence of symptoms once so familiar to us, we have
used the lancet—moderately, it is true, but with the most rapid success. The pain, the adhesive red expectoration, the state of the heart,
and the early appearance of the symptoms, were our chief guides.

The dreadful occurrence of sphacelus in consolidation of the lung
in typhus is to be met by the antiseptic and stimulant treatment.

That recovery is possible in this catastrophe I have already shown
you. The patient in question died after a lapse of some years from
the first attack. We found recent sphacelus in one lung, and a
cavity containing a dry slough, and with a firm lining membrane in
the other.

LECTURE XXXI.

TREATMENT OF INTESTINAL SECONDARY AFFECTIONS.—Two chief indications : (1) alleviation of symptoms, (2) modification of typhous deposition—Poulticing—Local depletion in early stage—Analogy in variolous eruption—Danger of alterative or
purgative treatment at the outset of Continued Fever—Necessity for caution—*Constipation—Diarrhœa*—Poultices, demulcents, sedative astringents, injections of flax-
seed tea—*Tympany*—Turpentine injection—*Diet* in diarrhœa—*Perforative peritonitis*
—Opium our sheet-anchor—Danger of the antiphlogistic method—Dr. Murchison
on the treatment of this accident—Bran poultices and warm fomentations—*Hemorrhage* from the intestine in fever—Not to be interfered with unless continued and
excessive—Treatment by astringents, opium—Illustrative case.

IN a case of enteric fever, or of a well-marked typhus with more or
less of intestinal affection, your efforts in reference to the treatment
of the local secondary disease will be directed less to the cure than to
the palliation of the symptoms, and to diminishing the activity of that
process under which the *mucous* membrane and glands become the
seat of the typhous deposit.

We seek to lessen the amount of change by modifying the specific
and afterwards the reactive irritation.

· Local bleeding and diligent poulticing are the measures on which
reliance is to be placed in the first instance, while everything which
might excite overaction or hypersecretion of the intestines is to be
avoided. The first of these remedial measures is best effected by
moderate leeching of the ileo-cæcal, and in some cases the epigastric
regions, due regard being paid to the strength of the patient and to

the period of the case at which the local symptoms become manifest. In the earlier periods from six to ten leeches may be applied first to one and then to the other situation, and this will be often followed by the relief of local suffering and—as regards the general symptoms—by the best effects. The repetition of this local bleeding will depend on circumstances. But if tenderness, local fulness, increased arterial action of the belly, or muscular rigidity be wholly or in part removed or modified, it is not often necessary to repeat the application. I need scarcely say that the presence of these symptoms affords an indication for this early use of local depletion.

I have shown you that Broussais, in defence of the doctrine that fever was only symptomatic of gastroenteritis, appealed to the fact of the relief which often follows local depletion, and I have suggested a more probable interpretation of the entire matter. Local depletion, if employed sufficiently early in the case, may prevent altogether, or greatly modify the development of intestinal symptoms. Here it would seem that the lessening of the blood supply interfered with the deposition of typhous material along the intestinal tract in the agminated and solitary glands. This is strikingly analogous to what is observed in certain cases of variola, where the local development of the secondary eruption on the face or elsewhere is largely under control by the application of leeches or by strapping the part at an early stage of the disease. This point I have already illustrated in a former lecture.

Again the analogy holds good with respect to the pustular eruption of variola, and the secondary typhous deposits of fever in the intestinal tract. For even where there is good reason for supposing that these deposits have already taken place, and are passing on to ulceration, it is found that local depletion may be of the greatest use in allaying irritation and so preventing the violence of a reactive inflammation.

All this goes to prove that the influence of local depletion cannot be taken as an evidence of the primary nature of the local malady ; for in the first place it receives a similar and easier explanation from the hypothesis of an essential disease with a secondary local affection ; and in the next place the argument from analogy is altogether in support of this hypothesis, and against the views of Broussais.

It is still necessary—I regret to say it—to warn you against following the routine practice of giving what is called "alterative," combined with purgative, medicine, in the early periods of fever—a course too commonly followed, even while the practitioner is unaware of the nature of the disease he is treating. In this way a threefold injury is inflicted. The strength of the patient is exhausted at a time when it should be husbanded ; the normal course of the fever is interfered with ; and, should there be any tendency to the intestinal affection, it is doubtless augmented and exasperated by measures which determine to the part of the economy most likely to be the seat of lesion. This is analogous to what is often observed in constitutional maladies. Thus, in cancerous cachexia the local organic change is frequently determined by the receipt of some injury. In acute essential diseases, again, the same thing is noticed, as for example in variola, where the application of rubefacients will be followed by an increased development of the eruption, while a contrary effect will, as we have seen in a former lecture, be produced by local depletive measures.

In a large proportion of our cases of perforative peritonitis, hypercatharsis by saline purgatives had been induced at an early period with the mistaken view of seeking to cut the fever short.

We have spoken of the use of leeches and of light poulticing. Should there be constipation, with swelling of the abdomen, to such an extent as to render it advisable to free the bowels, mild enemata may be employed, and turpentine fomentations applied to the surface. The enemata must be composed of the blandest fluids, to which, if there be any troublesome tympany, a little turpentine made into an emulsion with yolk of egg may be added.

I am ready to admit that cases will constantly present themselves, in which the practitioner will be at a loss to determine whether continued fever is threatening, or the symptoms are to be referred merely to the presence of a "feverish cold." Under these circumstances I would still inculcate the necessity for caution, and would recommend that the smallest doses of aperient medicines likely to effect the objects in view should be employed.

But when you have symptoms of irritation of the intestine attended by diarrhœa, the use of poultices and of demulcents may be combined with that of astringents of a sedative nature. I know no better remedy than the acetate of lead given with some preparation of opium. In the form of pill these two drugs may be conveniently given ; but if ordered in a mixture, it will be necessary to substitute the acetate of morphia for crude opium. I have never seen any bad result from lessening or checking the diarrhœa, or any symptoms of lead-poisoning, even when this medicine had been continued for many days.

Here I may allude to the fact, that, in the first two epidemics of cholera in this city, the use of the "pilula plumbi cum opio" was introduced by Dr. Graves, following the recommendation as to the value of the acetate of lead in the diarrhœa of Continued Fever by Sir

James Bardsley.[1] The remedy, in the hands of Dr. Graves and of many others, was employed in a vast number of cases, and I believe that during this great clinical experiment not a single case of lead-poisoning occurred either in the earlier stages of the case or in the later period of convalescence. We must, of course, remember that the acetate of lead is by no means so poisonous as the carbonate; but I would caution you against its possible change into this latter salt. If, for instance, it is compounded in a mixture with water containing carbonate of lime, it may be decomposed. This is still more likely to occur in the use of lead-lotions. The most violent and long-continued case of lead-colic I ever saw was that of a woman who had suffered from an extensive burn of the abdomen. Lead-lotion was applied to the injured surface for weeks together, and we must suppose that a considerable quantity of carbonate of lead was formed and absorbed, for symptoms of poisoning soon showed themselves.

To return—you are to use demulcents either by the mouth or in the form of injection. I remember, when a student, that a remedy called the "mistura olei et opii," was extensively employed in this hospital, and with the best effect. It was an emulsion of oil, gum arabic, and cinnamon water, to which a little laudanum was added. We used to believe that it acted mainly in lubricating the irritated surfaces. The injection which we have employed with greatest advantage in diarrhœa in fever has been one of flaxseed tea, to which a few drops of laudanum may be added. The infusion of flaxseed should be made with unbruised seed, and its effect in producing a sensation of general soothing, perceived throughout the intestinal tract, is most remarkable.

I have already spoken of the value of a turpentine injection in cases of constipation with tympany, but when this latter symptom accompanies diarrhœa, and becomes very extreme, the same remedy is often indicated. You might suppose that given by the mouth the turpentine would act as a purgative; but if it is given in small and repeated doses—as, for example, from 15 minims to half a drachm every two or three hours—the result may be just the opposite.

Nor is the mere symptom of tympany to be neglected, for although it is by no means commonly of much importance in the early stages of intestinal lesion in fever, it may assume dangerous proportions.

Some years ago a case occurred in these wards in which abdominal tympany seemed to be the direct cause of death. It resisted all

---

[1] Clinical Lectures on the Practice of Medicine, reprinted from the second edition, 1864, p. 317.

remedies, and we failed in the attempt to pass the long tube beyond the sigmoid flexure. On dissection the small intestine and the colon were found enormously distended—the large intestine being turned over and obstructed by the formation of a complete fold at the commencement of the sigmoid flexure.

Two points connected with the treatment of diarrhœa in fever remain to be considered. In the first place, we have to deal with the question of *diet*. We have already spoken of diet generally in fever, and you will remember the rules which were laid down for your guidance. It is occasionally found that beef-tea tends to increase the diarrhœa. Should this occur, we must either give it in smaller quantities, or suspend its administration. Chicken broth may be substituted, or farinaceous foods employed. Arrowroot with port wine, sago, tapioca, rice, rice milk, plain or boiled milk, and milk and lime-water in varying proportions are articles of diet to which recourse may be had. I have also used eggs, and have found them to agree perfectly. They may be boiled, or beaten up raw with milk sweetened with sugar. "Egg-flip," or the "mistura spiritus vini Gallici" of the "British Pharmacopœia," is one of the most valuable stimulant and nutritive preparations we possess.

The second point relates to the exhibition of other astringents than those already mentioned. These are "chalk mixture," gallic and tannic acids, the astringent tinctures (kino, rhatany, logwood, and so on), and dilute sulphuric acid. They are, I believe, all useful in their way. I have given pills of tannic acid combined with Dover's powder with good effect; but the most valuable of the remedies I have just named is undoubtedly the dilute sulphuric acid. It has a three-fold value—it allays thirst, acts as a tonic, and possesses powerfully astringent properties. It may be administered frequently, and in doses of from 15 to 25 or 30 minims well diluted; or the aromatic sulphuric may be substituted.

We shall now speak of peritonitis resulting from perforation of the intestine, the occurrence of which may be explained by that insusceptibility of the peritoneum to adhesive inflammation which we have already considered. Remember how rarely we meet with general adhesions of the peritoneum in comparison with the frequency of such a condition in the pleura. Now, it would appear that the violent symptoms of perforation depend, less on a localized serous inflammation corresponding to a perforating ulcer of the intestine, than on the fact that an effusion of the contents of the tube into the general cavity causes suddenly an extreme and commonly fatal inflammation. You may occasionally meet cases where, although the serous membrane is

perforated, no *general* inflammation occurs—the process is circumscribed, and is not attended with any effect on the constitutional
symptoms.   In fact, there is occlusion of the opening—the base of the
ulcer being formed by the serous membrane of the adjacent fold of
intestine, so that no effusion of the contents takes place.   And we
have seen that the effect of intense irritation in another cavity may
be to render latent even a general inflammation from effusion, as in
gastro-catarrhal fever or in cases of cerebral complication.

Dr. Murchison[1] gives a remarkable example of the latter.   A young
man aged 19, in enteric fever with acute delirium, suffered from profuse intestinal hemorrhage, but there were no symptoms of peritonitis.
After death, on the 19th day, there were found ulceration of the
intestine, perforation, and peritonitis.

Now, if we compare this terrible accident with the analogous condition of empyema and pneumothorax from perforation of the pleura,
it seems to be more rapidly and certainly fatal.   For, although in the
chest the accident is often attended by violent symptoms, these are
attributable rather to the frequently consequent and sudden collapse
of the lung than to the influence of the resulting pleuritis on the
nervous system.

It frequently happens in pneumothorax, that, after the first storm
of suffering is past, there comes an interval of calm—often prolonged
—while occasionally many of the vital symptoms of pulmonary disease disappear.   The condition of collapse and compression seems,
even for a long time, to suspend the diseased process in the lung, so
that its constitutional symptoms may actually subside and disappear
temporarily.

It was long believed, and is by some still held, that general peritonitis from perforation in fever is invariably fatal.   But we have in
this hospital arrived at a different conclusion.   It is now many years
since a female suffering from ascites, and under the care of Dr. Graves,
underwent the operation of paracentesis, soon after which she was
seized with symptoms of acute peritonitis.   In those days, I may tell
you, such an accident in the operation of tapping was not uncommon,
and no wonder.   A very large trocar and canula were employed, and
efforts made to get rid of every drop of fluid.   With this view the
abdomen, while the canula remained in the wound, was compressed
and kneaded in various places—the mouth of the hard instrument
thus scraping against the serous membrane of the intestines—and a
tight bandage afterwards applied.   Besides the effect of all this vio-

---

[1] Continued Fevers of Great Britain, second edition, page 571.

lence, the serous surfaces, long separated from the effusion, were rapidly brought into contact, so that you can easily understand the frequency of peritonitis. The accident is now comparatively rare.

In the case before us the strength was greatly reduced, and no remedial measure was proposed by the operator. The woman being in extreme pain, Dr. Graves administered a full opiate, with the best effect. Sleep soon followed, and after a few hours the patient awoke with the symptoms greatly alleviated. The opium was repeated in diminished doses, and after a few days all the symptoms of acute peritonitis had subsided. She made an excellent recovery.

The success in this case determined us to employ opium in free doses in the first example of perforative peritonitis which occurred, and the practice has since then proved in many instances successful.

The two great indications of relieving pain and of controlling the peristaltic action have been in these wards and in the practice of several of my friends fulfilled with the happiest effects, while the interesting result of the tolerance of opium in large quantities in acute peritonitis has been established. Thus a grain of opium, exhibited every hour, has been often given without any poisonous effect whatever.

A case occurred here which illustrates the danger which may follow any excitement of the peristaltic action even after recovery from the first access of peritonitis has ensued. A young man, in an enteric fever, was suddenly seized with the most violent symptoms of peritonitis. The pulse became small, rapid, and wiry—the abdomen swollen and exquisitely tender. No doubt was entertained as to the occurrence of a perforation, and the opium treatment was at once resorted to and continued for twenty-four hours. Next day the symptoms were greatly lessened in intensity, and we continued the remedy at longer intervals for a few days. All symptoms of peritonitis disappeared, the abdomen felt natural, and the pulse had returned almost to its normal standard. The patient's condition improved daily, he took nourishment freely, when, the bowels having been confined for many days, a very mild saline laxative was unfortunately given. It acted gently, when the former symptoms at once returned, and the patient sank in the course of some hours. On dissection, well-formed but recent adhesions were found in different portions of the peritoneum—evidently the result of the first, all-but-cured attack. The perforation was in the ascending colon. It was patulous, while bilious and feculent fluid existed in the serous cavity.

Now, that this patient would have been saved, had the laxative been withheld, there can be little doubt, and the case is full of instruction and warning.

There are few more interesting and important facts in therapeutics than the tolerance of opium in repeated doses in this form of peritonitis, and the remedy has been found applicable in other cases besides those of intestinal perforation. It has succeeded in a rupture from an over-distended bladder, in which immediately after the accident no urine could be found by the catheter. In a case in which an hepatic abscess had opened into the peritoneum, the inflammatory symptoms entirely subsided after a few days of the opium treatment. On dissection, after death from another abscess, numerous organized adhesions were observed between the convolutions of the intestine and the parietal peritoneum.

In connection with this subject of the treatment of perforative peritonitis, it may be well to remind you that this complication of fever, like the other secondary affections, varies in frequency according to the prevailing epidemic characters of the disease. Thus previously to 1827 Dr. Graves observed but one instance of the lesion out of more than 1000 cases of fever, while during the session of 1828–29 the occurrence was frequent in Dublin. At the present day, again, even though enteric fever has increased in prevalence, this terrible accident is comparatively rare.

Dr. Graves and I[1] have shown that the antiphlogistic method of treatment is not so applicable in these cases as in examples of idiopathic peritonitis. In the first place, the perforation occurs at an advanced period of some other disease, when the constitution is enfeebled, and, at the time you will be called on to interfere, the patient is suffering not merely from general peritonits but from the collapse which attends the accident. The disease runs its course with such rapidity that in a comparatively short time the patient is brought into the last stage. Under these circumstances the antiphlogistic plan only accelerates the fatal termination. No doubt in ordinary peritonitis bleeding may check the increase or extension of the disease; but in these cases the affection is immediately extensive and severe, and the indications are not to withdraw blood from the already enfeebled frame, but rather to relieve pain, control the peristaltic action of the bowel, and to support the strength until nature shall have completed the organization of the false membrane.

In the epidemic of 1827 the antiphlogistic method in these cases signally failed in our wards, while the exhibition of opium and wine,

[1] "Clinical Report of the Meath Hospital," Dublin Hospital Reports, vol. v.

or of opium in full doses, was attended by satisfactory results. More recent experience testifies largely to the truth of these observations.

Dr. Samuel Cusack, in speaking of puerperal fever, long ago bore witness to the efficacy of wine and opium in puerperal peritonitis, where the powers of life were greatly sunken, and any form of blood-letting or of depletion was inadmissible. His observations were fully confirmed by Dr. Gooch.

I would commend to your most attentive consideration the following admirable remarks by Dr. Murchison on the treatment of peritonitis in fever. He says:—[1]

"Although the cause of peritonitis cannot always be determined with certainty, in the great majority of instances it is perforation of the bowel. The case, though desperate, is not altogether hopeless. Opium is the only remedy to be relied on in such cases; but, to be of service, it must be given immediately and boldly. To an adult, two grains of solid opium may be given at once, followed by one grain every second or third hour, till slight stupor is induced. When the stomach is irritable, the subcutaneous injection of morphia is preferable to opium by the mouth. The doses will vary with the age and other conditions of the patient, but the amount of opium tolerated is often extraordinary; as much as sixty grains have been taken in three days with benefit. The opium is to be given alone, and not in combination with calomel, which brings down more bile into the lower bowel, and so excites peristaltic action. The object is not to produce absorption of lymph (even if the mercury had power to do this), but to paralyze the movements of the bowels, so as to prevent the escape of their contents into the peritoneum, and favour the formation of adhesions.

"Many writers have recommended the application of leeches to the abdomen on the supervention of peritonitis, but the extreme prostration, and the circumstance that the tendency is to death by asthenia, contraindicate such a practice. The pain and tension of the abdomen will also be relieved by warm fomentations, bran poultices, and turpentine stupes; but a much more certain method of subduing the inflammation is covering the abdomen with a bladder of ice, or with the ice poultice referred to under the treatment of tympanites. At the same time the patient must be kept in a state of absolute rest, and on no account raised in bed, and the ingesta ought to be liquid, and given in such small quantities at a time that they can be absorbed by the stomach. A tablespoonful of milk or of iced brandy and water may be given every hour, or every half-hour. The large quantities of food and stimulants sometimes given cannot fail, in my opinion, to be injurious."

He adds :—

"If the case does well, we must beware of interfering with the constipation induced by the opium : cases are recorded where the incautious administration of a purge appeared to break up the adhesions and produce a fresh and fatal attack of peritonitis."

HEMORRHAGE from the intestine in fever is not of very uncommon occurrence. It may sometimes be regarded as to some extent a *criti-*

[1] Loc. cit., page 655.

cal phenomenon, and it often produces a beneficial and curative effect, lessening the local determination and irritation. Under these conditions it should not be interfered with.

But cases are met with in which, from the amount, continuance, or recurrence of the bleeding, the patient's life is placed in jeopardy, and then we are called on to check the flow if possible.

The manner of the hemorrhage is twofold. Sometimes it consists in a *weeping* from the mucous membrane. More rarely a vessel of some size is opened by ulceration—this especially happens in the second or third week of enteric fever. Fortunately, the treatment likely to be of use is nearly the same in both cases. Rest is of paramount importance. Cold drinks and ice may be given. Turpentine, in small doses, is particularly useful where the hemorrhage is associated with much tympany. Acetate of lead and opium sometimes act well; or opium may be given in full doses if there are strong grounds for supposing that the source of the bleeding is an eroded artery. The points in favour of such a view will be the suddenness of the occurrence of the bleeding, its large amount, the advanced period of the illness, and the absence of hemorrhages in other parts of the body.

A man, of middle age, was almost convalescent from a comparatively mild enteric fever, when in the middle of the night he was seized with sudden diarrhœa. The resident clinical clerk was hastily summoned. He soon found that the motions consisted principally of blood, at first dark and tar-like, then of a more florid and arterial appearance. The quantity passing from the patient was so large that no time was to be lost. The clinical clerk accordingly at once administered a full opiate; in an hour he gave a grain of opium with acetate of lead, and he repeated this dose every two hours until the patient had taken 7 or 8 grains of crude opium. The hemorrhage was soon checked, and the curious thing is that the patient showed the same remarkable tolerance of the opium which we have already spoken of in connection with peritonitis. He made a good and rapid recovery. Of course the utmost caution should be employed in these cases, and the effect of every dose should be attentively watched.

Among other remedies in this complication may be mentioned tannin, tincture of the perchloride of iron, and ergot. The last is highly commended by such authorities as Dr. Murchison, and Dr. J. B. Russell, of Glasgow. The former has used it subcutaneously with excellent effect.

LECTURE XXXII.

TREATMENT OF THE NERVOUS SECONDARY SYMPTOMS OF FEVER—HEADACHE—Cold lotions, warm fomentations, moderate leeching, shaving the head, cold affusion, ice—DELIRIUM—Treatment depends on (1) period of case, (2) presence of hyperæmia of the brain, or otherwise—Ice, leeches, shaving the head, cold affusion in *active* delirium—Nourishment and wine in *passive* or anæmic delirium—SLEEPLESSNESS—Moderate leeching, cold affusion, ice—Turpentine in constipation and tympany—Catheterism in distended bladder—Sedatives—Opium, tartar emetic and opium, hyoscyamus, bromide of potassium, chloral, wine—CONVULSIONS—Most formidable in fever—Uræmic, due to (1) *retention* of urine: catheterism; (2) *suppression* of urine: dry-cupping and poulticing over kidneys, diluents, diuretics, aperient enemata, promotion of action of the skin.

AMONG the earliest, most frequent, and often most prominent of the nervous symptoms in fever is HEADACHE. At first it is seldom very violent, and no important or vigorous measures are required for its relief at this period. It is generally a symptom which subsides early in the case, and is rarely indicative of anything beyond functional derangement, or incipient or progressive affection of the brain. The intensity of the symptom is more marked in typhus than in typhoid; but in neither form of fever is it often accompanied by indications of active determination to the head, and in both it commonly subsides without any interference beyond the application of a cold lotion, such as vinegar and water, or chloride of ammonium (sal ammoniac) and water.

But should it be severe, and attended with more or less heat of the head, you may employ with advantage warm stuping of the forehead and temples. These warm fomentations may be repeated according to circumstances, and you have often seen the marked relief afforded by them. Should this measure fail, the application of two or three small leeches to the temples or behind the ears will be followed by relief—a relief out of proportion to the quantity of blood taken. You will, however, remember that the pain generally subsides by itself after the lapse of a few days. Yet it sometimes continues, and resists even the treatment I have suggested; and then, when it is severe and attended with heat and fulness of the head, you may adopt more active measures. You may apply a larger number of leeches in relays for two or three times. It used to be the practice in this city, when the pain was obstinate, with heat of the head, sleeplessness, and

commencing delirium, to open the temporal artery—a proceeding
often followed by excellent results. It should be remembered that I
speak of a time at the commencement of the change of type in
disease; yet the general adoption of this measure is not to be advised,
as the wearing of a tight ligature round the head is often distressing,
to say nothing of the accidental re-opening of the wound or the formation of a small traumatic aneurism. I should tell you that the
quantity of blood removed in this procedure was never excessive,
varying from six to ten or twelve ounces.

Now, I believe that by shaving the head, the cold affusion, and, if
necessary, the application of ice, you will do all that arteriotomy
could effect.

Yet *shaving the head* should not be a matter of routine, especially
among hospital patients. You must not forget that the poor convalescent cannot afford to purchase a wig, and that in consequence he
may become liable to otitis and other accidents, such as rheumatism
or neuralgia of the head. And this reminds me that in the epidemic
of 1826 and 1828 one of the physicians of our large temporary hospital adopted the routine practice of shaving the head of almost all
his patients. Dr. Graves and I, on the other hand, had very rarely
occasion to direct the operation, so that when the shorn and the
unshorn patients met in the convalescent wards the former became
greatly dissatisfied. But this was not all, for soon those whose heads
had escaped the routine razor turned on the shaved ones such a
battery of Irish satire on their appearance that on one occasion it
proved too much for endurance, and a general engagement took
place in the convalescent ward, which was quelled with the greatest
difficulty.

Cold affusion is best carried out in the following manner: The
patient's head is held over a basin, while cold water is allowed to
pour slowly from a jug holding a quart or two, and held at no great
height above the head. It is necessary to let the stream fall on
different parts of the head from time to time, for otherwise a very
painful sensation may be produced. The almost instantaneous relief
afforded in this way is often remarkable.

Now as to the *application of ice:* This is frequently most clumsily
and ineffectually performed. A bladder containing fragments of ice
is placed on the vertex and allowed to remain there. The effect of
the cold thus locally employed on the shaved head gives such distress
as to be at times intolerable until the ice is all melted, when you may
frequently find your patient's head covered for hours with a bag of
water at *fever heat.* Of course you will not permit such an error to

happen—the frequency of which showed how much we were in want of skilled nurse-tending. The proper method of proceeding is to place a piece of ice, rubbed smooth with the hand, in a cup-sponge of convenient size, and by inverting the sponge to bring the ice into contact with the shaved scalp, keeping it in gentle motion round the head. The sponge absorbs the water, and when it is saturated it can be squeezed out, the ice replaced, and the application recommenced. In this way no pain is caused, and the proceeding is grateful to the patient, while the entire head is cooled. Of course, in many cases the application must be renewed at shorter or longer intervals.

Before passing from the treatment of headache I wish to mention the influence for good on the general condition of the patient often observed on cooling of the head by some of the means I have described. At times, in advanced fever with continued determination to the head, you may see a rapid improvement (which continues to recovery) of the patient when the heat and fulness of the head have been allayed by appropriate measures. It seems as if the influence of periodicity, which had been interrupted by the local malady, was again permitted to act. There can be no doubt of the existence in fever of a condition more or less persistent, in which various influences may bring about a cessation or subsidence of the morbid phenomena. Thus we read of cases of camp fever subsiding on any forced removal of the patients. You will find marked benefit to follow the removal of a patient in protracted fever to another ward; and even crisis has been observed closely following a simpler proceeding, such as a change into a fresh bed, the washing and shaving of the patient's face, sponging the surface, and so on.

In considering DELIRIUM in fever, strive to keep the great pathological principle before you of the rarity of actual cerebritis in essential disease. Also that when it does occur it is in most cases specific and reactive, and as such, not to be treated as a simple primary inflammation. You will do well to study Dr. Collins' history of the epidemic of cerebro-spinal fever in Dublin—the so-called "cerebro-spinal arachnitis"—and you will perceive, I do not doubt, that the condition of the brain and spinal cord was strictly analogous to that of the ordinary secondary diseases in typhus and typhoid fevers; that it bore the same relation to the essential malady; and that in all things—treatment included—there was an analogy between the local and predominant affections of these forms of disease. They differed only as to symptoms referable to the organs which bore the weight of the secondary malady, and agreed in inconstancy of occurrence, variety in degree, and incompetency of the local phenomena to account for the general symptoms.

A key to the treatment of delirium is to be obtained by having regard mainly to two considerations. First, the period of the case at which this symptom is developed. The earlier the period, the greater the chance of relief by remedial measures, such as the cold affusion and leeching. Secondly, the presence, the degree, or the absence of signs of active hyperæmia of the brain.

Now, the symptom may be actively developed at an early period, making it probable that it is still of toxic and functional origin; or it may occur at a more advanced stage, when—if signs of active determination to the head be present—it may be supposed that reactive irritation is already set up. It is in this latter condition that Dr. Hudson advocates the practice of arteriotomy, but this measure is seldom necessary if leeches are judiciously used, and the cold affusion or the application of ice to the head properly carried out.

Ice is especially useful under such circumstances. I remember attending a professional man, who with a very large head was of a highly nervous and choleric temperament. He had a well-marked typhus fever with severe cerebral symptoms, such as frequently-violent delirium, long-continued want of sleep, and extreme heat of the head. Leeches had been freely applied, and followed by shaving the scalp and cold affusion. I recommended the application of ice in the way I have detailed to you. There had been no sleep for several days and nights. A proper supply of ice having been obtained, his wife commenced to move the sponge with ice slowly and steadily round and round and over the great head. The patient at once became quiet, and soon fell into tranquil sleep. So long as the application was continued he remained asleep, but awoke suddenly and delirious whenever from fatigue his wife rested her arm. In this way he used to get continuous sleep for half an hour or an hour. For three days and three nights she hardly ever intermitted her labour of love, and might be seen kneeling at the bedside while a cloud of vapour was rising from the head. Her unwearied efforts were rewarded, and her husband recovered.

The devotion of woman is truly wonderful. In another case—one of putrid typhus fever—the disease, from the condition of the skin and the discharges, was of a most loathsome nature, and the patient, also a medical man, in his wild delirium could not be kept in bed unless his wife undressed and lay down beside him. This, I ascertained, she continued to do during the long course of the disease, for in this way alone could any sleep be obtained. At our daily visit this lady received us in a fresh and elegant morning costume. She too had her well-earned reward, and we cannot doubt that her noble indifference to personal risk went far to protect her in the dreadful exposure to contagion. A lesson taught us is that contagion is one thing, the state of receptivity of the body another.

Gentlemen, you will learn many things in your future practice besides medicine, and will be taught what a woman will do when the object of her love lies prostrate in disease, in shame, in sorrow, or in madness. This is indeed the bravery of devotion. In one of the Ballads of the Cid, he is represented as rescuing from death by drowning a leper whom none of his train would approach. He mounts him on his horse, brings him to a place of refuge, and even shares his bed with him at night. He is awakened by a sensation as if a sword passed through him, to find his companion gone. Soon afterwards the room is suddenly filled with light, and the holy Lazarus stands effulgent by his side, bringing a message from the Throne of God, that all honour will be given to him in this world, death in victory, and life eternal in the world to come.

The form of delirium I have just been speaking of is that accompanied by high arterial tension and other active symptoms. If, on the other hand, such signs are wanting, you must be very cautious in bleeding locally, or even in the application of cold. An opposite line of treatment is in this case generally indicated. If we have delirium, even violent, without heat, fulness, or increased arterial action, the treatment by leeching and cold may be in the highest degree dangerous. This we have often witnessed in pure delirium tremens, and in the frequent affection in Dublin called "the whiskey-fever," when these are combated by depletion of the head.

It is now many years since I was called to see a Polish officer in an advanced stage of typhus fever. He had been very delirious, and at my visit I found him with his shaven head covered by a bladder of ice, while in each axilla a large mass of ice was fixed, and his hands were clasped as in prayer. He was perfectly pale, and with great feebleness of pulse; but he recognized me, and turning towards me he mournfully said, "I think I am one of the lost ones." I need not say the ice was all removed, warm and dry clothing supplied, while wine and nourishment were given. The result of the change of treatment was in every way satisfactory.

In administering stimulants in delirium you must in every case begin tentatively, watching their effect from hour to hour. The chief indications for their employment are the nature and the advanced period of the fever, the absence of signs of *active* determination to the head, the want of vigour in the heart as to its impulse and the intensity of its sounds, and, lastly, the age and previous history of your patient.

16

With regard to this last point, you will remember what I have said in a former lecture as to the sanative influence of stimulants so often observed in patients of previously temperate habits.

The question of the exhibition of sedatives in delirium may fitly be considered in connection with the treatment of INSOMNIA, or SLEEP-LESSNESS, to which I would now bespeak your attention. The symptom is frequently one of the most serious, troublesome, and unmanageable of the evidences of nervous derangement in fever. It is sometimes combated successfully by such measures as have been already considered—namely, moderate leeching, the cold affusion, and the application of ice. In cases where the bowels are confined with more or less tympany, Dr. Hudson states that the best effects were produced by the administration of a full dose of turpentine. I have myself observed a like result follow the relief of some local distress in a distant part of the body. A man in advanced fever, who had been sleepless and very delirious, was found to labour under a distended bladder. The catheter was at once passed, and an immense quantity of urine drawn off. Very shortly the delirium ceased and the patient fell asleep.

It remains for us to speak of sedatives in fever.

In seeking for a guide as to the exhibition of opium you will find assistance in observing the state of the eye, for the contracted or " pin-hole" pupil seems to be more closely related to active hyperæmia of the brain than the natural or dilated one. Still, the condition of the pupil is not an absolutely certain guide, and cases are recorded in which an opiate acted well notwithstanding its contraction. This sign also may be present in one eye and absent in the other. Speaking generally, it is far safer in fever to give opium in small and repeated doses than to venture upon a large single dose. It may be advantageously combined with antimony, as advocated by Dr. Graves, not so much as an antiphlogistic or eliminative agent, but as a direct means of increasing the hypnotic influence of opium. This appears to be one of those therapeutic results, the explanation of which, like that of many others relating to the action of medicine, is so far involved in obscurity. Dr. Graves used to prescribe a mixture containing four grains of tartar emetic and a drachm of tincture of opium in eight ounces of camphor water. A tablespoonful of this was given every second hour until the desired effect was produced. The efficacy of the remedy in his hands was most remarkable ; and in the number of the *Dublin Quarterly Journal* for August, 1849, Dr. Robert Law bears his testimony to the value of this treatment.[1]

[1] Second Series, vol. viii. p. 63.

Tartar emetic and opium are in general indicated in those cases of even high delirium, with sleeplessness, where the head is cool and the action of the heart is not vigorous.

Other sedatives which you will find of use in fever are the tincture of hyoscyamus, bromide of potassium, and chloral. With respect to the last-named remedy, I would caution you against giving too large a dose at once. In fever ten or fifteen grains of the hydrate of chloral are generally sufficient to produce the wished-for effect, and if this dose fails it can be repeated after a lapse of one or two hours. The remedy is of especial value in the management of many cases of simple delirium tremens. In this disease it may be employed in moderate and repeated doses if necessary.

You will occasionally find that wine has a well-marked calming and sedative effect in fever. A patient who has been restless, sleepless, and delirious will sometimes become quiet and fall asleep after the administration of a little wine. This occurs where the nervous symptoms are probably due to an anæmic or spanæmic condition of the brain associated with a weak heart and a flagging circulation.

CONVULSIONS in fever are among the most formidable complications of the disease, more particularly so when they occur in its advanced stages. Under the term "convulsions" may be included a group of phenomena varying from slight *subsultus tendinum* and *floccitatio*, or picking at the bed-clothes, to the most violent and general perturbation of the muscular system. These symptoms in a more advanced stage of the fever are often attributed to uræmic poisoning, and there can be no doubt that there is frequently disturbance referable to the urinary organs. You will see in Dr. Hudson's work[1] a quotation from Sir Dominic Corrigan in reference to the importance of attention to the relieving of the bladder. Sir Dominic shows that daily attention to the state of the bladder is imperatively necessary, and that the catheter should be employed in retention of urine with or without dribbling. In truth, you must not trust to any report from the nurse as to the existence or absence of retention, for often, although a large quantity of water may have been passed, the bladder will be found greatly distended. This state may have been preceded by suppression, and it sometimes happens that the return of the secretion is attended by an enormous flow, especially when this occurs at a critical time of the fever. In such a case it will be right for you to re-visit the patient within an hour or two after catheterism, when you may be surprised to find the bladder again over-distended.

[1] Lectures on the Study of Fever, second edition, p. 183.

The amount of distension is sometimes extraordinary. "I saw not long since, in private practice," says Sir Dominick Corrigan, in speaking of the necessity of attending to the bladder in fever, "another case illustrating the same point. In this case the patient was a lady under the care of a homœopath. You know a homœopath would not use a catheter. It was on the fifteenth or sixteenth day of fever. I found her in epileptic convulsions, which had continued for some hours, foaming at the mouth, insensible, unable to swallow, and, to all appearance, dying. On examining the abdomen, I felt the bladder extending up as high as the umbilicus. On introducing the catheter, it was scarcely possible to bear the intolerable ammoniacal smell of the urine, which must have been shut up for several days. It continued to flow until some large basinfuls were drawn off. This patient recovered, but she suffered much from the neglect. Subacute and then chronic cystitis followed, under which she continued to suffer for more than a year afterwards."

In connection with the presence of uræmia in fever we have observed the urine in such cases to effervesce briskly on adding a dilute acid, and I have already mentioned a case of extreme subsultus in which the cerebral sinuses and the veins of the pia mater contained air in considerable quantity.

The most long-continued and violent attack of convulsions I ever witnessed was in the case of a student of this hospital, who had gone on to the thirteenth day of fever. The distended bladder could be felt; but such was the violence of the convulsions, attended with extraordinary priapism, that all attempts at catheterism were futile. It was also impossible to get the patient to swallow anything, or to use an enema, and under these desperate circumstances we determined to employ chloroform inhalation. The greatest difficulties attended the administration, but at last the effect was produced. The convulsions ceased like magic, and suddenly a jet of urine sprang upwards to a great height from the still erect penis; the stream continuing to flow until the bladder was empty, when the priapism disappeared.

We see, therefore, that, where the uræmic condition and its accompanying convulsions depend on mere *retention* of urine, we have a ready and efficacious remedy in careful and judicious evacuation of the bladder by the catheter.

But in *suppression* of urine our treatment must be different. Dry-cupping freely employed over the kidneys, the diligent application of poultices and sinapisms in the same region, the use of diluents, and the exhibition of a combination of nitre with the spirit of nitrous ether, are the measures in which you are to place most confidence.

It is also necessary to keep the bowels open by turpentine enemata, and the action of the skin may be stimulated by sponging with tepid vinegar and water and subsequent rubbing with a dry towel.

LECTURE XXXIII.

PHLEGMASIA ALBA DOLENS—The swelling is not always painful, or white in appearance—Symmetry of the affected limb not lost—Professor Trousseau's views as to the etiology of the affection—Phlegmasia (1) of puerperal women, (2) in scrofulous and (3) cancerous cachexiæ—Pulmonary *embolism* caused by phlegmasia—Case of phlegmasia after typhus fever—TREATMENT of the affection—GENERAL CONCLUSION.

GENTLEMEN, you may remember my mentioning to you that a continued rapidity of pulse after the other constitutional symptoms of fever had subsided was to be taken, not—as suggested by Laennec —as a sign that the heart had been weakened, but rather as showing the existence of some acute organic change attended with irritation. I mentioned as examples of these changes two pathological conditions—one, the acute and sometimes general development of tubercle; and the other, that form of disease to which the name of PHLEGMASIA DOLENS, or PHLEGMASIA ALBA DOLENS, has been given.

We shall by-and-by examine how far the term "phlegmasia" is properly applied; and, although the disease is commonly more or less painful, it may occur so free from local suffering that its discovery is accidental; and so, as I have already shown, the adjective "dolens" is not always applicable. Again, in place of the swelling being colourless, the entire limb may be covered with deep purplish-blue arborescent stainings, so that the remaining portion of the term is not always appropriate. This, however, is less often met with than the absence of pain. The pain, too, may be singularly localized; thus, in a case which was under the care of an eminent physician, the pain was confined to the sciatic notch. The disease was held to be merely sciatica, and the actual cautery ordered to be applied over the nerve. In preparing to effect this the assistant accidentally exposed the opposite extremity, when he was struck by its comparative emaciation, and the real nature of the case was at once revealed.

This illustrates an interesting circumstance, which we have often observed—namely, that, though the swelling of the limb may be general, it has little if any effect on the symmetry of the part. The limb is simply larger and fuller than the opposite extremity, so that it is often only by comparison that the morbid enlargement is recognized. I detailed to you a case in which symptoms of intermittent fever, which, however, was then epidemic, were present and exasperated by the use of quinine. Here the discovery of the nature of the disease was due solely to an accidental comparison of the lower extremities. The patient was not conscious of the existence of any enlargement or pain in the limb.

It is probable that this remarkable appearance of symmetry of the affected limb occurs more frequently when the disease is a sequela of fever than in other cases. Thus Professor Trousseau,[1] in speaking of its occurrence in tubercular and cancerous cachexiæ, refers to the irregular form assumed by the painful œdema in these affections.

In his lectures the same great clinical teacher dwells on phlegmasia alba dolens as a result of puerperal fever, and also mentions its occurrence in typhus and in typhoid fevers.

He inclines to the opinion that it results rather from a condition of the blood predisposing to coagulation in the veins, and their consequent obstruction, than to primary phlebitis. The result is what he denominates "painful œdema," which disappears either by the establishment of a collateral circulation or by the resolution of the clot. He gives some important facts showing that the existence of a phlegmasia abla dolens may have an important influence in the diagnosis of visceral cancer.

You may now ask how far the term "phlegmasia" is applicable to this disease, or whether the coagulation of blood in the veins is not the first step of the local malady, while the inflammatory condition is secondary and reactive. Certain it is that when a cordy and painful state of the veins, such as the femoral or saphena, exists, the moderate use of leeches over the vessel is advisable. This is true at least in the case where the disease occurs as a sequela of fever, and it is on this that our observations are based.

Now, whether phlegmasia occurring in puerperal woman is or is not due to the presence of uterine phlebitis and the extension of inflammatory action along the veins, producing obstruction of them, may be a question ; but that actual primary or traumatic phlebitis is capable of obstructing a vein so as to cause painful œdema—in other words, phlegmasia dolens—appears from a case which occurred some years ago in our wards. It was of a patient labouring under an acute attack of visceral inflammation who was bled from the arm. The operator used a rusty and blunt lancet. The arm became painful and

[1] Clinical Medicine, vol. v. lect. xcv. New Syd. Soc. Translation.

tender along the course of the median basilic vein above and below the bend of the elbow. There was no swelling, but the type of fever changed to an asthenic form, attended by sweating and anxiety, so that the state of pyæmia was apprehended. This having continued for a few days, the arm suddenly swelled from above the elbow downwards, and presented all the characters of phlegmasia alba dolens. The constitutional symptoms subsided, and the patient gradually recovered.

Now, you know that ordinary phlegmasia dolens is seldom a fatal disease, a fact which may be accounted for by assuming that, as in the cachexiæ, the coagulation of the blood is the principal morbid condition, or that it acts in preventing the blood-poisoning by the localization of phlebitis. Be this as it may, it seems certain that the danger is inversely as the amount of swelling. I believe that in the case I have just now detailed suppurative inflammation of the vein was about to commence when coagulation put an end to further absorption.

In connection with this point I may notice that in certain forms of visceral irritation the bulk of the affected organ is greatly augmented. And it may be that this is caused by œdema, the result of venous obstruction. Thus in a case of croupous or plastic pneumonia which was brought before the Pathological Society of Dublin by Professor Robert William Smith the enlargement of the affected lung was so considerable as to simulate empyema ; the side was much dilated and the liver depressed. Every air-cell seemed to be filled with minute granular fibrinous bodies, of which thousands were obtainable by washing the cut surface of the lung.

Trousseau has shown that the principal condition in the phlegmasia dolens is coagulation of blood in some venous trunk, and not, as has been held, an affection of the lymphatics. In this hospital we have verified his statement of freedom of the lymphatics and glands in the groin. You will do well to study his 95th lecture, in which, in addition to an exhaustive pathological account of the disease, he shows that, in the cachexiæ generally, hæmatologists[1] have established that there is a diminution of the red globules and an augmentation of the fibrin and serum of the blood. This condition predisposes to a spontaneous coagulation, the tendency to which we may well suppose to be still further increased by the presence of any phlebitic irritation.

I have told you that Trousseau explains the frequency of phleg-

---

[1] Andral et Gaverret, Récherches sur les Modifications des Proportions des quelques Principes du Sang dans les Maladies. Paris, 1842.

masia in the cancerous and tubercular cachexiæ by a reference to this fibrinous and leucæmatous condition of the blood, and it is more than probable that its occurrence as a sequela of fever depends on the same cause. In further support of this view I may recall the fact, also noticed by Trousseau, that phlegmasia is more common after enteric than after typhus fever, the longer duration of the former tending to modify the constitution of the blood to a greater degree. There can be little doubt also that the local abdominal irritation so common in the advanced stages of enteric fever, like the uterine irritation in cases of *phlegmasia puerperarum*, acts as an exciting cause in the presence of such a deteriorated condition of blood.

Viewing the question again from another point, it may be held that the affection following fever is the result rather of a state of blood predisposing to coagulation than of an original phlebitis. It has been observed that there is often little, if any, increase of local temperature, and the disease appears to differ from the secondary affections of fever in not presenting any well-marked signs of periodic retrocession. Still, as I have said, in cases where at an early period a cordy state of the femoral or saphena veins—accompanied by tenderness—exists, the application of a few leeches along the course of the vessels, fomentations, poultices, and the moderate use of opium are followed by good effects.

Professor Trousseau also alludes to the occurrence of pulmonary *embolism* in phlegmasia dolens in the male subject, showing that spontaneous coagulation may be developed in the saphena, crural, or any other vein, and remain limited to a very small extent of the vessel. He observes that generally the migratory clot reaches the lung, causing dyspnœa and rapid death by apnœa; but he believes that in certain exceptional cases the clot may be arrested in the right auricle or ventricle of the heart. He says that, in accordance with the predisposition of the patient and the volume of the clot, the phenomena which belong to syncope will be observed; the heart, surprised, so to speak, by the arrival of the migratory clot, will at once cease to beat with regularity and power, and ere long contractions will entirely cease. In these cases death will take place by syncope—by "arrest" of the heart—in fact, the prolonged syncope leads to death.

I have sometimes thought that this form of syncope was induced less by the "surprise" of the heart than by the sudden cutting off of the blood supply from the left ventricle. A case was some years ago presented to the Pathological Society of Dublin in which symptoms of heart disease were at last followed by a sudden and fatal syncope.

An indurated coagulum of a spherical form had entered the funnel-shaped sinus described by Mr. Adams, and completely occluded the left auriculo-ventricular opening, thus absolutely and suddenly cutting off the blood supply from the left ventricle.

Before I conclude this lecture I will read the notes of a very interesting case of the affection which has been engaging our attention. The subject of it was a pupil of Dr. Graves and myself at this hospital, who for many years since has enjoyed an extensive practice in the country. The facts of the case are given in the gentleman's own words. He says :—

For a great part of the years 1827, 1828, and 1829, I acted as clinical clerk to you and our lamented friend Dr. Graves in the Meath Hospital, during the protracted continuance of an epidemic of typhus fever, which we cannot easily forget. My principal business was to ascertain, as far as possible, the critical days of the fever, in the investigation of which you and Dr. Graves were deeply interested at the time. In this occupation it was my duty to spend several hours every day at the bedside of patients in all stages of the fever, and my immunity from contagion for so long a period led me to imagine that I had become absolutely *fever-proof;* but I was destined to be undeceived.

One morning in June, 1829, Dr. Graves called the attention of the class to a remarkable instance of *calor mordax* in a female patient. Of course there was a rush of the pupils to witness this unusual phenomenon, myself amongst the foremost. I had no sooner laid my hand on the burning skin of the patient's arm than I was conscious, by a sudden thrill or shock through my whole frame, that I was stricken by fever. That day and the next constituted the period of incubation. I was not actually ill, but I was languid, uncomfortable, listless—out of sorts in every way. On the third day I had a rigor, followed by an intense pain in the head, with nearly all the usual characteristics of typhus, including a full crop of petechiæ. (It is worthy of notice, however, that neither in this nor in several subsequent fevers had I ever the slightest delirium.) On the twenty-first day from the rigor I appeared to have a crisis, and a terrible crisis it was. I was suddenly seized with violent pain, apparently in the left hip-joint, and gradually extending to the leg and foot. The whole limb became swollen and glazed, presenting all the appearance of a leg affected with *phlegmasia dolens*, as no doubt it was. The pain was excessive and almost intolerable. For fourteen nights the most powerful opiates which could be safely administered failed to procure sleep, though they served, in some degree, to alleviate pain.

After about three weeks of acute suffering—six weeks from the commencement of the fever—I was enabled to leave my bed. But the swelling of the limb remained, and it was evident that there was permanent hypertrophy of the cellular substance. In all likelihood I was doomed to have a thick leg for life. For many years, too, I continued to have more or less pain in the hip, always increased by exercise. Some short time after my recovery from the fever the veins of the affected leg became varicose, and I had a varicose ulcer which remained open for nearly two years. This, however, was healed under the influence of country air and consequently improved health, and it has never returned. Once—about twenty years ago—a vein burst, and I lost a considerable quantity of blood. Since then I have persistently worn a bandage, and the veins have given me little further trouble. No special remedies were adopted for the reduction of the swelling of the leg; but on one occasion Dr. Graves hesitatingly suggested a line of treatment to which, as it involved an undesirable contingency, I demurred.

I now come to a curious and interesting phase of the history of this thick leg. You recollect that the swelling of the leg appeared to be a sequela of *one* typhus fever. Exactly *thirty-one years* afterwards—that is to say, in June, 1860—I had *another* typhus fever, when you and Dr. Hudson kindly came to the country to visit me. (*How* I came to pick up this well-marked maculated typhus I never could divine. There was no epidemic fever of any description in the neighbourhood, nor had I seen a case of typhus for seven years.) Well, the result of *this* fever was to restore my thick leg to its original dimensions. There was no marked crisis. After two or three weeks of extreme danger, in which my life hung by a thread, the fever gradually subsided, and disappeared by the twenty-seventh or twenty-eighth day, leaving the affected leg as slim and emaciated as its fellow; and the hypertrophy has never since reappeared.

But this is not all. In the spring of the present year (1873) I had a severe attack of influenza, from the effects of which I have not even yet recovered. After two or three months of delicate health, during which my professional engagements prevented my having change of air, a blush of redness appeared over the middle third of the tibia of the varicose leg, accompanied by tingling pain, tenderness to the touch, and slight œdema of the leg. The redness gradually increased from day to day in extent and intensity, and from its upper margin a well-defined dark red line extended to the knee, where it abruptly terminated. Under the use of bark and iodide of potassium the redness and tumefaction subsided, and I then detected a hard ridge, apparently bony, and about three-fourths of an inch in length, on the inside surface of the tibia. At first I attributed these symptoms to *periostitis*; but when the œdema had almost entirely disappeared, I discovered that the "ridge" which I had believed to be bony was *not* bone at all, but a portion of obliterated vein like a piece of hard whip-cord and movable under the finger. Was this an attempt at a natural cure? I sometimes fancy that the varicose veins have diminished in fulness and bulk, though it may be *only* fancy.

Before I conclude I may be permitted to refer to a couple of facts which bear upon the vexed question of *a change of type* in fever and other diseases.

1. I was never strong or robust, and at the commencement of my first typhus fever, at the age of twenty-three, my health had been impaired by arduous study and close attendance on patients in a hospital atmosphere. And yet the treatment—which I maintain was *at that time* the correct and proper treatment—would not be adopted at the present day. After an unsuccessful attempt by poor Dan Pakenham (the worthy apothecary of the Meath Hospital) to open my temporal artery, a dozen leeches were applied for the relief of the pain of my head; and during the whole progress of this petechial fever I obstinately and successfully refused to swallow wine or any other stimulant whatever. Again, after twenty-one days' reduction of strength by typhus, and when phlebitis set in, I had a hundred leeches, in two relays, applied to the painful hip—without much apparent benefit, I admit, but still without killing me or causing any perceptible injury. What would happen under similar circumstances *now?*

2. I was placed under much more favourable circumstances when, at the age of fifty-four, I was attacked by my second typhus fever. I had previously been in good health, and was residing in pure country air. Never-

theless it was only by the continuous and lavish administration of stimulants —alcoholic and diffusive—that my life was saved. I offer no comment; is comment needed?

In this very remarkable case there are two circumstances of peculiar interest. One of these is the undoubted occurrence of a second typhus fever in the same individual after a long lapse of time, the malady setting in, in the absence of any of its presumed exciting causes; the other, the fact that the tumefaction of the limb, which had been of many years' standing, completely subsided during the second fever. It is also worthy of note that last year my friend's health had not been so good, as a result of which a cachectic condition of blood was established, and determined venous coagulation in the leg. At least this would seem to be the probable explanation of the recent attack of irritation and coagulation in the vein of the leg.

The treatment of this affection is sufficiently simple, and I have given you an outline of it as regards local measures. In the advanced stages the exhibition of iron is often most useful, the preparation on which I would specially place reliance being the "ferrum tartaratum."

In conclusion I would caution you against a possible error of diagnosis. In phlegmasia, when the œdema in lessening loses a certain condition of tension, the local sensation of fluctuation singularly simulates that of an abscess, even one near the surface. This is often more or less localized, and the surgeon who neglects the history of the case and the attending phenomena may commit the error of taking a diffused œdema for a localized purulent collection. I have known an operation to be performed in two situations in the same extremity ; fortunately no bad result followed. A similar condition more commonly observed is where parotid swellings form in connection with the eruptive fevers. I have seen deep incisions performed on the same occasion at both sides of the neck in cases where the sense of fluctuation solely was relied on. One patient died of oozing hemorrhage under these circumstances, the bleeding setting every treatment at defiance. A fact such as this will show you that the caution I give is not unnecessary.

GENTLEMEN,—We have now gone over the principal facts connected with the great subject of fever and its treatment, and have been much occupied with the local affections referable to one or more of the large cavities; but I trust that the junior members of the class will not imagine that, as a rule, they are to put all the recommendations given into force in any one case, or that I would encourage any meddlesome or complicated treatment in fever.   There are cases in which you will have to change your hand several times in the course of the disease; but the worst kind of physician is the man who, from his own timidity or want of confidence in himself, is constantly changing his treatment and interfering with his case.   You may still meet such practitioners—I regret to say it, too frequently—physicians, who have not learned to look at fever as a whole, who do not recognize the law of its spontaneous subsidence, or the great fact—especially as regards the nervous conditions—that the toxic state is to be looked to more than any supposed organic change.

I remember a case of bad cerebral typhus attended by a gentleman who every day made a new diagnosis, and who at last gravely assured me that he had come to the conclusion that there existed *acute inflammation of the hippocampus major !*

You must engrave on your minds that fever, although often showing secondary functional or organic anatomical change, may run its course without such complications.   In these simple, or so to speak normal, cases you have to see only that the patient is placed in the best condition as regards ventilation, cleanliness, and fitting nourishment; that stimulants are given when indicated; and that the state of the bladder and bowels is attended to.   Should symptoms of local suffering occur, you are to meet them—at least in the first instance—as signs of functional rather than of organic disease, and seek to relieve them at the least expense to the system.   You will remember what has been so often impressed on you here and in the wards—always to consider the *epidemic character;* and that in fever danger arises from debility—often an early effect of the poison; or, on the other hand, from the varied and inconstant forms of the secondary functional and organic conditions.

To conclude, it would appear that the more fever and its effects are studied—whether at the bedside or in the dead body—the less importance will be attached to anatomical change.   It is to the varying condition of innervation and of the chemico-vital states of the fluids that the great phenomena of Continued Fever are to be referred.

In relation to the weighty question of *prognosis,* you will ever remember that the course of a fever will be favourable in direct proportion to the absence of anomalous circumstances—even though individually these may indicate freedom from disease.

APPENDIX B.

The following observations have been furnished me by my colleague, Dr. A. W. Foot, as bearing upon the subject of the use of the thermometer in fever in our medical wards.

The thermometer has been in daily use in the medical wards of the Meath Hospital for many years. Its value as a reliable clinical aid in the diagnosis and prognosis of acute disease, especially in essential fever, has been established as fully as it has wherever else this instrument has been habitually employed.

During the past three years, 1871, 1872, 1873, 9248 observations on the temperature of the sick have been made in the medical wards. The observations are made twice daily, at or about 9 A. M , and 9 P. M., by the clinical assistants, the practising pupils in charge of the cases, or the physician on duty, and are recorded on the clinical charts of temperature published by Harvey and Reynolds of Leeds.

Of the 9248 observations 3696 were upon cases of typhoid and typhus fever; the remainder were upon cases of simple continued fever, scarlatina, measles, variola (1026 observations), lung diseases, erysipelas, cerebral fever, etc.

Of the 3696 observations on typhoid and typhus fever, 2649 were upon typhoid and 1047 on typhus fever. It has to be observed that there has been during the three years above mentioned—1871, 1872, 1873—much less demand than usual for the admission of " fever" patients—in part perhaps owing to the intercurrence of the smallpox epidemic.

The 2649 observations in typhoid fever were made upon 70 cases. The highest temperature registered among these was 107.2° Fahr., and the lowest temperature 94° Fahr.

On 27 occasions temperatures of 105° Fahr. or upwards were registered in typhoid fever in 15 patients, and of the 15 patients in whom the temperature, on one or more occasions reached 105° Fahr. or upwards, five died. On four of these cases whose illnesses had been marked by high temperature *post-mortem* examinations were made.

(*a*) A girl aged 16, temperature on 30th morning 107.2° Fahr., died on the 31st evening. Her mean temperature (51 observations) during the 26 days she was in hospital was 103.1° Fahr.

The morning temperature, 107.2°, was coincident with severe rigors, preceded by violent pain in the abdomen, ushering in peritonitis, not due to perforation, but to propagation outwards of the irritation arising from numerous and extensive ulcerations of the intestinal glands.

(*b*) A female, aged 24, who died on the afternoon of the 36th day. Her average temperature was 102.1° Fahr., but did not exceed 105.2° Fahr. There were 17 patches of ulceration in the last 53 inches of the ileum, pleuro-pneumonia of the right side with exudation of plastic lymph and sero-fibrinous fluid in the right pleural cavity.

(*c*) A female, aged 20, who died on the 36th day, with most extensive ulceration of both solitary and agminated follicles of the ileum. Her mean temperature (45 observations) during the 28 days she was in hospital was 102.3°.

(*d*) A lad, aged 16, who died on the 15th evening of his illness after repeated intestinal hemorrhages. The mean temperature (14 observations) during the seven days he was in hospital was 103.5°.

(*e*) A young man, aged 18, who died on the 15th evening. On the 9th evening his temperature reached 105.8°. He was of intemperate habits, and had albumen in the urine. The mean of 16 observations on his temperature during the eight days he was in hospital was 104° Fahr. In this case a *post-mortem* examination was not obtained.

Cases have proved fatal in which the mean temperature was not very high, especially under two circumstances—great protraction of the fever, and the collapse consequent upon perforation. Of this latter kind two examples have been verified by *post-mortem* examination.

(*a*) A man, aged 40, brought into hospital in collapse on the 10th day of illness, and who lived until the morning of the 16th day. The mean of 12 observations during the six days he was in hospital was 99.5° Fahr. His temperature on admission was 97° Fahr. ; the highest it reached in hospital was 100.8° Fahr.

(*b*) A man, aged 27, brought to hospital on the 8th day of illness, and who died on the 11th morning. His mean temperature during the four days, or part of four days, he was under observation was 100.2° Fahr.; the lowest point he reached was 97.7° Fahr.

In contrast with the two preceding cases is the case of a boy aged 18, who was brought to hospital in a state of collapse from perforation, and who only survived his admission 40 hours; the mean of three observations showed an average temperature of 103.7° Fahr.

In these three cases the intestinal perforation was discovered after death, and in each case fecal extravasation had taken place.

The extremely low temperature of 94° Fahr. was observed in a young woman, aged 24, upon the 24th morning of her illness. She was under observation during the whole course of her illness, as she got typhoid fever while under treatment in the medical wards for a different affection. She recovered, but had a long fever. Her chart was discontinued on the 46th day. She had during convalescence several abscesses over the sacro-iliac articulation, which were evacuated by aspiration.

Mistrusting the accuracy of the practising pupils' observation, I repeated it myself at 9½ A. M., and found the temperature of the axilla, with every precaution to secure accuracy, and with a correct instrument, to be 94°. The body felt cold and clammy like that of one taken out of water; cutis anserina was most strongly marked ; she had no new abdominal symptom ; the pulse was 88, regular, and easily felt at the wrist ; the respiration 26. The collapse came on early in the morning ; the temperature on the previous evening had been 101.6° Fahr., the pulse 101. She was quite conscious and sensible, felt cold, but had no pain anywhere ; there was a tendency to vomit. She had not been taking any antipyretic medicine. The temperature began to rise from noon, and by 9 P. M. had risen 6.2° Fahr. higher than it had been in the morning. This sudden collapse was never accounted for. The highest temperature recorded among 70 observations made on her case was 105.5° on the 12th evening.

Among 1047 observations made upon 43 cases of typhus the highest temperature recorded was 106° Fahr. On twelve occasions temperatures of

105° Fahr. or upwards were observed in the cases of eight patients, four males and four females. Of these eight cases in which temperatures of 105° Fahr. or upwards were observed, two died: one—that above alluded to—in which the temperature reached 106° on the 16th evening, was a man, aged 34, affected with well-marked sclerosis of the posterior columns of the spinal cord (autopsy made); the other was a man of bad constitution, and 43 years of age, who succumbed on the 14th day.

Deaths from typhus of course occurred in cases whose temperature did not reach 105° Fahr., other lethal conditions being in operation. For example, a boy, aged 17, died on the 10th evening of typhus caught during a convalescence from scarlatina, which in its turn had followed closely in the footsteps of typhoid fever. He had been exposed to infection in a fever hospital. He was brought to the Meath Hospital desquamating, but covered with a copious typhus eruption; he had epistaxis, hæmaturia, green vomiting, and died in convulsions. His temperature did not exceed 104° Fahr., and was twice in the six days he was under observation as low as 98° Fahr.

The employment of the thermometer has proved of great value in the diagnosis and prognosis of a given case, in distinguishing a factitious from a genuine convalescence, in estimating the severity of a case, in estimating the results of antipyretic treatment, in detecting imposition, as an indicator of complications. The students are soon firmly convinced of the great value and importance of medical thermometry, and the patients have never expressed themselves as in the slightest degree annoyed or fatigued by even the frequent use of the instruments. Its employment is general in the medical wards, and by no means confined merely to cases of acute disease.

INDEX.

ABDOMEN, affections of the, *see* Abdominal symptoms.

Abdominal symptoms in fever, 56, 62, 135 *seq.*, 142 *seq.*, 146 *seq.*
    swelling, 139
    tenderness, 139
    aorta, increased action of, 139
    abscess, 149

Abernethy's chylo-poietic theory of disease, 219

Aborted typhus, 91

Abscess, hepatic, 111, 157
    internal, in yellow fever of 1826–27, 111, 149
    splenic (?), 149
    simulated by the œdema in phlegmasia, 251

Absence of anatomical change in fever, 20
    of symptoms unfavourable, 207

Abuses of the antiphlogistic treatment, 9

Acetate of lead and opium, 229

Acland, Dr., on preventive medicine, 35
    on therapeutical research, 188

Affections, secondary, *see* Secondary affections.

Affusion, cold, 238

Age determining propriety of stimulation in fever, 197

Ague, *see* Intermittent fever.

Alison on change of type in disease, 12
    on coexistence of various species of fever, 52

Alteratives, danger of using, 228

Anœmic condition of organs in fever, 58
    murmurs, 131, 132, 133

Analogy between fevers and toxic diseases, 24 *seq.*
    and tubercle and syphilis, 32
    and increased arterial pulsations in various diseases, 140
    from effects of local depletion, 163, 164, 228

Anatomical character, diseases with an, 22
    change may be absent in fever, 20, 59 *seq.*
    expression for fever, wanting, 56
    local symptoms in fever, 58

Anatomical school, 182; errors of, 182, 183

Anatomy fails to solve the problem of healthy life, 19

Andral's description of French fevers, 67

Annesley, Mr., on adhesive peritonitis, 157

Anster's, Dr., translation of Goethe's Faust, quoted, 19

Anticipative stimulation in fever, 195, 215;
    rules for, 195
    in bronchial affection, 223

Antiphlogistic treatment not always called for in primary inflammation, 5
    abuses of the, 9
    contra-indicated in perforative peritonitis, 234

Aorta, increased action of abdominal, 139
    pulse in patency of the, 140

Aphonia in laryngo-typhus, 106

Appendix A, 40; Appendix B, 253

Arachnitis, cerebro-spinal, 165 *seq.*, 239

Armstrong's theory of fever, 218

Arteriotomy in delirium, 240
    in headache, 238

Asthenic pneumonia, 93

Astringents, 231

BANKS, Dr., on cerebro-spinal fever, 169

Bark, failure of, in intermittent fever, 6, 113

Beatty, Dr., on *frottement* of peritonitis, 158

Beaumont's, Dr., experiments on digestion, 190

Bed-sores, 209; treatment of, 212, 213
    subject to law of periodicity, 210

Belly, *see* Abdomen and Abdominal.

Black vomit, 147

Blane, Sir Gilbert, on mortality in the Peninsular War, 3

Blisters, 225, 226

Blood, characters of the, in phlegmasia dolens, 247

Blood-letting, local, 164, 226, 327, 237

Blood-waste in fever, 120; urohæmatin as a sign of, 120

Boston, North, New York, outbreak of enteric fever at, 46

Brain, Louis' researches on the, in fever, 60 *seq.*, 161
    inflammation of the, *see* Cerebritis.

Brennan's, Dr., receipt to make a fever, 220
    couplet on turpentine, 225

Brinkley, Bishop, problems on contagion, 30

Bromide of potassium, 175

Bronchial affection of fever, 68, 72 *seq.*

17

Bronchial affection of fever described, 73
    not primarily bronchitis. 75
    subject to law of periodicity, 77
    treatment of the, 77. 223 seq.
    simulating phthisis, 78, 79
    associated with weak heart, 223
    muscular fibre, paralysis of, 105, 223
Bronchitis. see Bronchial affection.
Broussais, theory of fever held by, 6, 218
    error of his school, 21 seq., 102, 137, 141, 161, 181, 218, 228
Buffed and cupped blood-clot, 16

CALCULI, bronchial, 83
    Camp fever, 45
Cancerous cachexia, phlegmasia dolens in, 246
Cardiac muscular fibre, weakening of, 105
    affections in fever, 106 seq.
    softening, 117
    excitement, 119, 200
    depression, 121, 200
    murmurs, 131. See Heart.
Catheterism in retention of urine, 243
Cause of fever, proximate, undiscovered, 23
Causes of fever, various, 32, 34, 48. 185
Cerebritis in fever, 162, 222
Cerebro-spinal complications, 159 seq., 165 seq., 178 seq.
    causes of, 164
    fever, 103, 160, 165 seq.; symptoms, 170
    an essential disease, 168
Change of practice in treatment of fever, 10
    of type in disease, 10
    Alison's views on, 12 seq.
    Christison's views on, 12 seq.
    the author's views on, 14 seq
    evidence from symptoms, 14 seq.
        from appearance of drawn blood, 16
        from pathological appearances, 16
        from isolated sthenic cases, 17
        from influence of treatment, 18
Change, anatomical, see Anatomical change.
Changes, local, in fever, nature of the, 64 seq.
Characteristics of fever, 54
Chest, effusion into the, 77, 105
Cheyne, Dr., on hysteria in fever, 177
    on intestinal ulceration in late stage of fever, 63, 79
Chloral in fever, 175, 243
Choice of food in fever, 189
Cholera, first invasion of, coincident with occurrence of change of type in disease, 18
Christison, Sir Robert, on change of type in disease, 12

Classification of diseases, 22 seq.
Clutterbuck's theory of fever, 218
Cold lotions, 237
    affusion, 238
Colles, Mr. Abraham, on simulative ague, 113
Collins, Dr. E., on epidemic of 1867, 166, seq., 239
Complications, see Secondary affections.
Congestions of the lung in fever, 89
Consolidation of lung, treatment of, 226
Consolidations of the lung in fever, 89; critical, 91
    ending in sphacelus, 96
    differential diagnosis of, 97
Constipation, treatment of, 229
Contagion, 23, 27 seq.
    implies essentiality in disease, 28
    arguments in favour of, 29 seq.
    problems on, 30, 31
    in enteric fever, 46
Continued fever, see Fever.
Continuity, diagnosis of internal solutions of, 154
Convalescence, imperfect, 79
Convertibility of zymotic diseases, 39
Convulsions, 243; uræmic, 244
Correlation of zymotic diseases, 39
Corrigan, Sir Dominic, cases of cerebritis in fever, 163
    on attention to the bladder, 243
Crepitus redux absent in resolution of typhous consolidation, 102
Crisis in fever, 92
Critical consolidation of lung, 91, 226
Croly, Mr., on cerebro-spinal fever, 171
Curative contrasted with preventive medicine, 34 seq.
Cusack, Mr., cases of tubercular fever, 88
Cusack, Dr. Samuel, on wine and opium in puerperal fever, 235

DANGER, sources of, to patient, 21, 188, 137
Deglutition, power of, retained, 205, 214
Delirium, Louis' investigations on, 60 seq., 103, 159, 161
    in fever 239; treatment of, 240 seq.
    toxic, 240
    asthenic, 241; stimulants in, 241
Depletion, local, 163, 226, 227, 237
Deposit, specific typhous, 64 seq.
Description of continued fever, 20, 217
Diagnosis in presence of fever, 56, 59, 98
    from want of accordance of phenomena, 82, 134
    of softening of the heart in fever, 134
    of intestinal perforation, 140
    of internal solutions of continuity, 154
Diarrhœa, treatment of, 229; diet in, 231
Digestion, Dr. Beaumont's experiments on, 190
    in fever, 191, 192; influence of rank on, 192
Disease, theories of, 5, 6

Disease, return to sthenic forms of, 17
  vital character of, 18
  sources of danger in, twofold, 21, 188, 195
  classification of, 22 *seq.*
  toxic, 25
  endemic, *see* Endemic disease.
  essential, 29; contagious, 33
    acute, two phases in history of, 33
    correlation of zymotic, 39
    convertibility of zymotic, 39
Dothinenteritis, 136, 137
Dry-cupping, 225, 244
Dublin, epidemics in, 37, 42, 44, 165, 172

ECCHYMOSES, 168
  Eclectic school, 183, 217
Edinburgh, epidemics of fever in, 13
Effusion into the chest, 77, 105
Embolism, pulmonary, in phlegmasia dolens, 248
Emetics in bronchial affections, 224
Empiric, 180
Empiricism, 180
Endemic disease arises independently of contagion, 28
Enemata, nutrient, 214
  aperient, 229
  of turpentine, 230, 245
Enteric fever, 45; contagious, 46
  and typhus contrasted, 45
  causes of, 38; Murchinson on, 38; Sir W. Jenner on, 38; author's views, 38, 39
  resemblances between, and typhus, 50 *seq.*, 135, 208
  and typhus, species, not genera, of fever, 51, 135
Epidemic character, 42, 44, 252
Epidemic of 1826–27, 44, 137, 143, 146
  of 1847, 52
  of 1847, 160, 165, *seq.*
  of 1846, 172
Epidemics of fever in Edinburgh, 13
  in Dublin, 37, 42, 44, 165, 172
  in Stockholm, 130
Epidemics within epidemics, 166
Eruption of rose-spots, 145
Eruptions, 145, 208
Essential disease, *see* Disease.
  fever, 55
Essentialism in fever proved, 44
État poisseux of heart, 107
Excitement of heart in fever, 119
Expectoration of calculi after fever, 83
Eye, condition of the, in fever, 61

FAMINE fever, 52 *seq.*
  Fatty degeneration of heart, slow pulse in, 129
Fear, physical, 3
Febris nigra, 166, 173
Fever, continued, importance of a practical knowledge of, 1

Fever, principle of treatment of, the same in all its forms, 2, 179 *seq.*
  mortality of, in the Peninsular War, 3
  may be the opposite of an inflammation, 5
  described, but not defined, 20, 217
  proximate cause of, as yet undiscovered, 23, 184
  nature of its secondary affections, 26 *seq.*
  causes of, are various, 32, 34 *seq.*, 48
  contagion a cause of, 27 *seq.*
  analogy between, and tubercle and syphilis, 33
  varieties of, dependent on epidemic character, 42
    observed in the same epidemic, 43, and in members of the same family, 43
  resemblances between forms of, 49, 50 *seq.*
  species, not genera, 51, 135
  characteristics of, 54
  no anatomical expression for, 56
  pathological conditions of, 66 *seq.*
  treatment of, change of practice in, 10, 121
  bronchial affection of, 72 *seq.*
  pulmonary affections of, 72 *seq.*
  cardiac affections of, 106 *seq.*; intestinal, 235 *seq.*
  cannot be cut short, 186
  intermittent, *see* Intermittent fever.
  temperatures in [Appendix B], 253
Fever-odour, 197
Fevers, distinctions between, and neuroses, 23
  analogies between, and toxic diseases, 24 *seq.*
  subject to law of periodicity, 23
  causing secondary affections, 23
  transmissible by contagion, 23
  knowledge of, negative, 122
Flint, Dr. Austin, on contagiousness of enteric fever, 46
Floccitatio, 243
Fœtal heart in fever, 124, 128, 199, 203
Food in fever, 188
  Dr. Graves on giving, 188 *seq.*
  choice of, 189; rules for giving, 190
Foot, Dr. A. W., a case of hysteria in fever, 174
  observations on temperature in fever [Appendix B], 253
Fordyce, Dr., definition of fever, 179
Foudroyante, Méningite, 167
Frottement of peritonitis, 158
Functional or nervous local symptoms in fever, 57, 59, 159, 165, 173

GANGRENE of lung, 96, 227
  in epidemic of 1826–27, 147
Gangrenous vesicles, 209
Gastro-catarrhal typhus, 73
Genera of fever do not exist, 51, 135

Geographical variation in form of fever, 67, 206

Goethe, Quotation from, 19; referred to, 184

Gordon, Dr., on cerebro-spinal fever, 166, 168, 171
  and coincident epidemic of measles, 173

Graves, Dr., on causes of epidemics of fever, 36
  of typhus, 37
  on temporary pneumothorax in pneumonia, 101
  on yellow fever of 1826–27, 111, 150, 172
  on treatment of fever, 182; on food in fever, 188
  on nutrient enemata, 214
  on value of turpentine, 225
  on acetate of lead and opium, 229
  on opium in intestinal perforation and peritonitis, 233
  opposed to treatment of perforative peritonitis by antiphlogistics, 234
  on tartar emetic and opium, 242

Grimshaw, Dr., on defective sanitary state of Dublin, 38

Gurgling in ileo-cœcal region, 141

HEMORRHAGE, intestinal, 235; treatment of, 236

Hemorrhagic smallpox, 173

Hardcastle, case of, 206 seq.

Harley, Dr. George, on urobrœmatin as an indication of blood-waste, 120

Harvey's, Dr., advice, 191

Haverty, Mr., on cerebro-spinal fever, 169

Hayden, Dr., observation of tympanitic resonance of lung, 101

Head symptoms in fever, 56, 59 seq., 159 seq.
  treatment of, 237 seq.
  absence of, an indication for use of stimulants, 215
  retraction of, 171
  shaving the, 238

Head-ache, 237; treatment of, 237

Heart, fatty degeneration of, slow pulse in, 129
  chronic failure of the, 196
  escape of, in fever, 200
  arrest of the, in phlegmasia dolens, 248
  in fever, 61, 106 seq., 114 seq., 121 seq., 127 seq., 198 seq.
    not altered except in rate, 115, 118
    weakened after a few days, 116, 199
    excited, 117, 119, 200
    softening of, 117
    depression of, 121, 200; more marked in typhus, 122
    diminution of impulse of, 122 seq., 199
    vermicular impulse of, 123

Heart in fever, diminution of sounds of, 125 seq., 199
  physical signs of, 126, 199
  murmurs of the, 131 seq.

"Heart, fœtal," 124, 128, 199, 203

Hepatic abscess, 111, 157

Hudson, Dr., on tympanitic resonance in typhous consolidation of lung, 99
  cerebritis in fever, 162, 163
  arteriotomy in delirium, 240
  on turpentine in tympanites and sleeplessness, 242

Humoral theory of disease, 5

Huss, Professor, on epidemic of 1841 at Stockholm, 130
  on value of turpentine, 225

Hypercatharsis, danger of, 229

Hysteria in fever, 178 seq.; Dr. Foot's case of, 174
  significance of, 173, 176
  masking diseases, 176
  outbreak of, in fever-ward, 177

ICE, 238; mode of applying, 238, 240

Idiopathic inflammation, 184
  pyœmia, 110; iritis, 184

Ileo-cœcal tenderness, 139
  gurgling, 141

Ileum, ulceration of, 143; latent, 139
  perforation of, 153

Impulse of heart, progressive diminution of, 122, 123, 124, 199
  "vermicular," 123
  effect of position on, 124

Indications for stimulation, 197

Inflammation, erroneous views as to the universality of, 4
  acute febrile diseases may be the opposite of, 5
  primary and antiphlogistic treatment of, 5
  erroneous ideas conveyed by the word, 8
  secondary, in fever, 103, 142, 224
  something the reverse of, 4, 180
  of brain rare in fever, 159
  a cause of nervous symptoms, 164

"Inflammation, healthy," 110

Inflammatory theory of disease, 5, 181
  symptoms in fever, 58

Insomnia, 242

Intermittent fever, 112
  failure of bark in, 6, 113; Mr. Colles on, 113
  mode of origin of, 28
  symptomatic of urinary disease, 113

Intestines, ulceration of the, indicated by quick pulse, 108
  perforation of the, 151 seq.

Intestinal affections, secondary, 135 seq., 142 seq., 146 seq., 227 seq.
  treatment of, 227 seq.
  perforation, 151 seq.; latent, 151
  intussusceptions, 148

Intestinal hemorrhage, 235
Intussusceptions in yellow fever of 1826-27, 148
Involuntary muscular tissue in fever, 117
Iritis, specific and idiopathic, 184

JAIL-FEVER, 45
Jaundice in fever of 1826-27, 147
Jenner, Sir William, causes of enteric fever, 39

KENNEDY, Dr. Henry, on coexistence of various species of fever, 52
on cerebro-spinal fever, 169

LAENNEC on waste of red blood in fever, 120
on phenomena of pneumonia, 95
on softening of the heart, "l'état poisseux," 107, 114
on muscular softening, 118
on error as to quick pulse in convalescence, 108, 245
Laryngeal muscles, paralysis of, 105
Laryngo-typhus of Rokitansky, 104 seq. ; aphonia in, 106
Larynx, inflammation of, 177
Latency of secondary affections, 74, 138
of intestinal perforation, 151
Law of periodicity, 1, 6, 21, 64, 77, 141, 187, 188, 210
interfered with by local irritation, 7, 141, 238
action restored, 238
Law, Dr. Robert, case of softening of spleen, 150
on tartar emetic and opium, 242
Lawrence, Dr., on yellow fever, 148
Leeching, see blood-letting, or depletion.
Levy on cerebro-spinal fever, 167
Liver, see Hepatic.
Local changes in fever are symptomatic, 64
are subject to periodicity, 64
symptoms in fever, 57
functional or nervous, 57
anatomical, 57
secondarily inflammatory, 57
due to anæmic condition of organs, 58
change masked by neighbouring irritation, 153
Lombard's, Dr., views on British fevers, 68
Louis, numerical system of, 29
investigations on delirium, 60 seq., 103, 159, 162
on softening of the heart, 114, 117, 122
Lyons, Dr., on tympanitic resonance of lung, 100
on cerebro-spinal fever, 169

MacDOWEL, Dr. E., affection of the joints, 168
Mackintosh, Dr., on emetics in bronchial affection, 224

MacSwiney, Dr., on cerebro-spinal fever, 169
Malaise in enteric fever, 138
Malignant fever, 45
purpuric fever, 166
smallpox, 173 ; measles, 173
Mayne, Dr., on cerebro-spinal fever of 1846, 172
Measles, malignant, 173
Medicine and surgery, hurtful effects of separation of, 7
preventive, contrasted with curative, 34 seq.
Membranes, mucous, in fever, 66
serous, in fever, 66
Méningite foudroyante, 167
Meningitis, epidemic cerebro-spinal, 166
Mental study, unfavourable effect of, 71, 215
Mistura olei et opii, 230
"Mixed" or "semi-involuntary" muscular fibre in fever, 118
Mucous membranes in fever, 66
Murchison, Dr., on causes of enteric fever, 38
on distinctions of fevers, 52
on rarity of cerebritis in fever, 160
on tentative stimulation, 216
on case of latent peritonitis, 232
on treatment of peritonitis, 235
Murmurs, cardiac, in fever, 131 seq.
more frequent in enteric than in typhus, 131
Muscular softening in fever, 105 seq., 117 seq
rigidity of abdomen, 141

NERVOUS local symptoms in fever, 58, 159, seq.
causes of, 222
Neuroses, 22
distinctions between, and fevers, 23
Nourishment, 188 ; see "Food."
Numerical system of Louis, 29
fallacies of, 216
Nurse-tending, skilled, 214
Nutrient enemata, 214
Nymphomania, 174, 175

ŒDEMA in phlegmasia, simulating abscess, 245
Opisthotonos, 172
Opium, 229, 233 seq., 242
in intestinal perforation, 233
mode of action of, 233
tolerance of, 234
wine and, in puerperal fever, 234

PAGET, Dr., on problems to establish existence of contagion, 31
Paralysis of laryngeal muscles, 105
of bronchial muscles, 105, 228
of cardiac muscles, 105
Parenchymatous structures in fever, 66, 94
Parr, Mr., on turpentine-punch, 225

Patency, aortic, "steel-hammer" pulse in, 140

Pathognomonic physical signs do not exist, 134

Pathological conditions in fever, 66 *seq.*
　of heart in fever, 127

Pathological school, 182

Perforation with peritonitis simulating poisoning, 219

Periodicity, law of, 6, 21, 64, 77, 141, 187, 188, 210

Peristaltic action in perforative peritonitis, 233

Peritoneum, insusceptibility of, to adhesion, 157, 231

Peritonitis, 151 *seq.*; limited, 152
　treatment of, 231
　from eruption of pus, 155, 156
　from perforation, 179

Phlebitis, question of, 246

Phlegmasia dolens, indicated by quick pulse in convalescence, 109, 245 *seq.*
　treatment of, 251
　symmetry of affected limb in, 245
　etiology of, 246
　cases of, 112, 248

Phthisis, rarity of intestinal perforation in, 151
　simulated by bronchial affection, 78, 79
　a sequela of fever, 80

Physical signs, no pathognomonic, 134
　of heart in fever, 126, 199; a guide in stimulation, 201

fear, 3

Physiological theory of disease, 5
　difference between pus and white-blood cell, 157

Physiological school, 182

Physiology, experimental, fallacies attending, 187

Pin-hole pupil, 242

Pneumonia, typhoid, 89
　croupous, or plastic, 247

Pneumonic complication of fever, 89, *seq.*
　forms, 89, 226
　treatment, 226

Pneumo-thorax, 232

Pneumo-typhus, 72

Points of resemblance between forms of continued fever, 49

Poison of fever, a cause of nervous symptoms, 164

Poisoning simulated by internal perforation, 219

Post-mortem appearances in yellow fever of 1826–27, 147

Poulticing, 225, 227

Practice, change of, in treatment of fever, 10

Pratt's, Dr., views on the causation of fever, 41

Preventive medicine, 34 *seq.*; object and scope of, 35
　Dr. Acland on, 35

Principle of treatment of continued fever, 179 *seq.*; the same in all its forms, 2

Prognosis, 252; influence of appearance of vesicles on, 211
　in cardiac affection of fever, 130, 145
　in cerebro-spinal fever, 159, 222

Proximate cause of fever undiscovered, 23

Puerperal women liable to simulative ague, 113
　fever, wine and opium in, 235
　phlegmasia dolens in, 246

Pulmonary affections of fever, 70, 72 *seq.*, 222
　treatment, 226
　embolism in phlegmasia dolens, 248

Pulse not always a guide in fever, 106, 198
　full and bounding, coincidently with weak heart, 107, 198
　slow in convalescence, 107, 129, 204;
　in fatty degeneration, 129
　rapid in convalescence, 108
　weak with excited heart, 119
　"steel-hammer," 140
　lessened rate of, sign of agreement of stimulants, 203

Pulsation, increased arterial, 139

Purpuric fever, 166; smallpox, 173

Pus, escape of, into peritoneum, 155, 156
　vital characters of, 157

Putrefaction, early, in cerebro-spinal fever, 171

Putrid fever, 45

Pyæmia idiopathic, 110; secondary, 142

Pythogenic fever, 39, 45

"QUACK" and "empiric" contrasted, 180
　Quick pulse in convalescence, 108, 245
　its significance, 108
　with tuberculosis, 108
　in secondary intestinal inflammation, 108
　in phlegmasia dolens, 109

RACE, influence of, 67, 206
　Rank, influence of, on symptoms, 71, 197; on choice of food, 192; on giving of stimulants, 215

"Rational school," 182

Reactive local inflammation, 142, 164, 224

"Receipt to make a fever," 220

Receptivity of disease, 26

Relapsing fever, 52 *seq.*
　of 1847–48, 53

Resemblances between forms of continued fever, 49
　typhus and enteric fevers, 50 *seq.*

Resonance, tympanitic, in typhous consolidation of lung, 99 *seq.*

Retention of urine, 178, 243

Retraction of head, 171

Rheumatism, local increased arterial action in, 140
　no specific treatment in, 2, 187

Rigidity of abdominal muscles, 140
　of neck in cerebro-spinal fever, 171

Rokitansky on reactive inflammation, 65
　on broncho-typhus, 69

Rokitansky on pneumo-typhus, 72
    on laryngo-typhus, 104 *seq.*
Rose-spots, 145
Routine systems of practice, 218
Routinism to be deprecated, 216
Rules for giving food in fever, 190
    stimulants in fever, 196, 351
Rutty, Dr., observation on treatment, 45

SANITARY science, 34 *seq*
    Secondary affections of essential dis-
        eases, 20, 21, 56
        of continued fever, 26, 67 *seq.*
            treatment of, 222 *seq.*
            nature of the, 56
        geographical variation of, 67
        seat of, influenced by locality, 70
            by social rank, 71
        alternating, 78
    bronchial affection, 72 *seq.* ; treatment
        of, 223 *seq*
    pneumonic affection, 89 *seq.* ; treat-
        ment of, 225 *seq.*
        its three forms, 95, 96
    cardiac affection, 106 *seq.* ; treatment
        of, 192 *seq.*
    intestinal affection, 135 *seq.* ; treat-
        ment of, 227 *seq.*
    cerebral and nervous affections, 159
        seq. ; treatment of, 63
Sedatives, 242, 243
Sequela of fever, tubercule a, 80, 108 *seq.*
Serous membranes in fever, 66
Shaving the head, 238
Sibson, Dr., on treatment of rheumatic
    fever, 1
Signs, physical, of heart in fever, 126, 199,
    201
Simulative ague, 113
Sleeplessness, 242
    treatment of, 242
Slow pulse in convalescence, 107, 129
        in fatty degeneration of heart,
            129
Smallpox, epidemic of hemorrhagic, 173
    local depletion in, 164
Smith, David, on coexistence of various
    species of fever, 52
Smith, Professor R. W., case of enlarge-
    ment of lung in croupous pneumonia,
    247
Social rank, influence of, on symptoms of
        fever, 71, 197
        on choice of food, 192
Softening of the heart in fever, 107, 114
        begins in left ventricle,
            115, 122
Solidist theory of disease, 5
Sound of heart, diminution of first, 124,
    199
        extinction of first, 125, 199
        relative augmentation of second,
            125
Sounds of heart, diminution of both, 125,
    199

Sounds of heart in fevers, phenomena at-
    tending the, 124 *seq.*
Spasms, 90
Species, not genera, of fever, 51, 135
Specific typhous deposit, 64 *seq.*
    treatment in disease not attainable, 2,
        185
Sphacelus of lung, 96 ; illustrative cases,
    97, 227
Spleen, enlargement of, in 1826-27, 148 ;
    softening of, 150
Splenic abscess, 149
Sponging of skin, 245
Spotted fever, 45, 166
"Steel-hammer" pulse, 140
Sthenic forms of disease, return to, 17
Stillé on nature of cerebro-spinal fever,
    168
Stimulants in fever, 116, 130, 188, 193 *seq.*,
        201 *seq.*, 212 *seq.*
    question of nutrient properties of, 194
    disagreement of, 195, 215
    anticipative use of, 195, 223
        dependent on age and habits,
            196, 215
        heart, 199 *seq*
    signs of agreement of, 202, 215
    necessity for persevering in use of,
        214
    should not be given by routine, 217
    in delirium, 241
Stockholm, epidemic of 1841 at, 130
Stokes, Dr. Whitley, his anecdote of Mr.
    West at Rosetta, 8
    researches on contagion, 30, 33,
        38
Subsultus tendinum, 243
Suppression of urine, 244
Surgery, exclusive study of, to be depre-
    cated, 2
Surgical student advised to study fever, 1
Swelling, abdominal, in fever, 139
        treatment of, 229
Symptoms, latent, 73, 138, 139, 151, 152
    of cerebro-spinal fever, 170
    absence of, an unfavourable feature,
        207
Symptomatic fever, 55, 141
Symptomological school, 6, 181
    theory of disease held by, 6, 181
Syncope, death by, in phlegmasia dolens,
    248
Syphilis, analogy between, and fever, 33
System, numerical, of Louis, 29

TARTAR emetic, dangers of, 224
        and opium, 242
Temperature increased, constant in fever,
    165
Temperatures in fever [Appendix B], 253
Temporal artery, opening of, 238, 240
Tenderness of abdomen, 139
Theories of disease, 5, 6, 218
Therapeutical research, 187
Thermometrical observations in fever, 253
Thirst, 139

Thoracic symptoms in fever, 56, 62, 72 seq., 89 seq.
Timidity from want of bedside experience of fever, 3
Todd, Dr., on secondary pyæmia, 142
  on stimulants in fever, 194
Tongue, the, in fever, 141
Tonics in fever, 130
Toxic diseases, 24
Transfusion of blood, 120
Treatment of fever based on general principles, 2, 131, 179 seq.
  antiphlogistic, not exclusively to be used in primary inflammation, 5
  of typhus and enteric fever, essentially the same, 48
  objects to be sought for in, 48
  of smallpox by local depletion, 164
  no specific treatment, 186
  of the local secondary affections, 222 seq.
  of bronchial affection, 77, 223 seq.
  of intestinal affection, 227 seq.
  of head affection, 237 seq.
  phlegmasia alba dolens, 251
  fever, change of practice in, 10
    by food and stimulants, 188 seq.
Treatment, anticipative, 195
Trousseau, Professor, on phlegmasia alba dolens, 246 seq.
Tubercle, analogy between, and fever, 33
  as a sequela of fever, 80, 108
  acute coexisting, 80
  acute consequent, 81
  consequent softened, 81
  indicated by quick pulse in convalescence, 108
Tubercular cachexia, phlegmasia dolens in, 246
Tubercular fever, 84 seq., 152; contagious, 88; an essential disease, 88
Tumefaction of belly, 139
Turpentine fomentations, 225
  injections, 229, 230
"Turpentine-punch," 225
Tussis clangosa, 104
  ferina, 174, 176
Tympanites, 139, 146, 230; treatment of, 229
Tympanitic resonance in typhous consolidation of lung, 99
  Dr. Hudson's view, 99
  Dr. Lyons' view, 100
  Dr. Hayden's view, 101
  author's view, 101
Type in disease, change of, 10; see Change of type.
  Alison on, 12
  Christison on, 12 seq.
  the author on, 14 seq.
Typhoid fever, see Enteric fever.
Typhoid pneumonia, 89; its forms, 90
  not dependent on gastritis, 98
Typhous deposit, specific, 64 seq.
  vital character of, 65

Typhus, 45; causes of, Dr. Graves on, 37
  and enteric contrasted, 45 seq.
  resemblances between, 50 seq., 136, 208
  species, not genera, of fever, 51, 135
  aborted, 91
  laryngo-, 104 seq.
  broncho-, 68; pneumo-, 72
Typhus abdominalis, 72
  gravior, 45
  malignant, 45

ULCERATION of the intestines indicated by quick pulse, 108
  latent, 139
  in epidemic of 1826–27, 143 seq.
Uræmia, 244
  a cause of nervous symptoms, 164, 243
Uræmic convulsions, 244
Urine, retention of, 178, 243
  effervescence of, in uræmia, 244
  suppression of, 244; its treatment, 244
Urohæmatin as an indication of blood-waste, 120, 121

VARIETIES of continued fever, 42; see Fever, continued.
Veins, cordy and painful state of, 246
Venesection in fever, 10, 15
Venienti occurrite morbo, 195
Venous irritation, 246
"Vermicular" impulse of heart, 123
Vesicles in fever, 209
  influence on prognosis, 211
Vis medicatrix naturæ, 218
Vital phenomena, study of, the basis of the healing art, 18
  character of disease, 19, 184
  typhous deposit, 65
  depression of the heart, 204
Voluntary muscular tissue in fever, 117, 118
Vomiting, black, 147

WANT of accordance of phenomena, diagnosis from, 82, 184
Warm stupes in headache, 237
Weakness of the heart, 116, 199
West, Mr., and his party, at the Rosetta Pest Hospital, 3
White blood cells and pus corpuscles, 157
Whitlow, increased arterial pulsation in, 139
Wine in fever, 213; see Stimulants.
  and opium in puerperal fever, 234
  sedative effect of, 242
Wolff, Mr. A., on the correlation of diseases (foot-note), 39

"YELLOW fever" of 1826–27, 111, 137, 146 seq., 166
Yellow fever, Dr. Lawrence on, 148

ZYMOTIC diseases, convertibility of, 40
  correlation of, 40

HENRY C. LEA'S

(LATE LEA & BLANCHARD'S)

CATALOGUE OF MEDICAL AND SURGICAL PUBLICATIONS.

In asking the attention of the profession to the works advertised in the following pages, the publisher would state that no pains are spared to secure a continuance of the confidence earned for the publications of the house by their careful selection and accuracy and finish of execution.

The printed prices are those at which books can generally be supplied by booksellers, who can readily procure for their customers any works not kept in stock. Where access to bookstores is not convenient, books will be sent by mail, with U. S. postage paid, on receipt of the prices, but no risks are assumed either on the money or the books, and no publications but my own are supplied. Gentlemen will therefore in most cases find it more convenient to deal with the nearest bookseller.

** No discounts or deductions are made from catalogue prices to buyers at retail.

An ILLUSTRATED CATALOGUE, of 64 octavo pages, handsomely printed, will be forwarded by mail, postpaid, on receipt of ten cents.

HENRY C. LEA.

Nos. 706 and 708 Sansom St., Philadelphia, April, 1876.

ADDITIONAL INDUCEMENT FOR SUBSCRIBERS TO

THE AMERICAN JOURNAL OF THE MEDICAL SCIENCES
FOR THE CENTENNIAL YEAR 1876.

THREE MEDICAL JOURNALS, containing over 2000 LARGE PAGES,
Free of Postage, for SIX DOLLARS Per Annum.

TERMS FOR 1876:

THE AMERICAN JOURNAL OF THE MEDICAL SCIENCES, and } Five Dollars per annum,
THE MEDICAL NEWS AND LIBRARY, both free of postage, } in advance.

OR

THE AMERICAN JOURNAL OF THE MEDICAL SCIENCES, published quarterly (1150 pages per annum), with } Six Dollars
THE MEDICAL NEWS AND LIBRARY, monthly (384 pp. per annum), and } per annum,
THE MONTHLY ABSTRACT OF MEDICAL SCIENCE (592 pages per annum), } in advance.

** Advance-paying subscribers for the current year can obtain cloth covers for each volume of the Journal (two annually), and of the Abstract (one annually), free by mail, on receipt of six cents in postage stamps for each cover.

SEPARATE SUBSCRIPTIONS TO

THE AMERICAN JOURNAL OF THE MEDICAL SCIENCES, when not paid for in advance, Five Dollars.

THE MEDICAL NEWS AND LIBRARY, free of postage, in advance, One Dollar.

THE MONTHLY ABSTRACT OF MEDICAL SCIENCE, free of postage, in advance, Two Dollars and a Half.

It is manifest that only a very wide circulation can enable so vast an amount of valuable practical matter to be supplied at a price so unprecedentedly low. The publisher, therefore, has much gratification in acknowledging the valuable assistance spontaneously rendered by so many of the old subscribers to the "JOURNAL," who have kindly made known among their friends the advantages thus offered, and have induced them to subscribe. Relying upon a continuance of these friendly exertions, he hopes to succeed in his endeavor to place upon the table of every reading practitioner in the United States the equivalent of three or four large octavo volumes, at the comparatively trifling cost of SIX DOLLARS *per annum.*

These periodicals are universally known for their high professional standing in their several spheres.

I.

THE AMERICAN JOURNAL OF THE MEDICAL SCIENCES,
EDITED BY ISAAC HAYS, M.D.,

is published Quarterly, on the first of January, April, July, and October. Each number contains nearly three hundred large octavo pages, appropriately illustrated wherever necessary. It has now been issued regularly for over FIFTY years, during

(For OBSTETRICAL JOURNAL, *see* p. 8.)

nearly the whole of which time it has been under the control of the present editor. Throughout this long period, among its Collaborators will be found a large number of the most distinguished names of the profession in every section of the United States, rendering the department devoted to

ORIGINAL COMMUNICATIONS

full of varied and important matter, of great interest to all practitioners. Thus, during 1875, articles have appeared in its pages from nearly one hundred gentlemen of the highest standing in the profession throughout the United States.*

Following this is the "REVIEW DEPARTMENT," containing extended and impartial reviews of all important new works, together with numerous elaborate "ANALYTICAL AND BIBLIOGRAPHICAL NOTICES" of nearly all the medical publications of the day.

This is followed by the "QUARTERLY SUMMARY OF IMPROVEMENTS AND DISCOVERIES IN THE MEDICAL SCIENCES," classified and arranged under different heads, presenting a very complete digest of all that is new and interesting to the physician, abroad as well as at home.

Thus, during the year 1875, the "JOURNAL" furnished to its subscribers 98 Original Communications, 95 Reviews and Bibliographical Notices, and 283 articles in the Quarterly Summaries making a total of about FIVE HUNDRED articles emanating from the best professional minds in America and Europe.

For the coming year a feature of special interest and value will be found in a series of CENTENNIAL REPORTS 'on the Progress of Medical Science in the United States since 1776. Of these there will be four prepared by gentlemen of the highest eminence in their several departments, as follows :—

On PRACTICAL MEDICINE, by EDWARD H. CLARKE, M.D., A.A.S., late Prof. of Mat. Med. in Harv. Univ.; and H. J. BIGELOW, M.D., Prof. of Surg. in Harv. Univ.

On SURGERY, by S. D. GROSS, M.D., D.C.L. Oxon., Professor of Surgery in Jefferson Med. College, Philadelphia.

On OBSTETRICS AND GYNÆCOLOGY, by T. GAILLARD THOMAS. M.D., Professor of Obstetrics, &c., in the Coll. Phys. and Surgeons, New York.

On MEDICAL LITERATURE, by J. S. BILLINGS, M.D., Asst. Surg. U.S.A., Librarian National Medical Library.

The permanent value of these records of the labors of the American medical profession during the last hundred years will be apparent to all.

That the efforts thus made to maintain the high reputation of the "JOURNAL" are successful, is shown by the position accorded to it in both America and Europe as a national exponent of medical progress :—

America continues to take a great place in this class of journals (quarterlies), at the head of which the great work of Dr. Hays, the *American Journal of the Medical Sciences*, still holds its ground, as our quotations have often proved.—*Dublin Med. Press and Circular*, Jan. 31, 1872.

Of English periodicals the *Lancet*, and of American the *Am. Journal of the Medical Sciences*, are to be regarded as necessities to the reading practitioner.—*N. Y. Medical Gazette*, Jan. 7, 1871.

The *American Journal of the Medical Sciences* yields to none in the amount of original and borrowed matter it contains, and has established for itself a reputation in every country where medicine is cultivated as a science.—*Brit. and For. Med.-Chirurg Review*, April, 1871.

This, if not the best, is one of the best-conducted medical quarterlies in the English language, and the present number is not by any means inferior to its predecessors.—*London Lancet*, Aug. 23, 1873.

Almost the only one that circulates everywhere, all over the Union and in Europe.—*London Medical Times*, Sept. 5, 1868.

And that it was specifically included in the award of a medal of merit to the Publisher in the Vienna Exhibition in 1873.

The subscription price of the "AMERICAN JOURNAL OF THE MEDICAL SCIENCES" has never been raised during its long career. It is still FIVE DOLLARS per annum; and when paid for in advance, the subscriber receives in addition the "MEDICAL NEWS AND LIBRARY," making in all about 1500 large octavo pages per annum, free of postage.

II.

THE MEDICAL NEWS AND LIBRARY

is a monthly periodical of Thirty-two large octavo pages, making 384 pages per annum. Its "NEWS DEPARTMENT" presents the current information of the day, with Clinical Lectures and Hospital Gleanings; while the "LIBRARY DEPARTMENT" is devoted to publishing standard works on the various branches of medical science, paged separately, so that they can be removed and bound on completion. In this manner subscribers have received, without expense, such works as "WATSON'S PRACTICE,"

---

* Communications are invited from gentlemen in all parts of the country. Elaborate articles inserted by the Editor are paid for by the Publisher.

"'Todd and Bowman's Physiology," "West on Children," "Malgaigne's Surgery," &c. &c. With Jan. 1875, was commenced the publication of Dr. William Stokes's new work on Fever (see p. 7), which will be continued to completion during 1876. New subscribers commencing with Jan. 1876 can obtain the portion printed in 1875 by remitting One Dollar to the publisher.

As stated above, the subscription price of the "Medical News and Library" is One Dollar per annum in advance; and it is furnished without charge to all advance paying subscribers to the "American Journal of the Medical Sciences."

III.

THE MONTHLY ABSTRACT OF MEDICAL SCIENCE.

The "Monthly Abstract" is issued on the first of every month, each number containing forty-eight large octavo pages, thus furnishing in the course of the year about six hundred pages. The aim of the Abstract will be to present a careful condensation of all that is new and important in the medical journalism of the world, and all the prominent professional periodicals of both hemispheres will be at the disposal of the Editors. To show the manner in which this plan has been carried out, a condensed summary of the contents of the numbers for the last half of the year 1875, will be found subjoined. In all, during 1875, it has contained—

> *42 Articles on Anatomy and Physiology.*
> *56 "   " Materia Medica and Therapeutics.*
> *204 "   " Medicine.*
> *183 "   " Surgery.*
> *118 "   " Midwifery and Gynæcology.*
> *18 "   " Medical Jurisprudence and Toxicology.*
> *8 "   " Hygiene—*

making in all Six Hundred and Twenty-nine articles per annum.

The subscription to the "Monthly Abstract," free of postage, is Two Dollars and a Half a year, in advance.

As stated above, however, it will be supplied in conjunction with the "American Journal of the Medical Sciences" and the "Medical News and Library," making in all more than Twenty-one Hundred pages per annum, the whole *free of postage*, for Six Dollars a year, in advance.

Those who desire to have complete sets, can still procure Vol. I. July to December, 1874, 1 vol. 8vo., cloth, of about 300 pages, for $1 50, and Vol. II. for 1875, 1 vol. 8vo. of about 600 pages, cloth, for $3 00.

In this effort to bring so large an amount of practical information within the reach of every member of the profession, the publisher confidently anticipates the friendly aid of all who are interested in the dissemination of sound medical literature. He trusts, especially, that the subscribers to the "American Medical Journal" will call the attention of their acquaintances to the advantages thus offered, and that he will be sustained in the endeavor to permanently establish medical periodical literature on a footing of cheapness never heretofore attempted.

PREMIUMS OFFERED TO SUBSCRIBERS.

Any gentleman who will remit the amount for two subscriptions for 1876, one of which must be for a *new subscriber*, will receive as a premium, free by mail, a copy of "Flints Essays on Conservative Medicine" (for advertisement of which see p. 17), or of "Sturges's Clinical Medicine" (see p. 28), or of the new edition of "Swayne's Obstetric Aphorisms" (see p. 27), or of "Tanner's Clinical Manual" (see p. 30), or of "Chambers's Restorative Medicine" (see p 13), or of "West on Nervous Disorders of Children" (see page 31).

* Gentlemen desiring to avail themselves of the advantages thus offered will do well to forward their subscriptions at an early day, in order to insure the receipt of complete sets for the year 1876, as the constant increase in the subscription list almost always exhausts the quantity printed shortly after publication.

☞ The safest mode of remittance is by bank check or postal money order, drawn to the order of the undersigned. Where these are not accessible, remittances for the "Journal" may be made at the risk of the publisher, by forwarding in registered letters. Address,

HENRY C. LEA,
Nos. 706 and 708 Sansom St., Philadelphia, Pa.

CONTENTS

OF THE

MONTHLY ABSTRACT OF MEDICAL SCIENCE,

FOR SIX MONTHS, FROM JULY TO DECEMBER, 1875.

Anatomy and Physiology.

On a Pharyngeal Diverticulum. By Prof. Watson 289
On the Consequences of Section of the Optic Nerve in the Frog. By W. Krenchel . 289
On Heart-Sounds. By M. Dezautière . . 290
Ligature of the Bile-duct, and on the Blood in Diffuse Hepatitis. By Messrs. Feltz and Ritter 290
Atmospheric Pressure on the Joints. By Prof. Ch. Aeby and Dr. Fr. Schmid . . . 337
Anomalies of the Infraorbital Canal and Nerve. By Prof. Luigi Calori 337
Case of Twin Monstrosity. By Prof. von Buhl. 338
On some Bursæ Mucosæ corresponding to the Trachea, Larynx, and certain Adjacent Parts. By Prof. Luigi Calori 385
Bilateral Irritation of the Pneumogastrics in Man. By Dr. Thanhoffer 386
On the Canals which are supposed to connect the Bloodvessels with the Lymphatics. By J. Tarchanoff 433
Experiments on the Brains of Monkeys, with especial reference to the Localization of Sensory Centres in the Convolutions. By Dr. David Ferrier 433
The Chemistry of the Blood. By M. Gauthier 434
On the Distribution of the Fibres of the Optic Nerve in the Human Retina. By Prof. Michel. 481
A Case of Apparent Hermaphrodism. By Dr. Schœneberg 481
Complete Transposition of the Viscera. By Dr. Schule 482
On the Migrations and Metamorphoses of the White Corpuscles of the Blood. By Ch. Rouget 482
Absence of the Clavicle. By O. Kappeler . 529
The Lymphatics of the Lung. By Dr. Klein . 529
Anatomy and Physiology of the Liver. By Mons. G. Asp 531

Materia Medica and Therapeutics.

The Local Use of Chloral Hydrate. By Charles A. Peabody 291
Conium and its Use in Diseases of the Eye. By Dr. Edward Curtis 292
Chloroform and Nitrite of Amyl. By Dr. F. A. Burrall 293
On the Hemp and Gypsum Splint. By Dr. Beely 294
The Action of Ammonia on the Animal Organism. By Lange 339
Therapeutic Action of the Oleum Aleuritis Triloba. By Dr. Calixto Oxamendi . . 339
Thymol an Antiseptic and Antifermentative Substance. By Prof. Lewin . . . 340
Impermeable Caoutchouc Dressings. By Dr. Besnier 341
The Continued and the Frequent Dose. By Dr. Edward H. Clarke 387
Jaborandi. By Dr. Ambrosoli . . . 389
Action of Aconitina upon the Heart. By Lewin 390
Damiana—a powerful Aphrodisiac. By Drs. J. J. Caldwell and Charles McQuestin . 391
The Action of Certain Drugs on the Secretion of Bile. By Prof. Rutherford . . . 435
Diuretics 435
Raw Onion as a Diuretic. By Dr. G. W. Balfour 438
Bromide of Camphor. By M. Pathault . 439
Nitric Acid as a Caustic in Uterine Practice, and its superiority as such to Nitrate of Silver. By Dr. James Braithwaite 439
On the Action of Salicylic Acid. By Dr. Winter 482
On the Phenate and Salicylate of Quinia. By M. Maury 483
Cucurbitaceous Anthelmintics. By M. Heckel 483
The Actual Cautery; its Uses and Powers. By Dr. C. E. Brown-Séquard 484
Physiological and Therapeutic Properties of Nitrite of Amyl. By M. Bourneville . . 531

Salicylic Acid as an Antiseptic. By Mr. Callender 532

Medicine.

On Two Interesting Cases of Variola. By Dr. Emmanuel Kramer 295
On Eserine as a Remedy for Chorea. By M. Bouchut 295
The Pathology of Progressive Muscular Atrophy. By Dr. Troisier 296
On a Case of Atrophy of the Right Thenar Eminence with Lesion of the Spinal Cord. By J. L. Prevost and C. David 297
On Auditory Vertigo. By Drs. Brown-Séquard and Labadie-Lagrave 298
On Unilateral Paralysis of the Velum Palati of Central Origin. By Dr. Dumenil . . 300
On Ipecacuanha Spray in Winter Cough and Bronchitic Asthma. By Dr. Sydney Ringer and Mr Wm. Murrell 301
Jaborandi in Pleuritic Effusion. By M. Créquy 302
A Case of Paracentesis of the Pleura, Abdomen, and Pericardium. By MM. Ferari-Bravo and Valcosta 302
A Case of Dilated Heart from Valvular Lesion, in which the Right Ventricle was Tapped by Error, not only without Harm, but with Relief of Symptoms. By Dr. George Evans . 304
On the Mode in which the Circulation of Fecal Matters is Re-established after Ligature of Intestine. By Sales-Girons . . . 305
Paroxysmal Hæmaturia. By Drs. Legg and Warburton Begbie 306
Electricity in the Asphyxia of New-Born Infants. By Dr. Zaunschirm 307
A New Test for Waxy Degeneration. By M. Cornil 307
On Diabetes. By C. Bock and F. A. Hoffmann 342
Treatment of Diabetes Insipidus by Ergot. By Dr. J. M. Da Costa 342
On Melanæmia. By Dr. W. Kornmüller . 344
Cholera treated with Subcutaneous Injection of Morphia. By Dr. F. Milford . . 345
The Sensibility of the Skin in Acute Rheumatism. By Dr. V. Drosdoff 346
Gout in some of its Surgical Relations. By Sir James Paget 347
The Treatment of Typhoid Fever by Quinine. By Dr. Corral 350
Gangrene of the Lower Extremity after Diphtheria. By Dr. Moroni 350
The Condition of the Spinal Cord in a Case of Talipes Equinus. By M. Dejerine . . 351
The Influence of Amyl-Nitrite in Melancholia. By Dr. Schramm 352
On the Use of Chloral in the Treatment of Whooping-Cough. By Dr. Greslou . . 352
On the Nature, Varieties, and Etiology of Pulmonary Consumption in the Army. By Mr. Welch 353
Pathogeny of Spontaneous Aneurism. By Prof. Köster 354
Phlebitis following the Hypodermic Use of Ergot in the Treatment of a Fibroid Tumour of the Uterus. By Dr E P. Allen . . 355
Sudden Death from Puncture of a Hydatid Cyst. By M. Martineau 535
Intestinal obstruction successfully treated by Gaseous Enemata Dr. Bernardino Torres . 355
On Herpes Zoster. By M. Bucquoy . . 356
The Cause of some of the Eruptions which have been classed as Hydroa. By Mr. Hutchinson 356
Pernicious Progressive Anæmia By Prof. Immermann 393
A Typhoid Epidemic, apparently arising from Infected Milk. By Dr. Alexander Ogston . 393
Modus Operandi of the Yellow Fever Poison. By Dr. George M. Sternberg . . . 394
Bromide of Potassium in the Treatment of Epilepsy. By Dr. J. Warburton Begbie . . 394

Contents of Monthly Abstract of Med. Science, July—Dec. 1875—(Continued.)

Intermittent Spinal Paralysis. By H. Hartwig . 395
Thoracentesis in the Pneumothorax incident to Empyema. By Dr. Austin Flint . . . 395
On a Case of Unusually Rapid Action of the Heart. By Dr. Robert Farquharson . . 396
Remarkable Retardation of Pulse. By Mr. Pugin Thornton and M. Cornil . . . 399
Hyperidrosis excited by change of Posture By Dr. David Inglis 401
Three Cases of Dilatation of Lymphatic Radicles. By Mr. C. Handfield Jones . . 402
Kamesla as a Remedy for Tapeworms. By M. Blondean 406
Congenital Deficiency of the Peritoneum resulting in Intestinal Obstruction, and simulating an Abdominal Tumour. By Mr. Lawson Tait 407
Molluscum Contagiosum. By Dr. C. Boeck . 407
Nasal Lupus. By Mr Gay 408
On the Cure of Splenic Leukhæmia by means of Phosphorus. By Dr. Wilson Fox . . 440
Treatment of Sea-sickness by Chloral. By Dr. L. C. Obet 440
Nitrite of Amyl in Sea-sickness. By Mr. Crochley Clapham 441
Successful Treatment of Locomotor Ataxy. By Dr. G. W. Balfour 442
Peripheric Traumatic Epilepsy. By Dr. Briand 442
Hystero-Epilepsy with Anuria. By M. Bourneville 442
Case of Abnormal Disposition to Sleep alternated with Choreic Movements. By Dr. W. T. Gairdner 443
Electrical Chorea. By Dr. Stefanini . . 444
On an Imperfectly Recognized Combination of Spinal Symptoms. By Dr. Erb . . . 445
Case of Hysteria in a Male. By Dr. Bonnemaison 446
Ménière's Disease. By Dr. Ladreit de Lacharrière 447
Autumnal Catarrh. By Dr. Morrill Wyman . 448
Tracheotomy and Croup in Diphtheria. By Prof. Syme 450
Tincture of Eucalyptus in Gaugrene of the Lungs. By M. Bucquoy 451
The Presystolic Murmur 451
Unusually Rapid Action of the Heart. By Dr. John Cavafy 452
Case of Dissecting Aneurism of the Thoracic Aorta. By P. Hedenius 453
Embolic Aneurisms and their analogy to Acute Cardiac Aneurism. By Prof Pontick . 454
A Remarkable Case of Periodical Venesection. By Dr. E Warren Sawyer 454
Tabetic Arthritis. By M. Charcot . . 455
Hydrophobia treated by Chloral By Dr. V. Grazi 486
On the Successful Use of Jaborandi in Diabetes Insipidus. By Dr. Laycock . . . 487
On the Use of Tepid Baths in the Febrile Disorders of Infants. By Dr. Meyer . . 488
Treatment of Acute Rheumatism by Tincture of the Perchloride of Iron. By Dr. J. Russell Reynolds 489
On the Use of Cold Baths in Cerebral Rheumatism By M. Féréol 492
Alterations in the Brain Typhoid and Typhus Fever. By Dr. Leo Popoff . . . 493
Intra-Cranial Aneurism diagnosticated during Life. By Dr William E Hamble . . 493
On Hypodermic Injection of Ergotine in Certain Cases of Acute Mania. By Dr. A. H. Van Andel 495
On Some Points in the Diagnosis of Sclerosis of the Nervous System. By M. Mollière . 496
Nitrite of Amyl in Facial Neuralgia. By Dr. George H. Evans 497
On the Relation between Exophthalmic Goitre and Vitiligo. By Dr. Raynaud . . 498
Auscultation of the Œsophagus. By Dr. Clifford Allbutt 499
On the Significance of Prolonged Expiration, and on Tenderness on Percussion. By Dr. Sulger 500
On Whooping-Cough. By Dr. Nöel Gueneau de Mussy 501
On a Case of Pulsating Empyema. By Dr. Lorenzo Lorenzutti 501
Large Pleuritic Effusions in Phthisis. By M. Leudet 503
On a Case of Puncture of the Pericardium. By M. Villeneuve 504

Chronic Aortitis. By M. Jousset . . . 505
Treatment of Chronic Dysentery. By Dr. Handfield Jones 505
Differential Diagnosis of Intestinal Invagination. By Dr. O. Lachenstein . . . 506
Intestinal Diseases healed by Introduction into the Intestinal Tract of large quantities of Fluid. By Prof. Mosler 507
Presence of a Bruit of Fluctuation and Metallic Tinkling in Abdominal Tumours. By M. Laboulbène 508
Amyloid Disease of the Liver without preceding Purulent Discharge. By Dr. Hayden . 509
Splenic Tumours treated by Injection. By Prof. Mosler 509
On Recurrent Zona. By Dr. Kaposi . . 511
Veruca Senilis. By Dr. I. Neumann . . 512
Papular Erythema related to Rheumatism. By M. Coulard 512
Malarial Hematuria. By Mr. C. R. Francis . 533
Paralysis Agitans and Insular Sclerosis . . 531
Case of Paralysis of the Serratus Magnus. By Dr. Samuel Woodman 511
On the Morbid Changes in the Sympathetic in Constitutional Syphilis. By Dr. P. Petrow 515
Disease of the Sympathetic Nerve in the Neck. By Dr. Paul Guttman 546
A New Method of treating Strictures of the Larynx. By Dr. Michael Grossmann . . 547
Rheumatoid Disease in Dilatation of the Bronchi. By C Gerbardt 547
Gelseminum Sempervirens as a Remedy for Cough. By Dr. J. Roberts Thomson . . 548
On a Case of Suppurative Pneumonia successfully treated by Carbolic Acid and Essential Oil of Turpentine. By Dr. Angelo Cianciosi 548
Treatment of Aneurism of the Arch of the Aorta by means of Galvano-Puncture. By Dr. T. McCall Anderson 548
On a Case of Perforating Ulcer of the Duodenum. By Levertin and Axel Key . . . 550
Treatment of Intestinal Obstruction by Electricity. By Dr. Fleuriot 551
On a Case of Embolism and Disintegrated Thrombus of the Portal System. By G. Bolling 551
Primary Cancer of the Gall-Bladder. By M. Lamétine 552
Treatment of Catarrh of the Urinary Organs accompanied by Ammoniacal Fermentation of the Urine. By Gosselin and Robin . . 553

Surgery.

The Least Sacrifice of Parts as a Principle of Surgical Practice. By Mr. Bryant . . 308
Acute Tetanus treated by Nitrite of Amyl. By Dr. William S. Forbes 309
On a Case of Encephalitis and Interstitial Myelitis with Ulceration of both Corneæ. By Dr. Jacusiel 310
On Sympathetic Ophthalmia. By Dr. Grossman 310
Extirpation of the Tongue. By Dr. Von Langenbeck 311
Removal of a Growth from the Larynx with the Aid of Local Anæsthesia. By Dr. Massei . 311
Intestinal Obstruction; Laparotomy. By Dr. Erskine Mason 312
Removal of the Os Coccygis for Coccyodynia. By Dr. J. C. Irish 312
Statistics of Amputations performed in the Glasgow Royal Infirmary during the Twenty-five Years ending 31st December, 1873. By Dr. Moses Thomas 313
Monstrosity by Inclusion; Successful Excision. By Dr. W. W. Miner 314
Dumreicher's Method of treating Ununited Fracture. By Dr. Carl Nicoladoni . . 315
Treatment of Ununited Fracture by Transplantation of Bone. By Prof. Nussbaum . . 316
The Treatment of False Joint. By Dr. Volkmann 316
Fracture of the Clavicle. By M. Delens . . 318
Sequel to a Paper on Excision of the Ankle-Joint. By Mr. Lee 319
Excessive and Long-maintained High Temperature after Injury to the Spine; Recovery. By Mr. J W. Teale 320
On a Case of Ligature of the Internal Iliac Artery for Wound of a Branch of the Gluteal. By Dr. Landi 323

Contents of Monthly Abstract of Med. Science, July—Dec. 1875—(Continued.)

Precocious Secondary Traumatisms. By Prof. Verneuil 324

New Forceps for keeping the Eustachian Catheter in position. By Dr. Delstanche-Sohn 325

Transplantation of Skin. By Dr. Clemens . 358

Conjunctival Grafting. By Dr. Masselon . 358

Gonorrhœal Ophthalmia. By Prof. Hirschberg 359

Imperfect Teeth and Zonnlar Cataract. By Mr. Jonathan Hutchinson 360

On Disease of the Choroid consequent on the Use of Chloral Hydrate. By Dr Steinheim . 361

On Nystagmus as the Result of Hemeralopia. By Dr. Nieden 362

On Phthisical Otitis. By M. Bellière . . 364

On Anthrax and Furunculus of the Face. By Dr. J. Labatut 364

On Adenoid Vegetations in the Pharyngeal Space. By Prof. Politzer . . . 365

Laparotomy for Intussusception. By Mr. Jos. Bell 365

The Proper Time for Aspiratory Puncture in the Treatment of Strangulated Hernia. By Dr Bonisson 365

Extirpation of a Tumour of the Bladder. By Dr. Carl Gussenbauer 366

Chylocele. By Dr. C. H. Mastin . . . 367

Arthritis Deformans. By Dr. Duplay . . 368

Five Cases of Resection of the Sternum and Ribs. By Prof. Mazzoni 369

Resection of the Knee after Gunshot Wound. By Dr. Mensel 370

Fracture of Spine; Compression of the Cord; Removal of the Depressed Bone. By Dr H. A. Clark 371

On the Use of Adhesive Plaster in Fracture of the Patella. By Dr. John Neill . . 372

Histogenesis of Cancer. By Dr. Creighton . 409

Mr. Teale's Case of High Temperature . 410

On Extraction of Cataract by a Median Section through the Cornea. By Dr. Vicente Chiralt 411

An Improved Method of treating certain Cases of Cataract requiring Extraction. By Mr. J. Vose Solomon 411

On Concussion of the Retina, and on Foreign Bodies in the Eyeball. By Dr. Hirschberg . 412

Chronic Inflammation of the Lachrymal Sac. By Dr. Sigmund Bacher . . . 413

On a Case of nearly complete Deafness of one Ear after an Apoplectic Seizure. By Dr. J. Hughlings-Jackson 413

On a Slight Modification of the Operation for Closing Fissures of the Soft Palate. By Mr. Edward Bellamy 414

Cyst of the Thyroid Gland cured by Electrolysis after Injections had failed. By Dr. Andrew H. Smith 415

Lithotrity 416

Strangulated Hernia reduced by Taxis through the Colon. By Dr. Alexander Hadden . 417

A Combination of the Cutaneous and Musculo-Cutaneous Plans of Amputation. By Dr. D. Hayes Agnew 418

A New Operation for the Cure of certain cases of Aggravated "Knock-knee." By Mr. Thomas Annandale 419

Duration of Bloodless Operations. By Prof. Langenbeck 420

An Antiphlogistic Method of Dressing Operation Wounds. By Mr. Jonathan Hutchinson 455

The Subperiosteal Method. By Prof. Spence . 455

On a new Operation for the Obliteration of Depressed Cicatrices after Glandular Abscesses or Exfoliation of Bone. By Mr. William Adams 458

On the Origin and Treatment of Purulent Ophthalmia. By Prof. Arlt . . . 459

On Iridectomy as an Aid to the Extraction of Cataract. By Dr. Dezanncau . . 460

Statistical Review of Operations for Tumours of the Superior Maxilla. By Dr. Ohlemann 461

Excision of the Thyroid Gland. By Dr. P. Heron Watson 461

Case of Recovery after Complete Division of the Larynx and Œsophagus. By S Henschen . 463

A Century of Operations for Stone. By Prof. Dittel 464

Treatment of Ununited Fractures. By Prof. Spence 466

On the Treatment of Club-Foot. By Dr. W. J. Little 466

Removal of Tumours. By Mr. Jas. Spence . 513

Coexistence of Lupus and Carcinoma. By Prof. E. Lang 51

On the Occurrence of Carcinoma after Lupus. By Baron von Langenbeck . . . 515

Notes on the Modern Methods of Extracting Cataract. By Mr. C. B. Taylor . . 516

Tracheotomy in Cases of Impending Suffocation by Pressure on Trachea or Laryngeal Nerves. By Mr. Spence 517

Case of Gonorrhœal Epididymitis occurring before the Appearance of the Discharge. By Dr. Fred. R. Sturgis 517

Two Cases of Removal of Omental Tumour from the Scrotum. By Prof. J. F. Miner . 518

A Case of Avulsion of the Tuberosity of the Tibia. By Dr. F. Parona . . . 519

Fracture of the Humerus at its Anatomical and Surgical Neck. By Mr. Gustavus Foote . 520

New Operation for Ununited Fractures. By Mr. Matthew Hill 521

On the Analogies of Dislocation of the Shoulder and Hip-joints, and the Methods of Reducing them. By Dr Kocher . . . 521

Ligature of the Common Femoral Artery; and especially on Ligature by an Antiseptic Material. By Mr. Oliver Pemberton . . 522

Angioma and its Galvano Caustic Treatment. By Alfred Battig 523

Esmarch's Bloodless Method. By Mr. James Spence 524

Pathology of Carcinoma. By Prof Beneke . 554

Nitrite of Amyl in Acute Tetanus. By Mr. Wagstaffe 556

Disinfecting Treatment of Corneal Ulcers. By Dr. Horner 556

A Method of performing Iridectomy for the Improvement of Sight. By Mr. Brudenell Carter 557

Subcutaneous Injection of Nitrate of Strychnia in Nervous Deafness and in Disturbance of Innervation of the Intrinsic Muscles of the Ear. By Dr. R. Hagen . . . 557

A New Mode of treating certain Tumours of the Lymphatic Glands. By Mr. S. Messenger Bradley 558

The Treatment of Patent Urachus. By Dr. J. J. Charles 559

Treatment of the Complications of Gonorrhœa. By M. Ricord 560

The Wire Compress as a Substitute for the Ligature. By Mr. John Dix . . . 560

On Ligature of the Common Femoral Artery, and especially on Ligature by an Antiseptic Material. By Mr. Oliver Pemberton . 561

Spina Bifida treated by Excision. By Dr. Matthews Duncan 562

Section of Nerves in Neuralgia. By MM. Arloing and Tripier 563

On the Reparation of Fractures. By Dr H. Leboucq 564

On a Case of Avulsion of the Forearm, attended with Severe Hemorrhage. By Dr. Parona . 565

Pathogeny of Knock knee. By M. Léon Tripier 565

Midwifery and Gynæcology.

Use of the Hand to correct Unfavourable Presentations and Positions of the Head during Labour. By Dr. John S. Parry . . 326

Extra-Uterine Pregnancy. By Dr. Conrad . 327

Indian Hemp in the Post-Partum Hemorrhage By Mr. William Donovan . . . 328

Ergot as an Antidote for an Excessive Secretion of Milk and Inflammation of the Breast. By Dr. Schtscherbinenkoff. . . . 328

The Non-existence of Puerperal Fever. By Dr. Sirédey 329

Erysipelas and Puerperal Fever. By Mr. Spencer Wells and S. N. Squire . . . 330

On a Case of Complete Congenital Closure of the Vagina and of the External Os Uteri, with consequent Hæmatometra and Acute Peritonitis. By Herr Krumptmane 331

On the Evacuation of Hæmatometra through the Bladder after Dilatation of the Urethra. By Prof. Simon 331

Electricity in Cases of Auteflexion and Retroflexion. By M. Tripier . . . 332

Case of Complete Inversion of the Uterus. By Dr. A. Voelkel 333

The Internal and External Application of Chloral Hydrate in Carcinoma Uteri. By Herr Fleischer 333

Contents of Monthly Abstract of Med. Science. July—Dec. 1875—(Continued.)

On Adhesion of the Placenta. By Dr. J. G. Swayne 373
Diminution of the Uterus after Delivery. By Dr. Ar. Serdukoff 374
On the Causation of Puerperal Fever. By Dr. A. L. Galabin 375
Some Practical Hints concerning the Care of New-born Children. By Dr. Charles E. Buckingham 376
Case of Sterility from Anteflexion of the Uterus, and Constriction of the Internal Os Uteri, cured. By Dr. Heywood Smith . . 377
Stoltz's Operation for Cystocele. By Dr. Heywood Smith 378
Emphysematous Cysts of the Vaginal Mucous Membrane 378
The Diagnosis of Ovarian Cysts and the Indications for their Treatment. By Dr. Rheinstaedter 378
Dermoid Cyst of the Ovary. By M. Terrier . 379
On Serous Ovarian Cysts. By Dr. Panas . 380
Treatment of Fibrous Tumours of the Uterus by Ergot. By Dr. W. H. Byford . . 380
On the Use of Salicylic Acid in Obstetric and Gynæcological Practice. By Professor Crede 381
Gastro-Elytrotomy. By Dr. T. Gaillard Thomas 421
A Case of Extra-Uterine Pregnancy; successful Operation. By Dr. G. Dresselhuys . 421
Galactorrhœa. By Dr. A. Puech . . 423
Case of Hirsuties Gestationis. By Dr. Chas. E. Slocum 424
Ovariotomy complicated with Pregnancy; Cæsarean Operation; Cure. By Mr. Thos. Hillas 424
A Fibroma Molluscum Cysticum Abdominale. By Prof. Virchow 425
Follicular Dropsy of the Ovary. By Dr. J. Matthews Duncan 427
Perovarian Cysts. By Dr. J. Matthews Duncan 427
On the Management of the Lying-in Woman. By Mr. Thomas Whiteside Hime . . 468
Notes on a Case of Triplets, complicated by Double Uterus. By Dr. A. G. Duncan . 469
Extra-Uterine Peritoneal Pregnancy. By Prof. Depaul 469
Extra-Uterine Gestation terminating by the Ovum becoming Encysted. By M. Polaillon 469
On Laceration of the Navel-String. By Dr. William Pfannkuch 470
Rupture of the Symphysis Pubis during Parturition. By Dr. Eidam 471
Syphilitic Placenta. By Dr. Augus MacDonald 471
The Cephalotribe; its Inconveniences and its Dangers. By Dr. Boissarie . . 472
Discussion on Puerperal Fever before the Obstetrical Society of London . . . 472
On the Employment of Chloral in Puerperal Convulsions. By Dr. Portal . . . 473
Complete Atresia of the Female Genital Organs, or Unilateral Hæmatometra. By Dr. Albert Puech 473
Tetanus following Menorrhagia, with Purpura Hemorrhagica and Vaginal Diphtheria; Hypodermic Injection of Chloral; Cure. By Dr. Ribell

On Metrorrhagia arrested by the Application of Heat to the Lumbar Region. By Dr. Noel Gueneau de Mussy 475
Performance of Ovariotomy twice in the same Patient. By Mr. Spencer Wells . . 475
On Drainage of Douglas's Cul-de-sac in Ovariotomy. By Prof. Schroeder . . 476
Crayons of Iodoform. By Dr. Leblond . 478
Influence of Chloroform upon the Fœtus in Utero. By Dr. Zweifel 478
On the Absorption of Medicaments by Infants from the Mother's Milk. By Dr. Lewald . 478
Treatment of cases of Labor with Contracted Pelvis. By Prof. Taylor . . . 525
On Temperature in Puerperal Eclampsia and the Clinical Indications it furnishes. By Dr. Bourneville 525
Case of Double Vagina and Uterus, with Pregnancy of the Right Uterus and Delivery through the Left Vagina. By Dr A E Hoadley 526
On a Modification of the Ordinary Forceps to enable Traction to be applied to the Centre of the Blades. By M. Laroyenne . . 566
On Uterine Hemorrhages consecutive to Parturition. By M. Bouchacourt . . 567
On the Genesis of an Epidemic of Puerperal Fever. By Prof. W. T. Lusk . . . 567
Epidemic Puerperal Fever. By Dr. Fordyce Barker 569
Distension of the Urinary Bladder mistaken for an Ovarian Cyst. By M. Jaccoud . 571

Medical Jurisprudence and Toxicology.

What constitutes a Live Birth? By Dr. John J. Reese 333
On Microscopic Examination of Blue Lines on the Gums supposed to be due to Lead Poisoning. By Dr. Gras 335
A Case of Poisoning by Oil of Wintergreen. By Dr. Allan McLane Hamilton . . 381
On the Antagonism between Strychnia and Monobromide of Camphor. By Dr. Valenti y Vivo 383
Responsibility in Mental Disease . . 428
Case of Chronic Lead Poisoning, the result of using Flake-white as a cosmetic. By Dr. Geo. Johnson 479
On Poisoning by Santonin, and its Treatment. By Becker 572

Hygiene.

Enteric Fever and Milk Supply. By Dr. E. Duncan 430
Epidemic of Typhoid Fever propagated through the Milk-supply. By Mr. John Spear . 527
Defective House Sewerage and Disease produced by it. By Dr. James D. Trask . . 572
Means of rendering healthy, Workshops where Phosphorus is manipulated . . . 575
Maternities 575

Publishing in the "Medical News and Library" for 1875-1876.

Stokes (William), M.D., D.C.L., F.R.S.,

Regius Professor of Physic in the Univ. of Dublin, etc.

LECTURES ON FEVER, delivered in the Theatre of the Meath Hospital and County of Dublin Infirmary. Edited by JOHN WILLIAM MOORE, M D., Assistant Physician to the Cork St. Fever Hospital. To form one neat octavo volume.

The publication of this work was commenced in the "MEDICAL NEWS AND LIBRARY" for Jan. 1875. It can thus be obtained from the commencement by subscribers to the Am. Journ. Med. Sciences. (See p. 3.)

The great value of Dr. Stokes's lectures lies in the fact that they embody the views which have been formed by a physician acute in observation, and unsurpassed in reflective power—after looking on during half a century at the various visitations of epidemic disease which have passed over this country.—*Dublin Journ. of Med. Sciences,* June, 1874.

The lectures on treatment ought to be studied by every practitioner of medicine. They teem with practical instructions, which could only emanate from an acute and observant physician, who has had a life-long experience of fever on the largest scale. We would particularly direct attention to the rules which Dr. Stokes lays down for the feeding of fever patients, and the indications for the use of stimulants derived from those morbid phenomena of the heart and arteries in fever, to which he was the first to call attention. Altogether, the volume is one which will further enhance the great reputation of its author, as well as that of the Dublin School of Medicine.—*Brit'sh Med. Journ.,* Aug. 29, 1874.

The Obstetrical Journal. (*Free of postage for* 1876.)

THE OBSTETRICAL JOURNAL of Great Britain and Ireland; Including MIDWIFERY, and the DISEASES OF WOMEN AND INFANTS. With an American Supplement, edited by J. V. INGHAM, M.D. A monthly of ninety-six octavo pages, very handsomely printed. Subscription, Five Dollars per annum. Single numbers, 50 cents each.

Commencing with April, 1873, the "OBSTETRICAL JOURNAL" consists of Original Papers and Lectures by British and Foreign Contributors; Transactions of the Obstetrical Societies in Great Britain and abroad; Reports of Hospital Practice; Reviews and Bibliographical Notices; Selections from Journals; Correspondence; Editorial Articles and Notes, Historical, Forensic, and Miscellaneous. The leading representatives of British Obstetrics and Gynæcology have pledged to it their support, and it numbers among its contributors such men as LOMBE ATT. HILL, J. H. AVELING, ROBERT BARNES, J. HENRY BENNET, THOMAS CHAMBERS, FLEETWOOD CHURCHILL, CHARLES CLAY, JOHN CLAY, J. MATTHEWS DUNCAN, ARTHUR FARRE, ROBERT GREENHALGH, W. M. GRAILY HEWITT, J. BRAXTON HICKS, WILLIAM LEISHMAN, ALFRED MEADOWS, ALEX. SIMPSON, J. G. SWAYNE, LAWSON TAIT, EDWARD J. TILT, T. SPENCER WELLS, and many other distinguished practitioners. Under such auspices it has amply fulfilled its object of presenting to the physician all that is new and interesting in the rapid development of obstetrical and gynæcological science.

In order to render the "OBSTETRICAL JOURNAL" fully adequate to the wants of the profession in this country, each number contains an "AMERICAN SUPPLEMENT." This portion is under the charge of Dr. J V. INGHAM, to whom all communications, Exchanges, Books for Review, &c., may be addressed, to the care of the undersigned. Articles have appeared in it from Professors R. A. F. PENROSE, D. WARREN BRICKELL, WILLIAM GOODELL, ALBERT H. SMITH, WILLIAM F. JENKS, and other distinguished American obstetricians, and others of equal eminence have promised it their support in the future.

The "OBSTETRICAL JOURNAL," with the "SUPPLEMENT," during the past year has contained over One Thousand Pages, very handsomely printed, with numerous wood-cuts and plates, plain, and colored. Its contents have consisted of—

	Articles.			Articles.
ORIGINAL COMMUNICATIONS	34	In American Supplement.		
REPORTS OF HOSPITAL PRACTICE	14			
GENERAL CORRESPONDENCE	11	ORIGINAL COMMUNICATIONS		8
LEADING ARTICLES	10	MONTHLY SUMMARY, MIDWIFERY		26
REVIEWS OF BOOKS	9	" " DISEASES OF WOMEN		30
IN PROCEEDINGS OF SOCIETIES	105	" " CHILDREN		15
IN MONTHLY SUMMARY, OBSTETRIC	20	BIBLIOGRAPHICAL NOTICES		5
" " GYNECIC	36			
" " PEDIATRIC	12	IN ALL		352
NOTICES	17			

Thus presenting an amount and variety of valuable practical information which it would be difficult to find elsewhere in so convenient and accessible a form.

Subscriptions can commence with January, 1876, but sets for 1875 can no longer be supplied.

We cannot withhold the expression of the admiration this elegant journal excites.—*Western Lancet,* March, 1875.

This is certainly a very excellent journal. It

gives us the best obstetrical literature from across the water, while the Supplement supplies the latest of interest in this country.—*Indiana Journ. of Med.,* Nov. 1874.

Ashhurst (John, Jr.), M.D.,
Surgeon to the Episcopal Hospital, Philadelphia.

THE PRINCIPLES AND PRACTICE OF SURGERY. In one very large and handsome octavo volume of about 1000 pages, with nearly 550 illustrations, cloth, $6 50; leather, raised bands, $7 50. (*Lately Published.*)

The object of the author has been to present, within as condensed a compass as possible, a complete treatise on Surgery in all its branches, suitable both as a text-book for the student and a work of reference for the practitioner. So much has of late years been done for the advancement of Surgical Art and Science, that there seemed to be a want of a work which should present the latest aspects of every subject, and which, by its American character, should render accessible to the profession at large the experience of the practitioners of both hemispheres. This has been the aim of the author, and it is hoped that the volume will be found to fulfil its purpose satisfactorily.

Its author has evidently tested the writings and experiences of the past and present in the crucible of a careful, analytic, and honorable mind, and faithfully endeavored to bring his work up to the level of the highest standard of practical surgery. He is frank and definite, and gives us opinions, and generally sound ones, instead of a mere *résumé* of the opinions of others. He is conservative, but not hide-bound by authority. His style is clear, elegant, and scholarly. The work is an admirable text-book, and a useful book of reference. It is a credit to American professional literature, and one of the first ripe fruits of the soil fertilized by the blood of our late unhappy war. —*N. Y. Med. Record,* Feb. 1 1872.

Indeed, the work as a whole must be regarded as an excellent and concise exponent of modern surgery, and as such it will be found a valuable text-book for the student, and a useful book of reference for the general practitioner.—*N Y. Med. Journal,* Feb 1872.

It gives us great pleasure to call the attention of the profession to this excellent work. Our knowledge of its talented and accomplished author led us to expect from him a very valuable treatise upon subjects to which he has repeatedly given evidence of having profitably devoted much time and labor, and we are in no way disappointed.—*Philadelphia Med. Times,* Feb. 1, 1872.

Attfield (John), Ph.D.,
Professor of Practical Chemistry to the Pharmaceutical Society of Great Britain, &c.

CHEMISTRY, GENERAL, MEDICAL, AND PHARMACEUTICAL; including the Chemistry of the U. S. Pharmacopœia. A Manual of the General Principles of the Science, and their application to Medicine and Pharmacy   Fifth Edition, revised by the author. In one handsome royal 12mo. volume; cloth, $2 75; leather, $3 25; (*Lately Issued.*)

No other American publication with which we are acquainted covers the same ground, or does it so well. In addition to an admirable exposé of the facts and principles of general elementary chemistry, the author has presented us with a condensed mass of practical matter, just such as the medical student and practitioner needs.—*Cincinnati Lancet*, Mar. 1874.

This work is characterized as much by its rich contents and its great originality, as by its simple intelligibleness and the skilful manner in which theory and practice are combined.—*Neues Repertorium, für Pharmacie.*

We commend the work heartily as one of the best text-books extant for the medical student.—*Detroit Rev. of Med. and Pharm.*, Feb. 1872.

The best work of the kind in the English language.—*N. Y. Psychological Journal*, Jan. 1872.

The work is constructed with direct reference to the wants of medical and pharmaceutical students; and, although an English work, the points of difference between the British and United States Pharmacopœias are indicated, making it as useful here as in England. Altogether, the book is one we can heartily recommend to practitioners as well as students.—*N. Y. Med. Journal*, Dec. 1871.

It differs from other text books in the following particulars: first, in the exclusion of matter relating to compounds which, at present, are only of interest to the scientific chemist; secondly, in containing the chemistry of every substance recognized officially or in general, as a remedial agent. It will be found a most valuable book for pupils, assistants, and others engaged in medicine and pharmacy, and we heartily commend it to our readers.—*Canada Lancet*, Oct. 1871.

When the original English edition of this work was published, we had occasion to express our high appreciation of its worth, and also to review, in considerable detail, the main features of the book. As the arrangement of subjects, and the main part of the text of the present edition are similar to the former publication, it will be needless for us to go over the ground a second time; we may, however, call attention to a marked advantage possessed by the American work—we allude to the introduction of the chemistry of the preparations of the United States Pharmacopœia, as well as that relating to the British authority.—*Canadian Pharm. Journ.*, Nov. 1871.

Chemistry has borne the name of being a hard subject to master by the student of medicine, and chiefly because so much of it consists of compounds only of interest to the scientific chemist; in this work such portions are modified or altogether left out, and in the arrangement of the subject-matter of the work, practical utility is sought after, and we think fully attained. We commend it for its clearness and order to both teacher and pupil.—*Oregon Med. and Surg. Reporter*, Oct. 1871.

Anderson (McCall), M.D.,
Physician to the Dispensary for Skin Diseases, Glasgow, &c.

ON THE TREATMENT OF DISEASES OF THE SKIN. With an Analysis of Eleven Thousand Consecutive Cases. In one vol. 8vo. $1. (*Lately Published.*)

Ashton (T. J.).
ON THE DISEASES, INJURIES, AND MALFORMATIONS OF THE RECTUM AND ANUS; with remarks on Habitual Constipation. Second American, from the fourth and enlarged London edition. With handsome illustrations. In one very beautifully printed octavo volume of about 300 pages, cloth, $3 25.

ANATOMICAL ATLAS.—SMITH AND HORNER. (See p. 27.)

ASHWELL'S PRACTICAL TREATISE ON THE DISEASES PECULIAR TO WOMEN. Third American, from the Third and revised London edition. 1 vol. 8vo., pp. 528, cloth, $3 50.

BARLOW'S MANUAL OF THE PRACTICE OF MEDICINE. With Additions by D. F. Condie, M.D. 1 vol. 8vo., pp. 600, cloth, $2 50.

Bellamy (E.), F.R.C.S,
THE STUDENT'S GUIDE TO SURGICAL ANATOMY; a Text-Book for Students preparing for their Pass Examination. With Engravings on wood. In one handsome royal 12mo. volume. Cloth, $2 25. (*Just Issued.*)

We welcome Mr. Bellamy's work, as a contribution to the study of regional anatomy, of equal value to the student and the surgeon. It is written in a clear and concise style, and its practical suggestions add largely to the interest attaching to its technical details.—*Chicago Med. Examiner*, March 1, 1874.

We cordially congratulate Mr. Bellamy upon having produced it.—*Med. Times and Gaz.*

We cannot too highly recommend it.—*Student's Journal.*

Mr. Bellamy has spared no pains to produce a really reliable student's guide to surgical anatomy—one which all candidates for surgical degrees may consult with advantage, and which possesses much original matter.—*Med. Press and Circular.*

Blandford (G. Fielding), M.D., F.R.C.P.,
Lecturer on Psychological Medicine at the School of St. George's Hospital, etc.

INSANITY AND ITS TREATMENT; Lectures on the Treatment, Medical and Legal, of Insane Patients. With a Summary of the Laws in force in the United States on the Confinement of the Insane. By Isaac Ray, M.D. In one very handsome octavo volume of 471 pages: cloth, $3 25.

This volume is presented to meet the want, so frequently expressed, of a comprehensive treatise, in moderate compass, on the pathology, diagnosis, and treatment of insanity. To render it of more value to the practitioner in this country, Dr. Ray has added an appendix which affords information, not elsewhere to be found in so accessible a form, to physicians who may at any moment be called upon to take action in relation to patients.

Barnes (Robert), M.D., F.R.C.P.,

Obstetric Physician to St. Thomas's Hospital, &c.

A CLINICAL EXPOSITION OF THE MEDICAL AND SURGICAL

DISEASES OF WOMEN. In one handsome octavo volume of about 800 pages, with 169 illustrations. Cloth, $5 00; leather, $6 00. (*Just Issued.*)

Embodying the long experience and personal observation of one of the greatest of living teachers in diseases of women, it seems pervaded by the presence of the author, who speaks directly to the reader, and speaks, too, as one having authority. And yet, notwithstanding this distinct personality, there is nothing narrow as to time, place, or individuals, in the views presented, and in the instructions given; Dr. Barnes has been an attentive student, not only of European, but also of American literature, pertaining to diseases of females, and enriched his own experience by treasures thence gathered; he seems as familiar, for example, with the writings of Sims, Emmet, Thomas, and Peaslee, as if these eminent men were his countrymen and colleagues, and gives them a credit which must be gratifying to every American physician.— *Am. Journ. Med. Sci.,* April, 1874.

Throughout the whole book it is impossible not to feel that the author has spontaneously, conscientiously, and fearlessly performed his task. He goes direct to the point, and does not loiter on the way to gossip or quarrel with other authors. Dr. Barnes's book will be eagerly read all over the world, and will everywhere be admired for its comprehensiveness, honesty of purpose, and ability.— *The Obstet. Journ. of Great Britain and Ireland,* March, 1874.

Dr. Barnes is not only a practitioner of exceptionally large opportunities, which he has used well, but he has kept informed of what has been said and done by others; and he has in the present volume judiciously used this knowledge. We can strongly recommend Dr. Barnes's work to the gynæcological student and practitioner. — *N. Y. Med. Record,* June 15, 1874.

There has seldom appeared in the English language a more complete, thorough, and exhaustive treatise

on any medical subject than the one now under notice. Dr. Barnes had already established for himself, by his writings and his practice, a position second to none as an obstetric authority. He has had probably the largest operative midwifery experience of any living practitioner, and his name is associated with some of the most important improvements in midwifery practice. The work which has just issued from his pen will go far to establish him as an equal authority in the special department of practice of which he treats. We can only repeat that, as a thoroughly sound, practical, clinical treatise, we know of no English work which can compare to this of Dr. Barnes. To the so-called specialist, as well as to the general practitioner, it will prove a most useful guide.— *London Lancet,* Jan. 10, 1874.

In conclusion, we must express our conviction that, in view of the wide range of subjects compressed into a single volume, this book is admirable for the conciseness and clearness with which practical points are treated, and evidently from a large experience. For students, and, indeed, for a good many of those who for want of time cannot, or for want of inclination will not, be students, it is a safe and satisfactory guide, and no one who attempts to treat the diseases peculiar to women can afford to be without it. The volume is profusely illustrated; many of the cuts are new to gynæcological literature, and most of them are essential adjuncts to the text. — *Boston Med. and Surg. Journ.,* April 17, 1874.

Dr. Barnes's present work is a magnificent contribution to the literature of that branch of the profession with which his name has so long been honorably connected. To attempt, however, an exhaustive analysis of so voluminous a treatise would carry us far beyond all reasonable bounds.— *Glasgow Med. Journ.,* July, 1874.

Bryant (Thomas), F.R.C.S.,

Surgeon to Guy's Hospital.

THE PRACTICE OF SURGERY. With over Five Hundred Engravings

on Wood. In one large and very handsome octavo volume of nearly 1000 pages, cloth, $6 25; leather, raised bands, $7 25. (*Lately Published.*)

Again, the author gives us his own practice, his own beliefs, and illustrates by his own cases, or those treated in Guy's Hospital. This feature adds joint emphasis, and a solidity to his statements that inspire confidence. One feels himself almost by the side of the surgeon, seeing his work and hearing his living words. The views, etc., of other surgeons are considered calmly and fairly, but Mr. Bryant's are adopted. Thus the work is not a compilation of other writings; it is not an encyclopædia, but the plain statements, on practical points, of a man who has lived and breathed and had his being in the richest surgical experience. The whole profession owe a debt of gratitude to Mr. Bryant, for his work in their behalf. We are confident that the American profession will give substantial testimonial of their feelings towards both author and publisher, by speedily exhausting this edition. We cordially and heartily commend it to our friends, and think that no live surgeon can afford to be without it.— *Detroit Review of Med. and Pharmacy,* August, 1873.

As a manual of the practice of surgery for the use of the student, we do not hesitate to pronounce Mr. Bryant's book a first-rate work. Mr. Bryant has a good deal of the dogmatic energy which goes with

the clear, pronounced opinions of a man whose reflections and experience have moulded a character not wanting in firmness and decision. At the same time he teaches with the enthusiasm of one who has faith in his teaching; he speaks as one having authority, and herein lies the charm and excellence of his work. He states the opinions of others freely and fairly, yet it is no mere compilation. The book combines much of the merit of the manual with the merit of the monograph. One may recognize in almost every chapter of the ninety-four of which the work is made up the acuteness of a surgeon who has seen much, and observed closely, and who gives forth the results of actual experience. In conclusion we repeat what we stated at first, that Mr. Bryant's book is one which we can conscientiously recommend both to practitioners and students as an admirable work. — *Dublin Journ. of Med Science,* August, 1873.

This is, as the preface states, an entirely new book, and contains in a moderately condensed form all the surgical information necessary to a general practitioner. It is written in a spirit consistent with the present improved standard of medical and surgical science.— *American Journal of Obstetrics,* August, 1873.

Bigelow (Henry J.), M.D.,

Professor of Surgery in the Massachusetts Med. College.

ON THE MECHANISM OF DISLOCATION AND FRACTURE OF

THE HIP With the Reduction of the Dislocation by the Flexion Method. With numerous original illustrations. In one very handsome octavo volume. Cloth, $2 50.

Bumstead (Freeman J.), M.D.,

Professor of Venereal Diseases at the Coll. of Phys. and Surg., New York, etc.

THE PATHOLOGY AND TREATMENT OF VENEREAL DISEASES. Including the results of recent investigations upon the subject. Third edition, revised and enlarged, with illustrations. In one large and handsome octavo volume of over 700 pages, cloth, $5 00; leather, $6 00.

In preparing this standard work again for the press, the author has subjected it to a very thorough revision. Many portions have been rewritten, and much new matter added, in order to bring it completely on a level with the most advanced condition of syphilography, but by careful compression of the text of previous editions, the work has been increased by only sixty-four pages. The labor thus bestowed upon it, it is hoped, will insure for it a continuance of its position as a complete and trustworthy guide for the practitioner.

It is the most complete book with which we are acquainted in the language. The latest views of the best authorities are put forward, and the information is well arranged—a great point for the student, and still more for the practitioner. The subjects of visceral syphilis, syphilitic affections of the eyes, and the treatment of syphilis by repeated inoculations, are very fully discussed.—*Lond. Lancet*, Jan. 7, 1871.

Dr. Bumstead's work is already so universally known as the best treatise in the English language on venereal diseases, that it may seem almost superfluous to say more of it than that a new edition has been issued. But the author's industry has rendered this new edition virtually a new work, and so merits as much special commendation as if its predecessors had not been published. As a thoroughly practical book on a class of diseases which form a large share of nearly every physician's practice, the volume before us is by far the best of which we have knowledge.—*N. Y. Med. Gazette*, Jan. 28, 1871.

It is rare in the history of medicine to find any one book which contains all that a practitioner needs to know; while the possessor of "Bumstead on Venereal" has no occasion to look outside of its covers for anything practical connected with the diagnosis, history, or treatment of these affections.—*N. Y. Med. Journal*, March, 1871.

Cullerier (A.), and Bumstead (Freeman J.),

Surgeon to the Hôpital du Midi.

Professor of Venereal Diseases in the College of Physicians and Surgeons, N. Y.

AN ATLAS OF VENEREAL DISEASES Translated and Edited by FREEMAN J. BUMSTEAD. In one large imperial 4to. volume of 328 pages, double-columns, with 26 plates, containing about 150 figures, beautifully colored, many of them the size of life; strongly bound in cloth, $17 00; also, in five parts, stout wrappers for mailing, at $3 per part.

Anticipating a very large sale for this work, it is offered at the very low price of THREE DOLLARS a Part, thus placing it within the reach of all who are interested in this department of practice. Gentlemen desiring early impressions of the plates would do well to order it without delay.

A specimen of the plates and text sent free by mail, on receipt of 25 cents.

We wish for once that our province was not restricted to methods of treatment, that we might say something of the exquisite colored plates in this volume. —*London Practitioner*, May, 1869.

As a whole, it teaches all that can be taught by means of plates and print.—*London Lancet*, March 13, 1869.

Superior to anything of the kind ever before issued on this continent.—*Canada Med. Journ.*, March, '69.

The practitioner who desires to understand this branch of medicine thoroughly should obtain this, the most complete and best work ever published.—*Dominion Med. Journ.*, May, 1869.

This is a work of master hands on both sides. M. Cullerier is scarcely second to, we think we may truly say is a peer of the illustrious and venerable Ricord, while in this country we do not hesitate to say that Dr. Bumstead, as an authority, is without a rival. Assuring our readers that these illustrations tell the whole history of venereal disease, from its inception to its end, we do not know a single medical work

which for its kind is more *necessary* for them to have. —*California Med. Gaz.*, March, 1869.

The most splendidly illustrated work in the language, and in our opinion far more useful than the French original.—*Am. Journ. Med. Sci.*, Jan. 1869.

The fifth and concluding number of this magnificent work has reached us, and we have no hesitation in saying that its illustrations surpass those of previous numbers.—*Boston Med. and Surg. Journ.*, Jan. 14, 1869.

Other writers besides M. Cullerier have given us a good account of the diseases of which he treats, but no one has furnished us with such a complete series of illustrations of the venereal diseases. There is, however, an additional interest and value possessed by the volume before us; for it is an American reprint and translation of M. Cullerier's work, with incidental remarks by one of the most eminent American syphilographers, Mr. Bumstead.—*Brit. and For. Med.-Chir. Rev.*, July, 1869.

Bowman (John E.), M.D.

PRACTICAL HANDBOOK OF MEDICAL CHEMISTRY. Edited by C. L. BLOXAM, Professor of Practical Chemistry in King's College, London. Sixth American, from the fourth and revised English Edition. In one neat volume, royal 12mo., pp. 351, with numerous illustrations: cloth, $2 25.

By the same Author. (*Lately Issued.*)

INTRODUCTION TO PRACTICAL CHEMISTRY, INCLUDING ANALYSIS. Sixth American, from the sixth and revised London edition. Edited by C. L. BLOXAM, Prof. of Practical Chemistry in King's College, London. With numerous illustrations. In one neat vol., royal 12mo., cloth, $2 25.

Basham (W. R.), M.D.

Senior Physician to the Westminster Hospital, etc.

RENAL DISEASES: a Clinical Guide to their Diagnosis and Treatment. With illustrations. In one neat royal 12mo. volume of 304 pages: cloth, $2 00.

Bloxam (C. L.),
Professor of Chemistry in King's College, London.

CHEMISTRY, INORGANIC AND ORGANIC. From the Second London Edition. In one very handsome octavo volume, of 700 pages, with about 300 illustrations. Cloth, $4 00; leather, $5 00. (*Lately Issued.*)

It has been the author's endeavor to produce a Treatise on Chemistry sufficiently comprehensive for those studying the science as a branch of general education, and one which students may use with advantage in pursuing their chemical studies in the colleges or medical schools. The special attention devoted to Metallurgy and some other branches of Applied Chemistry renders the work especially useful to those who are being educated for employment in manufacture.

We have spoken of the work as admirably adapted to the wants of students; it is quite as well suited to the wants of practitioners who wish to review their chemistry, or have occasion to refresh their memories on any point relating to it. In a word, it is a book to be read by all who wish to know what is the chemistry of the present day.—*Am. Practitioner,* Nov. 1873.

We cordially welcome this American reprint of a work which has already won for itself so substantial a reputation in England. Professor Bloxam has condensed into a wonderfully small compass all the important principles and facts of chemical science. The details of illustrative experiment have been worked up with especial care, and many of the experiments described are both new and striking.—*Detroit Rev. of Med. and Pharm.*, Nov. 1873.

It would be difficult for a practical chemist and teacher to find any material fault with this most admirable treatise. The author has given us almost a cyclopedia within the limits of a convenient volume, and has done so without penning the *useless* paragraphs too commonly making up a great part of the bulk of many cumbrous works. Altogether, it is seldom you see a text book so nearly faultless.—*Cincinnati Lancet,* Nov. 1873.

Professor Bloxam has given us a most excellent and useful practical treatise. His 666 pages are crowded with facts and experiments, nearly all well chosen, and many quite new, even to scientific men. . . . It is astonishing how much information he often conveys in a few paragraphs. We might quote fifty instances of this.—*Lond. Chemical News*

Brinton (William), M.D., F.R.S.

LECTURES ON THE DISEASES OF THE STOMACH; with an Introduction on its Anatomy and Physiology. From the second and enlarged London edition. With illustrations on wood. In one handsome octavo volume of about 300 pages: cloth, $3 25.

Bristowe (John Syer) M.D., F.R.C.P.,
Physician and Joint Lecturer on Medicine, St. Thomas's Hospital.

A MANUAL OF THE PRACTICE OF MEDICINE. Edited, with Additions, by JAMES H. HUTCHINSON, M.D., Physician to the Penna. Hospital. In one handsome octavo volume. (*Nearly Ready.*)

Carter (R. Brudenell), F.R.C.S.,
Ophthalmic Surgeon to St. George's Hospital, etc.

A PRACTICAL TREATISE ON DISEASES OF THE EYE. Edited, with Additions, by JOHN GREEN, M.D. (of St. Louis, Mo). With test-types and numerous illustrations. In one handsome octavo volume. (*Nearly Ready.*)

The object of the author has been to produce, within a moderate compass, a work which should serve the purposes of the general practitioner by giving, "in a concise and readable form, a general view of the present state of knowledge with regard to the nature and treatment of the more important diseases of the eye." That he has fully succeeded in his effort is shown by the commendation which the volume has received wherever its merits have become known.

It would be difficult for Mr. Carter to write an uninstructive book, and impossible for him to write an uninteresting one. Even on subjects with which he is not bound to be familiar, he can discourse with a rare degree of clearness and effect. Our readers will therefore not be surprised to learn that a work by him on the Diseases of the Eye makes a very valuable addition to ophthalmic literature. . . . The book will remain one useful alike to the general and the special practitioner. Not the least valuable result which we expect from it is that it will to some considerable extent despecialize this brilliant department of medicine.—*London Lancet*, Oct. 30, 1875.

It is with great pleasure that we can endorse the work as a most valuable contribution to practical ophthalmology. Mr. Carter never deviates from the end he has in view, and presents the subject in

a clear and concise manner, easy of comprehension, and hence the more valuable. We would especially commend, however, as worthy of high praise, the manner in which the therapeutics of disease of the eye is elaborated, for here the author is particularly clear and practical, where other writers are unfortunately too often deficient. The final chapter is devoted to a discussion of the uses and selection of spectacles, and is admirably compact, plain, and useful, especially the paragraphs on the treatment of presbyopia and myopia. In conclusion, our thanks are due the author for many useful hints in the great subject of ophthalmic surgery and therapeutics, a field where of late years we glean but a few grains of sound wheat from a mass of chaff.—*N. Y. Med. Record*, Oct. 23, 1875.

Condie (D. Francis), M.D.

A PRACTICAL TREATISE ON THE DISEASES OF CHILDREN. Sixth edition, revised and augmented. In one large octavo volume of nearly 800 closely printed pages, cloth, $5 25; leather, $6 25.

Chambers (T. K.), M.D.,

Consulting Physician to St. Mary's Hospital, London, &c.

A MANUAL OF DIET IN HEALTH AND DISEASE. In one handsome octavo volume, cloth, $2 75. (*Now Ready.*)

The aims of this handbook are purely practical, and therefore it has not been thought right to increase its size by the addition of the chemical, botanical, and industrial learning which rapidly collects round the nucleus of every article interesting as an eatable. Space has been thus gained for a full discussion of many matters connecting food and drink with the daily current of social life, which the position of the author as a practising physician has led him to believe highly important to the present and future of our race.—(*Preface.*)

In compliing this small but comprehensive manual, Dr. Chambers has laid the profession under a debt of gratitude to him. He writes on the subject like one who has given his mind to it, and therefore is entitled to speak with authority. As a pioneer Dr. Chambers deserves much credit: he has opened up a new field of which others will no doubt avail themselves. Taken altogether this work is one which gives, in an agreeable form, much valuable information on a most important subject, and ought to have a large sale both in the profession and out of it.—*London Med. Record*, May 19, 1875.

In thorough mastery of the subjects upon which he writes, and in the happy command of language to convey his meaning in the fewest possible words, he is certainly unexcelled and rarely equalled by any writer in the English language. It is altogether a work of rare excellence and should, as it doubtless will, speedily find a place on the table of every physician.—*The N. Y. Sanitarian*, June, 1875.

This work is a substantial addition to our standard works, and not only should the neat little volume find a place in the most restricted libraries, but its contents ought to be read, marked, learned, and inwardly digested by each practitioner, until they have become woven into the web of the ordinary every day thought of all medical men who truly love their profession.—*Lond. Practitioner*, June, '75.

By the same Author. (*Lately Published.*)

RESTORATIVE MEDICINE. An Harveian Annual Oration. With Two Sequels. In one very handsome volume, small 12mo., cloth, $1 00.

Cullerier (A.), and Bumstead (Freeman J.)

AN ATLAS OF VENEREAL DISEASES. (*See p 11.*)

Carpenter (William B.), M.D., F.R.S.,

Examiner in Physiology and Comparative Anatomy in the University of London.

PRINCIPLES OF HUMAN PHYSIOLOGY; with their chief applications to Psychology, Pathology, Therapeutics, Hygiene, and Forensic Medicine. A new American from the last and revised London edition. With nearly nine hundred illustrations. Edited, with additions, by FRANCIS GURNEY SMITH, M D., Professor of the Institutes of Medicine in the University of Pennsylvania, &c. In one very large and beautiful octavo volume, of about 900 large pages, handsomely printed; cloth, $5 50; leather, raised bands, $6 50.

CARPENTER'S PRIZE ESSAY ON THE USE OF ALCOHOLIC LIQUORS IN HEALTH AND DISEASE. New edition, with a Preface by D. F. CONDIE, M.D., and explanations of scientific words. In one neat 12mo. volume, pp. 178, cloth. 60 cents.

COOPER'S LECTURES ON THE PRINCIPLES AND PRACTICE OF SURGERY. In 1 vol. 8vo., cloth, 750 pp., $200.

CHURCHILL'S ESSAYS ON THE PUERPERAL FEVER, AND OTHER DISEASES PECULIAR TO WOMEN. 1 vol. 8vo., of 450 pages. Cloth, $2 50

CHURCHILL ON THE THEORY AND PRACTICE OF MEDICINE. A new American, from the fourth revised and enlarged London edition. With notes and additions by D. FRANCIS CONDIE, M.D. With one hundred and ninety-four illustrations. In one very handsome octavo volume of nearly 700 pages. Cloth, 4 00; leather, $5 00.

CHRISTISON'S DISPENSATORY. With copious additions, and 213 large wood engravings. By R. EGLESFELD GRIFFITH, M.D. One vol. 8vo., pp. 1000; cloth, $4 00.

Davis (Nathan S.),

Prof. of Principles and Practice of Medicine, etc., in Chicago Med. College.

CLINICAL LECTURES ON VARIOUS IMPORTANT DISEASES. Being a Collection of the Clinical Lectures delivered in the Medical Wards of Mercy Hospital, Chicago. Edited by FRANK H. DAVIS, M.D. Second Edition, enlarged. In one handsome royal 12mo. volume: cloth, $1 75. (*Now Ready.*)

Chicago is such a wonderful place that we are prepared to hear almost anything of it, but we were scarcely prepared to receive from it such an excellent little volume of clinical lectures as we have here, and which we commend to all clinical students and

practitioners. We commend Dr. Davis's lectures to the attention of our readers. The whole book, we repeat, is valuable as the outcome of thirty years of intelligent practice.—*London Lancet*, May 29, 1875.

Dunglison, Forbes, Tweedie, and Conolly.

THE CYCLOPÆDIA OF PRACTICAL MEDICINE: comprising Treatises on the Nature and Treatment of Diseases, Materia Medica and Therapeutics, Diseases of Women and Children, Medical Jurisprudence, etc. etc. In four super-royal octavo volumes, of 3254 double-columned pages, strongly and handsomely bound in leather, $15; cloth, $11.

Dunglison (Robley), M.D.,

Late Professor of Institutes of Medicine in Jefferson Medical College, Philadelphia.

MEDICAL LEXICON ; A DICTIONARY OF MEDICAL SCIENCE ; Containing a concise explanation of the various Subjects and Terms of Anatomy, Physiology, Pathology, Hygiene, Therapeutics, Pharmacology, Pharmacy, Surgery, Obstetrics, Medical Jurisprudence, and Dentistry. Notices of Climate and of Mineral Waters ; Formulæ for Officinal, Empirical, and Dietetic Preparations ; with the Accentuation and Etymology of the Terms, and the French and other Synonymes; so as to constitute a French as well as English Medical Lexicon. A New Edition. Thoroughly Revised, and very greatly Modified and Augmented. By RICHARD J. DUNGLISON, M.D. In one very large and handsome royal octavo volume of over 1100 pages. Cloth, $6 50; leather, raised bands, $7 50. (*Just Issued.*)

The object of the author from the outset has not been to make the work a mere lexicon or dictionary of terms, but to afford, under each, a condensed view of its various medical relations, and thus to render the work an epitome of the existing condition of medical science. Starting with this view, the immense demand which has existed for the work has enabled him, in repeated revisions, to augment its completeness and usefulness, until at length it has attained the position of a recognized and standard authority wherever the language is spoken.

Special pains have been taken in the preparation of the present edition to maintain this enviable reputation. During the ten years which have elapsed since the last revision, the additions to the nomenclature of the medical sciences have been greater than perhaps in any similar period of the past, and up to the time of his death the author labored assiduously to incorporate everything requiring the attention of the student or practitioner. Since then, the editor has been equally industrious, so that the additions to the vocabulary are more numerous than in any previous revision. Especial attention has been bestowed on the accentuation, which will be found marked on every word. The typographical arrangement has been much improved, rendering reference much more easy, and every care has been taken with the mechanical execution. The work has been printed on new type, small but exceedingly clear, with an enlarged page, so that the additions have been incorporated with an increase of but little over a hundred pages, and the volume now contains the matter of at least four ordinary octavos.

A book well known to our readers, and of which every American ought to be proud. When the learned author of the work passed away, probably all of us feared lest the book should not maintain its place in the advancing science whose terms it defines. Fortunately, Dr. Richard J. Dunglison, having assisted his father in the revision of several editions of the work, and having been, therefore, trained in the methods and imbued with the spirit of the book, has been able to edit it, not in the patchwork manner so dear to the heart of book editors, so repulsive to the taste of intelligent book readers, but to edit it as a work of the kind should be edited—to carry it on steadily, without jar or interruption, along the grooves of thought it has travelled during its lifetime. To show the magnitude of the task which Dr. Dunglison has assumed and carried through, it is only necessary to state that more than six thousand new subjects have been added in the present edition. Without occupying more space with the theme, we congratulate the editor on the successful completion of his labors, and hope he may reap the well-earned reward of profit and honor.—*Phila. Med. Times,* Jan. 3, 1874.

A work to which there is no equal in the English language.—*Edinburgh Med. Journal.*

About the first book purchased by the medical student is the Medical Dictionary. The lexicon explanatory of technical terms is simply a *sine qua non.* In a science so extensive, and with such collaterals as medicine, it is as much a necessity also to the practising physician. To meet the wants of students and most physicians, the dictionary must be condensed while comprehensive, and practical while perspicacious. It was because Dunglison's met these indications that it became at once the dictionary of general use wherever medicine was studied in the English language. In no former revision have the alterations and additions been so

great. More than six thousand new subjects and terms have been added. The chief terms have been set in black letter, while the derivatives follow in small caps; an arrangement which greatly facilitates reference. We may safely confirm the hope ventured by the editor "that the work, which possesses for him a filial as well as an individual interest, will be found worthy a continuance of the position so long accorded to it as a standard authority."—*Cincinnati Clinic,* Jan. 10, 1874.

With a history of forty years of unexampled success and universal indorsement by the medical profession of the western continent, it would be presumption in any living medical American to essay its review. No reviewer, however able, can add to its fame ; no captious critic, however caustic, can remove a single stone from its firm and enduring foundation. It is destined, as a colossal monument, to perpetuate the solid and richly deserved fame of Robley Dunglison to coming generations. The large additions made to the vocabulary, we think, will be welcomed by the profession as supplying the want of a lexicon fully up with the march of science, which has been increasingly felt for some years past. The accentuation of terms is very complete, and, as far as we have been able to examine it, very excellent. We hope it may be the means of securing greater uniformity of pronunciation among medical men.—*Atlanta Med and Surg Journ,* Feb. 1874.

Few works of the class exhibit a grander monument of patient research and of scientific lore. The extent of the sale of this lexicon is sufficient to testify to its usefulness, and to the great service conferred by Dr. Robley Dunglison on the profession, and indeed on others, by its issue.—*London Lancet.*

It has the rare merit that it certainly has no rival in the English language for accuracy and extent of references.—*London Medical Gazette.*

By the same Author.

HUMAN PHYSIOLOGY. Eighth edition. Thoroughly revised and extensively modified and enlarged, with five hundred and thirty-two illustrations. In two large and handsomely printed octavo volumes of about 1500 pages : cloth, $7 00.

By the same Author.

NEW REMEDIES: WITH FORMULÆ FOR THEIR PREPARATION AND ADMINISTRATION. Seventh edition, with extensive additions. 1 vol. 8vo., pp. 770 : cloth, $4 00.

Dalton (J. C.), M.D.,

Professor of Physiology in the College of Physicians and Surgeons, New York, etc.

A TREATISE ON HUMAN PHYSIOLOGY. Designed for the use of

Students and Practitioners of Medicine. Sixth Edition, thoroughly revised and enlarged. In one very beautiful octavo volume of 830 pages. With 316 illustrations on wood. cloth, $5 50; leather, $6 50. (*Now Ready.*)

In the preparation of this edition the author has spared no pains to render it worthy a continuance of the very remarkable favor which it has thus far enjoyed. Every portion has been subjected to a careful revision for the purpose of making it a clear and accurate exposition of the most advanced condition of scientific knowledge in so far as its results can be stated with certainty. To accomplish this has required a considerable increase in the amount of the text, resulting, in spite of the author's efforts at condensation, in an enlargement equivalent to fully one-half of the previous edition. A change in the typographical arrangement, however, has accommodated these extensive additions without rendering the volume unwieldy in size. The series of illustrations has also been very greatly improved, not only by the introduction of additional figures, but by the substitution of new and more perfect ones for others which were deemed unsatisfactory. Every care has been taken in the mechanical execution of the volume, and it is confidently presented as one of the handsomest productions of the American press.

During the past few years several new works on physiology, and the new editions of old works, have appeared, competing for the favor of the medical student, but none will rival this new edition of Dalton. As now enlarged, it will be found also to be, in general, a satisfactory work of reference for the practitioner — *Chicago Med. Journ. and Examiner*, Jan. 1876

Prof. Dalton has discussed conflicting theories and conclusions regarding physiological questions with a fairness, a fulness, and a conciseness which lend freshness and vigor to the entire book. But his discussions have been so guarded by a refusal of admission to those speculative and theoretical explanations, which at best exist in the minds of observers themselves as only probabilities, that none of his readers need be led into grave errors while making them a study.—*The Medical Record*, Feb. 19, 1876.

The revision of this great work has brought it forward with the physiological advances of the day, and renders it, as it has ever been, the finest work for students extant.—*Nashville Journ. of Med. and Surg.*, Jan. 1876.

For clearness and perspicuity, Dalton's Physiology commended itself to the student years ago, and was a pleasant relief from the verbose productions which it supplanted. Physiology has, however, made many advances since then—and while the style has been preserved intact, the work in the present edition has been brought up fully abreast of the times. The new chemical notation and nomenclature have also been introduced into the present edition. Notwithstanding the multiplicity of text books on physiology, this will lose none

of its old time popularity. The mechanical execution of the work is all that could be desired.—*Peninsular Journ. of Med.*, Dec. 1875.

This popular text-book on physiology comes to us in its sixth edition with the addition of about fifty per cent. of new matter, chiefly in the departments of pathological chemistry and the nervous system, where the principal advances have been realized. With so thorough revision and additions, that keep the work well up to the times, its continued popularity may be confidently predicted, notwithstanding the competition it may encounter. The publisher's work is admirably done.—*St. Louis Med. and Surg. Journ.*, Dec. 1875.

We heartily welcome this, the sixth edition of this admirable text-book, than which there are none of equal brevity more valuable. It is cordially recommended by the Professor of Physiology in the University of Louisiana, as by all competent teachers in the United States and wherever the English language is read, this book has been appreciated. The present edition, with its 316 admirably executed illustrations, has been carefully revised and very much enlarged, although its bulk does not seem perceptibly increased.—*New Orleans Medical and Surgical Journal*, March, 1876.

The present edition is very much superior to every other, not only in that it brings the subject up to the times, but that it does so more fully and satisfactorily than any previous edition. Take it altogether, it remains in our humble opinion the best text-book on physiology in any land or language.—*The Clinic*, Nov 6, 1875.

Druitt (Robert), M.R.C.S., &c.

THE PRINCIPLES AND PRACTICE OF MODERN SURGERY. From

the eighth enlarged and improved London edition. Illustrated with four hundred and thirty-two wood engravings. In one very handsome octavo volume of nearly 700 large and closely printed pages: cloth, $4 00; leather, $5 00.

All that the surgical student or practitioner could desire.—*Dublin Quarterly Journal.*

It is a most admirable book. We do not know when we have examined one with more pleasure.—*Boston Med. and Surg. Journal.*

In Mr. Druitt's book, though containing only some seven hundred pages, both the principles and the

practice of surgery are treated, and so clearly and perspicuously, as to elucidate every important topic. We have examined the book most thoroughly, and can say that this success is well merited. His book, moreover, possesses the inestimable advantages of having the subjects perfectly well arranged and classified, and of being written in a style at once clear and succinct.—*Am. Journ. of Med. Sciences.*

DEWEES ON THE PHYSICAL AND MEDICAL TREATMENT OF CHILDREN. Eleventh edition. 1 vol. 8vo. of 548 pages. Cloth, $2 80

De JONGH ON THE THREE KINDS OF COD LIVER OIL, with their Chemical and Therapeutic Properties, 1 vol. 12mo., cloth. 75 cents.

DEWEES'S TREATISE ON THE DISEASES OF FEMALES. With illustrations. Eleventh Edition, with the Author's last improvements and corrections. In one octavo volume of 536 pages, with plates, cloth. $3 00.

Ellis (Benjamin), M.D.

THE MEDICAL FORMULARY; being a Collection of Prescriptions derived

from the writings and practice of many of the most eminent physicians of America and Europe. Together with the usual Dietetic Preparations and Antidotes for Poisons. The whole accompanied with a few brief Pharmaceutic and Medical Observations. Twelfth edition, carefully revised and much improved by ALBERT H. SMITH, M.D. In one volume 8vo. of 376 pages: cloth, $3 00.

Erichsen (John E.),
Professor of Surgery in University College, London, etc.

THE SCIENCE AND ART OF SURGERY; being a Treatise on Surgical
Injuries, Diseases, and Operations. Revised by the author from the Sixth and enlarged English Edition. Illustrated by over seven hundred engravings on wood. In two large and beautiful octavo volumes of over 1700 pages: cloth, $9; leather, $11. (*Lately Issued.*)

From the Author's Preface to the New American Edition.

"The favorable reception with which the 'Science and Art of Surgery' has been honored by the Surgical Profession in the United States of America has been not only a source of deep gratification and of just pride to me, but has laid the foundation of many professional friendships that are amongst the most agreeable and valued recollections of my life.

"I have endeavored to make the present edition of this work more deserving than its predecessors of the favor that has been accorded to them. In consequence of the delays that have unavoidably occurred in the publication of the Sixth British Edition, time has been afforded to me to add to this one several paragraphs which I trust will be found to increase the practical value of the work."

LONDON, Oct. 1872.

On no former edition of this work has the author bestowed more pains to render it a complete and satisfactory exposition of British Surgery in its modern aspects. Every portion has been sedulously revised, and a large number of new illustrations have been introduced. In addition to the material thus added to the English edition, the author has furnished for the American edition such material as has accumulated since the passage of the sheets through the press in London, so that the work, as now presented to the American profession, contains his latest views and experience.

The increase in the size of the work has seemed to render necessary its division into two volumes. Great care has been exercised in its typographical execution, and it is confidently presented as in every respect worthy to maintain the high reputation which has rendered it a standard authority on this department of medical science.

These are only a few of the points in which the present edition of Mr. Erichsen's work surpasses its predecessors. Throughout there is evidence of a laborious care and solicitude in seizing the passing knowledge of the day, which reflects the greatest credit on the author, and much enhances the value of his work. We can only admire the industry which has enabled Mr. Erichsen thus to succeed, amid the distractions of active practice, in producing emphatically THE book of reference and study for British practitioners of surgery.—*London Lancet*, Oct. 26, 1872.

The entire work, complete, as the great English treatise on Surgery of our own time, is, we can assure our readers, equally well adapted for the most junior student, and, as a book of reference, for the advanced practitioner.—*Dublin Quarterly Journal.*

This excellent standard work on surgery has for many years deservedly been the favorite text-book with the vast mass of American as well as English medical students. The present is a thoroughly revised and enlarged edition. No effort has been spared to make it a complete exposition of the Science and Art of Surgery, and no work on the subject is better adapted, either for a text-book for students, or work of reference for practitioners.—*St. Louis Med. Archives*, May, 1873.

For years past American students have regarded "Erichsen" as *the* surgical text-book *par excellence*. To the general practitioner the present edition is decidedly more valuable than its predecessors, although its main features of course are the same.—*Cincinnati Clinic*, March 22, 1873.

The present edition places the work fully abreast of the times in all improvements in modern surgery. Many chapters are rewritten and re-arranged, and much useful matter has been added. The work has always been held in high estimation in the past, and the present edition fully entitles it to the confidence and support of the profession as a work of reference. —*Chicago Med. Examiner*, April 15, 1873.

Fownes (George), Ph.D.

A MANUAL OF ELEMENTARY CHEMISTRY; Theoretical and
Practical. With one hundred and ninety-seven illustrations, A new American, from the tenth and revised London edition. Edited by ROBERT BRIDGES, M.D. In one large royal 12mo. volume, of about 850 pages: cloth, $2 75; leather; $3 25. (*Lately Issued.*)

This work is so well known that it seems almost superfluous for us to speak about it. It has been a favorite text-book with medical students for years, and its popularity has in no respect diminished. Whenever we have been consulted by medical students, as has frequently occurred, what treatise on chemistry they should procure, we have always recommended Fownes', for we regarded it as the best. There is no work that combines so many excellences. It is of convenient size, not prolix, of plain, perspicuous diction, contains all the most recent discoveries, and is of moderate price.—*Cincinnati Med. Repertory*, Aug. 1869.

Large additions have been made, especially in the department of organic chemistry, and we know of no other work that has greater claims on the physician, pharmaceutist, or student, than this. We cheerfully recommend it as the best text-book on elementary chemistry, and bespeak for it the careful attention of students of pharmacy.—*Chicago Pharmacist*, Aug. 1869.

Here is a new edition which has been long watched for by eager teachers of chemistry. In its new garb, and under the editorship of Mr. Watts, it has resumed its old place as the most successful of text-books.—*Indian Medical Gazette*, Jan. 1, 1869.

It will continue, as heretofore, to hold the first rank as a text-book for students of medicine.—*Chicago Med. Examiner*, Aug. 1869.

Fox (Wilson), M.D.,
Holme Prof. of Clinical Med., University Coll., London.

THE DISEASES OF THE STOMACH: Being the Third Edition of
the "Diagnosis and Treatment of the Varieties of Dyspepsia." Revised and Enlarged. With Illustrations. In one handsome octavo volume: cloth, $2 00. (*Now Ready*)

Dr. Fox has put forth a volume of uncommon excellence, which we feel very sure will take a high rank among works that treat of the stomach.—*Am. Practitioner*, March, 1873.

Flint (Austin), M.D.,
Professor of the Principles and Practice of Medicine in Bellevue Med. College, N. Y.

A TREATISE ON THE PRINCIPLES AND PRACTICE OF MEDICINE; designed for the use of Students and Practitioners of Medicine. Fourth edition, revised and enlarged. In one large and closely printed octavo volume of about 1100 pages: cloth, $6 00; or strongly bound in leather, with raised bands, $7 00. (*Just Issued.*)

By common consent of the English and American medical press, this work has been assigned to the highest position as a complete and compendious text-book on the most advanced condition of medical science. At the very moderate price at which it is offered it will be found one of the cheapest volumes now before the profession.

This excellent treatise on medicine has acquired for itself in the United States a reputation similar to that enjoyed in England by the admirable lectures of Sir Thomas Watson. It may not possess the same charm of style, but it has like solidity, the fruit of long and patient observation, and presents kindred moderation and eclecticism. We have referred to many of the most important chapters, and find the revision spoken of in the preface is a genuine one, and that the author has very fairly brought up his matter to the level of the knowledge of the present day. The work has this great recommendation, that it is in one volume, and therefore will not be so terrifying to the student as the bulky volumes which several of our English text-books of medicine have developed into. —*British and For. Med.-Chir. Rev.*, Jan. 1875.

It is of course unnecessary to introduce or eulogize this now standard treatise. All the colleges recommend it as a text-book, and there are few libraries in which one of its editions is not to be found. The present edition has been enlarged and revised to bring it up to the author's present level of experience and reading. His own clinical studies and the latest contributions to medical literature both in this country and in Europe, have received careful attention, so that some portions have been entirely rewritten, and about seventy pages of new matter have been added. —*Chicago Med. Journ.*, June, 1873.

Has never been surpassed as a text-book for students and a book of ready reference for practitioners.

The force of its logic, its simple and practical teachings, have left it without a rival in the field.—*N. Y. Med. Record*, Sept. 15, 1874.

Flint's Practice of Medicine has become so fixed in its position as an American text-book that little need be said beyond the announcement of a new edition. It may, however, be proper to say that the author has improved the occasion to introduce the latest contributions of medical literature together with the results of his own continued clinical observations. Not so extended as many of the standard works on practice, it still is sufficiently complete for all ordinary reference, and we do not know of a more convenient work for the busy general practitioner.—*Cincinnati Lancet and Observer*, June, 1873.

Prof. Flint, in the fourth edition of his great work, has performed a labor reflecting much credit upon himself, and conferring a lasting benefit upon the profession. The whole work shows evidence of thorough revision, so that it appears like a new book written expressly for the times. For the general practitioner and student of medicine, we cannot recommend the book in too strong terms.—*N. Y. Med. Journ.*, Sept. 1873.

It is given to very few men to tread in the steps of Austin Flint, whose single volume on medicine, though here and there defective, is a masterpiece of lucid condensation and of general grasp of an enormously wide subject. —*London Practitioner*, Dec. 1873.

By the same Author. (*Just Issued.*)

PHTHISIS: ITS MORBID ANATOMY, ETIOLOGY, SYMPTOMATIC EVENTS AND COMPLICATIONS, FATALITY, AND PROGNOSIS, TREATMENT AND PHYSICAL DIAGNOSIS: in a series of Clinical Studies. In one handsome octavo volume. $3 50.

This book contains an analysis, in the author's lucid style, of the notes which he has made in several hundred cases in hospital and private practice. We commend the book to the perusal of all interested in the study of this disease.—*Boston Med. and Surg. Journ.*, Feb. 10, 1876.

It is a rich contribution to the study of the most destructive of diseases, and should be in the hands of every medical practitioner.—*Pacific Med. and Surg. Journ.*, Feb 1876.

The name of the author is a sufficient guarantee that this book is of practical value to both student and practitioner. While the author takes issue with many of the leading minds of the day on important questions arising in the study of phthisis, the strong testimony of experience and authority will have great weight with the seeker after truth. As the result of clinical study, the work is unequalled.—*St. Louis Med. and Surg. Journ.*, March, 1876.

By the same Author.

ESSAYS ON CONSERVATIVE MEDICINE AND KINDRED TOPICS. In one very handsome royal 12mo. volume. Cloth, $1 38. (*Just Issued.*)

By the same Author.

A PRACTICAL TREATISE ON THE DIAGNOSIS, PATHOLOGY, AND TREATMENT OF DISEASES OF THE HEART. Second revised and enlarged edition. In one octavo volume of 550 pages, with a plate; cloth, $4 00.

The author has sedulously improved the opportunity afforded him of revising this work. Portions of it have been rewritten, and the whole brought up to a level with the most advanced condition of science. It must, therefore, continue to maintain its position as the standard treatise on the subject.

By the same Author.

A PRACTICAL TREATISE ON THE PHYSICAL EXPLORATION OF THE CHEST AND THE DIAGNOSIS OF DISEASES AFFECTING THE RESPIRATORY ORGANS. Second and Revised Edition. In one handsome octavo volume of 595 pages: cloth, $4 50.

Dr. Flint's treatise is one of the most trustworthy guides which we can consult. The style is clear and distinct, and is also concise, being free from that tendency to over-refinement and unnecessary minuteness which characterizes many works on the same subject.—*Dublin Medical Press*, Feb. 6, 1867.

Fenwick (Samuel), M.D.,
Assistant Physician to the London Hospital.

THE STUDENT'S GUIDE TO MEDICAL DIAGNOSIS. From the
Third Revised and Enlarged English Edition. With eighty-four illustrations on wood. In one very handsome volume, royal 12mo., cloth, $2 25. (*Just Issued.*)

The very great success which this work has obtained in England, shows that it has supplied an admitted want among elementary books for the guidance of students and junior practitioners. Taking up in order each portion of the body or class of disease, the author has endeavored to present in simple language the value of symptoms, so as to lead the student to a correct appreciation of the pathological changes indicated by them. The latest investigations have been carefully introduced into the present edition, so that it may fairly be considered as on a level with the most advanced condition of medical science.

Of the many guide-books on medical diagnosis, claimed to be written for the special instruction of students, this is the best. The author is evidently a well-read and accomplished physician, and he knows how to teach practical medicine. The charm of simplicity is not the least interesting feature in the manner in which Dr. Fenwick conveys instruction. There are few books of this size on practical medicine that contain so much and convey it so well as the volume before us. It is a book we can sincerely recommend to the student for direct instruction, and to the practitioner as a ready and useful aid to his memory.—*Am. Journ. of Syphilography*, Jan. 1874.

It covers the ground of medical diagnosis in a

concise, practical manner, well calculated to assist the student in forming a correct, thorough, and systematic method of examination and diagnosis of disease. The illustrations are numerous, and finely executed. Those illustrative of the microscopic appearance of morbid tissue, &c., are especially clear and distinct.—*Chicago Med. Examiner*, Nov. 1873.

So far superior to any offered to students, that the colleges of this country should recommend it to their respective classes.—*N. O. Med. and Surg. Journ.*, March, 1874.

This little book ought to be in the possession of every medical student.—*Boston Med. and Surgical Journ.*, Jan. 15, 1874.

Fuller (Henry William), M.D.,
Physician to St. George's Hospital, London.

ON DISEASES OF THE LUNGS AND AIR-PASSAGES. Their Pathol-
ogy, Physical Diagnosis, Symptoms, and Treatment. From the second and revised English edition. In one handsome octavo volume of about 500 pages: cloth, $3 50.

Gray (Henry), F.R.S.,
Lecturer on Anatomy at St. George's Hospital, London.

ANATOMY, DESCRIPTIVE AND SURGICAL. The Drawings by
H. V. CARTER, M.D., late Demonstrator of Anatomy at St. George's Hospital ; the Dissections jointly by the AUTHOR and DR CARTER A New American, from the fifth enlarged and improved London edition. In one magnificent imperial octavo volume, of nearly 900 pages, with 465 large and elaborate engravings on wood. Price in cloth, $6 00 ; leather, raised bands, $7 00. (*Just Issued.*)

The author has endeavored in this work to cover a more extended range of subjects than is customary in the ordinary text-books, by giving not only the details necessary for the student, but also the application of those details in the practice of medicine and surgery, thus rendering it both a guide for the learner, and an admirable work of reference for the active practitioner. The engravings form a special feature in the work, many of them being the size of nature, nearly all original, and having the names of the various parts printed on the body of the cut, in place of figures of reference, with descriptions at the foot. They thus form a complete and splendid series, which will greatly assist the student in obtaining a clear idea of Anatomy, and will also serve to refresh the memory of those who may find in the exigencies of practice the necessity of recalling the details of the dissecting room ; while combining, as it does, a complete Atlas of Anatomy, with a thorough treatise on systematic, descriptive, and applied Anatomy, the work will be found of essential use to all physicians who receive students in their offices, relieving both preceptor and pupil of much labor in laying the groundwork of a thorough medical education.

Notwithstanding the enlargement of this edition, it has been kept at its former very moderate price, rendering it one of the cheapest works now before the profession.

The illustrations are beautifully executed, and render this work an indispensable adjunct to the library of the surgeon This remark applies with great force to those surgeons practising at a distance from our large cities, as the opportunity of refreshing their memory by actual dissection is not always attainable.—*Canada Med. Journal*, Aug. 1870.

To commend Gray's Anatomy to the medical profession is almost as much a work of supererogation as it would be to give a favorable notice of the Bible in the religious press. To say that it is the most complete and conveniently arranged text-book of its kind, is to repeat what each generation of students has learned as a tradition of the elders, and verified by personal experience.—*N. Y. Med Gazette*, Dec. 17, 1870.

The new edition of this very valuable treatise is in many respects an improvement upon the editions which have preceded it. Those already familiar with the work will be struck at a glance with the more systematic arrangement of the subjects em-

braced in it. General Anatomy, for instance, has been isolated from the departments of Descriptive and Surgical Anatomy, with which it had been previously incorporated, and now occupies an important position in an elaborate and instructive introductory chapter of eighty-three pages. Much labor has evidently been expended in the preparation of the very recent English edition, of which this is a transcript, and new cuts and a large amount of matter have been added, to keep this useful work thoroughly up to the requirements of the day, and to preserve its reputation as the best exponent of the present state of anatomical science, which the student can consult. The advantages presented in the method of copious illustration by large cuts, abundantly lettered on the block itself, on the very point of interest described in the text, whether it be process, muscle, tendon, artery, or nerve, have long since been recognized by teacher and student alike, and have contributed largely to the wide-spread popularity which this anatomical text book has attained on both sides of the Atlantic.—*Am. Journ. Med. Sci.*, July, 1870.

Gross (Samuel D.), M.D.,
Professor of Surgery in the Jefferson Medical College of Philadelphia.

A SYSTEM OF SURGERY : Pathological, Diagnostic, Therapeutic, and Operative. Illustrated by upwards of Fourteen Hundred Engravings. Fifth edition, carefully revised, and improved In two large and beautifully printed imperial octavo volumes of about 2300 pages, strongly bound in leather, with raised bands, $15. (*Just Issued.*)

The continued favor, shown by the exhaustion of repeated large editions of this great work, proves that it has successfully supplied a want felt by American practitioners and students. In the present revision no pains have been spared by the author to bring it in every respect fully up to the day. To effect this a large part of the work has been re-written, and the whole enlarged by nearly one-fourth, notwithstanding which the price has been kept at its former very moderate rate. By the use of a close, though very legible type, an unusually large amount of matter is condensed in its pages, the two volumes containing as much as four or five ordinary octavos. This, combined with the most careful mechanical execution, and its very durable binding, renders it one of the cheapest works accessible to the profession. Every subject properly belonging to the domain of surgery is treated in detail, so that the student who possesses this work may be said to have in it a surgical library.

We have now brought our task to a conclusion, and have seldom read a work with the practical value of which we have been more impressed. Every chapter is so concisely put together, that the busy practitioner, when in difficulty, can at once find the information he requires. His work, on the contrary, is cosmopolitan, the surgery of the world being fully represented in it. The work, in fact, is so historically unprejudiced, and so eminently practical, that it is almost a false compliment to say that we believe it to be destined to occupy a foremost place as a work of reference, while a system of surgery like the present system of surgery is the practice of surgeons. The printing and binding of the work is unexceptionable; indeed, it contrasts, in the latter respect, remarkably with English medical and surgical cloth-bound publications, which are generally so wretchedly stitched as to require re-binding before they are any time in use.—*Dublin Journ. of Med. Sci.*, March, 1874.

Dr. Gross's Surgery, a great work, has become still greater, both in size and merit, in its most recent form. The difference in actual number of pages is not more than 130, but, the size of the page having been increased to what we believe is technically termed "elephant," there has been room for considerable additions, which, together with the alterations, are improvements.—*Lond. Lancet*, Nov. 16, 1872.

A complete system of Surgery—not a mere text-book of operations but a scientific account of surgical theory and practice in all its departments.—*Brit. and For. Med.-Chir. Review*, Jan. 1873.

It combines, as perfectly as possible, the qualities of a text book and work of reference We think this last edition of Gross's "Surgery" will confirm his title of "*Primus inter Pares.*" It is learned, scholar-like, methodical, precise, and exhaustive. We scarcely think any living man could write so complete and faultless a treatise, or comprehend more solid, instructive matter, in the given number of pages. The labor must have been immense, and the work gives evidence of great powers of mind, and the highest order of intellectual discipline and methodical disposition. and arrangement of acquired knowledge and personal experience.—*N. Y. Med. Journ.*, Feb. 1873.

As a whole, we regard the work as the representative "System of Surgery" in the English language.—*St. Louis Medical and Surg. Journ.*, Oct. 1872.

Among the many valuable medical works which the American press has been freely issuing in the last five years, there is none that can compare with the last edition of Gross's Surgery for completeness of details, comprehensiveness of facts, and general usefulness of subject matter. The first edition has proven so invaluable to practitioners and students that they will not be satisfied without this one.—*Va. Clinical Record*, Nov. 1872.

The two magnificent volumes before us afford a very complete view of the surgical knowledge of the day. Some years ago we had the pleasure of presenting the first edition of Gross's Surgery to the profession as a work of unrivalled excellence; and now we have the result of years of experience, labor, and study, all condensed upon the great work before us. And to students or practitioners desirous of enriching their library with a treasure of reference, we can simply commend the purchase of these two volumes of immense research.—*Cincinnati Lancet and Observer*, Sept. 1872.

By the same Author.

A PRACTICAL TREATISE ON FOREIGN BODIES IN THE AIR-PASSAGES. In 1 vol. 8vo., with illustrations, pp. 468, cloth, $2 75.

Green (T. Henry), M.D.,
Lecturer on Pathology and Morbid Anatomy at Charing-Cross Hospital Medical School.

PATHOLOGY AND MORBID ANATOMY. Second American, from the Third and Enlarged English Edition. With numerous illustrations. In one very handsome octavo volume. (*Nearly Ready.*)

This useful and convenient manual has already reached a third edition, and we are glad to find that, although it has grown somewhat larger, it still remains a little book, and we are inclined to forgive the increase in size on account of the valuable additions which the author has made both to the printed matter and to the illustrations. The new illustrations, drawn by Mr. Collings from preparations by Dr. Green himself, are very good, and the care and trouble expended by the author in the preparation of this edition will no doubt increase the popularity of his book, great though it already is.—*The London Practitioner*, Feb. 1876.

We observe that the whole has been carefully revised, that a considerable addition has been made to the illustrations, and that much new matter has been added. We have not space for noting each of the additions that have been made, and it is quite unnecessary to attempt this, for a work which has already gained a deservedly solid reputation. It is enough to say that it has been brought thoroughly up to the knowledge of the present day, and that the student can have no better or safer guide to pathology and morbid anatomy than Dr. Green's book.—*Lond. Times and Gaz.*, Sept. 1875.

Galloway (Robert), F.C.S.,
Prof. of Applied Chemistry in the Royal College of Science for Ireland etc.

A MANUAL OF QUANTITATIVE ANALYSIS. From the Fifth London Edition. In one neat royal 12mo. volume, with illustrations: cloth, $2 50. (*Just Issued.*)

Griffith (Robert E.), M.D.

A UNIVERSAL FORMULARY, Containing the Methods of Preparing and Administering Officinal and other Medicines. The whole adapted to Physicians and Pharmaceutists. Third edition, thoroughly revised, with numerous additions, by JOHN M MAISCH, Professor of Materia Medica in the Philadelphia College of Pharmacy. In one large and handsome octavo volume of about 800 pp., cloth, $4 50; leather, $5 50. (*Just Issued.*)

This work has long been known for the vast amount of information which it presents in a condensed form, arranged for easy reference. The new edition has received the most careful revision at the competent hands of Professor Maisch, who has brought the whole up to the standard of the most recent authorities. More than eighty new headings of remedies have been introduced, the entire work has been thoroughly remodelled, and whatever has seemed to be obsolete has been omitted As a comparative view of the United States, the British, the German, and the French Pharmacopœias, together with an immense amount of unofficinal formulas, it affords to the practitioner and pharmaceutist an aid in their daily avocations not to be found elsewhere, while three indexes, one of "Diseases and their Remedies," one of Pharmaceutical Names, and a General Index, afford an easy key to the alphabetical arrangement adopted in the text.

The young practitioner will find the work invaluable in suggesting eligible modes of administering many remedies.—*Am. Journ. of Pharm.*, Feb. 1874.

Our copy of Griffith's Formulary, after long use, first in the dispensing shop, and afterwards in our medical practice, had gradually fallen behind in the onward march of materia medica, pharmacy, and therapeutics, until we had ceased to consult it as a daily book of reference. So completely has Prof. Maisch reformed, remodelled, and rejuvenated it in the new edition, we shall gladly welcome it back to our table again beside Dunglison, Webster, and Wood & Bache. The publisher could not have been more fortunate in the selection of an editor. Prof. Maisch

is eminently the man for the work, and he has done it thoroughly and ably. To enumerate the alterations, amendments, and additions, would be an endless task; everywhere we are greeted with the evidences of his labor. Following the Formulary, is an addendum of useful Recipes, Dietetic Preparations, List of Incompatibles, Posological table, table of Pharmaceutical Names, Officinal Preparations and Directions, Poisons, Antidotes and Treatment, and copious Indices. which afford ready access to all parts of the work. We unhesitatingly commend the book as being the best of its kind within our knowledge. —*Atlanta Med. and Surg. Journ.*, Feb. 1874.

GIBSON'S INSTITUTES AND PRACTICE OF SURGERY. Eighth edition, improved and altered. With thirty-four plates. In two handsome octavo volumes, about 1000 pp.: leather, raised bands, $6 50.

GLUGE'S ATLAS OF PATHOLOGICAL HISTOLOGY. Translated, with Notes and Additions, by JOSEPH LEIDY, M.D. In one volume, very large imperial quarto, with 320 copper-plate figures, plain and colored: cloth, $4 00.

HILLIER'S HANDBOOK OF SKIN DISEASES, for

Students and Practitioners. Second American Edition. In 1 royal 12mo. vol. of 358 pp. With Illustrations. Cloth, $2 25.

HORNER'S SPECIAL ANATOMY AND HISTOLOGY. Eighth edition, extensively revised and modified. In 2 vols., 8vo., of over 1000 pages, with more than 300 wood-cuts: cloth, $6 00.

HUDSON'S LECTURES ON THE STUDY OF FEVER. 1 vol. 8vo., cloth, $2 50

HOLLAND'S MEDICAL NOTES AND REFLECTIONS. 1 vol. 8vo., pp. 600, cloth, $3 50.

Hamilton (Frank H.), M.D.,
Surgeon to Bellevue Hospital, New York.

A PRACTICAL TREATISE ON FRACTURES AND DISLOCATIONS. Fifth edition, revised and improved. Illustrated with 344 wood-cuts. . In one large and handsome octavo volume of 831 pages: cloth, $5 75; leather, $6 75. (*Just Issued.*)

This work is well known, abroad as well as at home, as the highest authority on its important subject—an authority recognized in the courts as well as in the schools and in practice—and again manifested, not only by the demand for a fifth edition, but by arrangements now in progress for the speedy appearance of a translation in Germany. The repeated revisions which the author has thus had the opportunity of making have enabled him to give the most careful consideration to every portion of the volume, and he has sedulously endeavored, in the present issue, to perfect the work by the aid of his own enlarged experience and to incorporate in it whatever of value has been added in this department since the issue of the fourth edition. It will therefore be found considerably improved in matter, while the most careful attention has been paid to the typographical execution, and the volume is presented to the profession in the confident hope that it will more than maintain its very distinguished reputation.

There is no better work on the subject in existence than that of Dr. Hamilton. It should be in the possession of every general practitioner and surgeon.—*The Am. Journ. of Obstetrics*, Feb. 1876.

The value of a work like this to the practical physician and surgeon can hardly be over-estimated, and the necessity of having such a book revised to the latest dates, not merely on account of the practical importance

of its teachings. but also by reason of the medico-legal bearings of the cases of which it treats, and which have recently been the subject of useful papers by Dr. Hamilton and others, is sufficiently obvious to every one. The present volume seems to amply fill all the requisites. We can safely recommend it as the best of its kind in the English language. and not excelled in any other.—*Journ. of Nervous and Mental Disease*, Jan. 1876.

Hoblyn (Richard D.), M.D.

A DICTIONARY OF THE TERMS USED IN MEDICINE AND THE COLLATERAL SCIENCES. Revised, with numerous additions, by ISAAC HAYS, M.D., Editor of the "American Journal of the Medical Sciences." In one large royal 12mo. volume of over 500 double-columned pages: cloth, $1 50; leather, $2.

It is the best book of definitions we have, and ought always to be upon the student's table —*Southern Med. and Surg. Journal.*

Holmes (Timothy),

Surgeon to St. George's Hospital, London.

SURGERY, ITS PRINCIPLES AND PRACTICE. In one large and handsome octavo volume of nearly 1000 pages, with 411 illustrations on wood. Cloth, $6; leather, $7. (*Now Ready.*)

The distinguished position of Mr. Holmes, his large practical experience, and his familiarity with surgical literature, have enabled him to condense within a moderate compass a complete view of all the departments of surgery in their most modern aspect. The labors of American surgeons will be found fully represented in its pages, and it is presented as a compact and convenient manual for the use of both student and practitioner.

From ROBERT REYBURN, M.D., Prof. of Principles of Surgery and Microscopic Anat., Medical Dept. Georgetown Univ.

"I believe it to be the best epitome of surgery for the use of the student and busy practitioner of medicine that I have yet seen."

From HUNTER McGUIRE, M.D., Prof. of Surgery in the Medical College of Va., Richmond.

"It is an admirable book, and one which I can conscientiously recommend both to students and practitioners."

From T. R. BROWN, M.D., Prof. of Surgery, College of Physicians and Surgeons, Baltimore.

"I have made a cursory examination only, but enough to satisfy me it is a most excellent work. I have made up my mind sufficiently as to its especial adaptation to students to warrant me in placing it in a foremost place among the text-books."

We believe it to be by far the best surgical text-book that we have, inasmuch as it is the completest, and the one most thoroughly brought up to the knowledge of the present day. All who will give this book the careful perusal that it deserves and requires, whether student or practitioner, will agree with us that from the happy way in which justice is done, both to the principles and practice of surgery, from the care with which its pages are brought up to modern date, from the respect which is paid all along to the opinions of others, it deserves to take the first place among the text-books on surgery. — *British Med. Journ.*, Dec. 25, 1875.

Mr. Holmes, in the work before us, seems to have exactly hit the happy mean, and to have produced, in a convenient form, a most complete and accurate text-book. It is also necessary in such a work to give an impartial judgment upon many disputed questions and opposed methods of treatment; and no one is more competent to do this than Mr. Holmes, whose writings are notably distinguished by their clearness of thought and judicial accuracy. The book is an extremely fair exposition of British surgery. and its illustrations are, of course, largely drawn from the case books and museum of St. George's Hospital; but it exhibits, also, a thorough knowledge of, and gives abundant references to, the works of American and Continental surgeons. We have no hesitation in recommending this as by far the best of existing surgical text-books: it is well up to the time; it exhibits a thorough acquaintance with surgical literature and practice; is characterized by the most impartial fairness, and written in excellent English.—*Lond. Med. Times and Gaz.*, Jan. 8, 1876.

Taken as a whole, the work of Mr. Holmes gives very high promise. If he can only prevent it from getting too large in successive editions, it seems a work which, from its completeness, generally admirable arrangement, judicious illustrations, and copious index, will prove a most useful one, containing, as it does, accounts of special branches—eye, ear, syphilis, operative surgery, and bandaging—it will be useful for the type of student who may be described as *homo unius libri*, at least during his first year of surgery. If Mr. Holmes succeeds in getting over all the ground he travels in this work, during a winter course of systematic lectures, all we can say is, he is a fortunate and wonderful man.—*Edin. Med. Journ.*, March, 1876.

Hodge (Hugh L.), M.D.,

Emeritus Professor of Midwifery, &c., in the University of Pennsylvania, &c.

THE PRINCIPLES AND PRACTICE OF OBSTETRICS. Illustrated with large lithographic plates containing one hundred and fifty-nine figures from original photographs, and with numerous wood-cuts. In one large and beautifully printed quarto volume of 550 double-columned pages, strongly bound in cloth, $14.

The work of Dr. Hodge is something more than a simple presentation of his particular views in the department of Obstetrics; it is something more than an ordinary treatise on midwifery; it is, in fact, a cyclopædia of midwifery. He has aimed to embody in a single volume the whole science and art of Obstetrics. An elaborate text is combined with accurate and varied pictorial illustrations, so that no fact or principle is left unstated or unexplained.—*Am. Med. Times*, Sept. 3, 1864.

It is very large, profusely and elegantly illustrated, and is fitted to take its place near the works of great obstetricians. Of the American works on the subject it is decidedly the best.—*Edin. Medical Journ.*, Dec. 1864.

*** Specimens of the plates and letter-press will be forwarded to any address free, by mail, on receipt of six cents in postage stamps.

By the same Author.

ON DISEASES PECULIAR TO WOMEN; including Displacements of the Uterus. With original illustrations. Second edition, revised and enlarged. In one beautifully printed octavo volume of 531 pages, cloth, $4 50.

Heath (Christopher), F.R.C.S.,

Teacher of Operative Surgery in University College, London.

PRACTICAL ANATOMY: A Manual of Dissections. From the Second revised and improved London edition. Edited, with additions, by W. W. KEEN, M.D., Lecturer on Pathological Anatomy in the Jefferson Medical College, Philadelphia. In one handsome royal 12mo. volume of 578 pages, with 247 illustrations. Cloth, $3 50; leather, $4 00. (*Lately Published.*)

HODGE'S PRACTICAL DISSECTIONS. 2d edition, thoroughly revised. In 1 royal 12mo. vol., half bound, $2.

HILL ON SYPHILIS AND LOCAL CONTAGIOUS DISORDERS. In 1 handsome 8vo vol. Cloth, $3 25.

Hartshorne (Henry), M.D.,
Professor of Hygiene in the University of Pennsylvania.

ESSENTIALS OF THE PRINCIPLES AND PRACTICE OF MEDI-CINE. A handy-book for Students and Practitioners. Fourth edition, revised and improved. With about one hundred illustrations. In one handsome royal 12mo. volume, of about 550 pages : cloth, $2 63; half bound, $2 88. *(Just Issued.)*

The thorough manner in which the author has labored to fully represent in this favorite handbook the most advanced condition of practical medicine is shown by the fact that the present edition contains more than 250 additions, representing the investigations of 172 authors not referred to in previous editions. Notwithstanding an enlargement of the page, the size has been increased by sixty pages. A number of illustrations have been introduced, which it is hoped will facilitate the comprehension of details by the reader, and no effort has been spared to make the volume worthy a continuance of the very great favor with which it has hitherto been received.

The work is brought fully up with all the recent advances in medicine, is admirably condensed, and yet sufficiently explicit for all the purposes intended, thus making it by far the best work of its character ever published.—*Cincinnati Clinic,* Oct. 24, 1874.

We have already had occasion to notice the previous editions of this work. It is excellent of its kind. The author has given a very careful revision, in

view of the rapid progress of medical science.—*N. Y. Med. Journ.,* Nov. 1874.

Without doubt the best book of the kind published in the English language.—*St. Louis Med. and Surg. Journ.,* Nov. 1874.

As a handbook, which clearly sets forth the ESSENTIALS of the PRINCIPLES AND PRACTICE OF MEDICINE, we do not know of its equal.—*Va. Med. Monthly.*

By the same Author.

A CONSPECTUS OF THE MEDICAL SCIENCES; containing Handbooks on Anatomy. Physiology, Chemistry, Materia Medica, Practical Medicine, Surgery, and Obstetrics. Second Edition, thoroughly revised and improved. In one large royal 12mo. volume of more than 1000 closely printed pages, with 477 illustrations on wood. Cloth, $4 25 ; leather, $5 00. *(Lately Issued.)*

The favor with which this work has been received has stimulated the author in its revision to render it in every way fitted to meet the wants of the student, or of the practitioner desirous to refresh his acquaintance with the various departments of medical science. The various sections have been brought up to a level with the existing knowledge of the day, while preserving the condensation of form by which so vast an accumulation of facts has been brought within so narrow a compass. The series of illustrations has been much improved, while by the use of a smaller type the additions have been incorporated without increasing unduly the size of the volume.

The work before us has already successfully asserted its claim to the confidence and favor of the profession ; it but remains for us to say that in the present edition the whole work has been fully overhauled and brought up to the present status of the science.—*Atlanta Med. and Surg. Journ.,* Sept. 1874.

This work is intended as an aid to the medical student, and as such appears to admirably fulfil its object by its excellent arrangement, the full compilation of facts, the perspicuity and terseness of

language, and the clear and instructive illustrations in some parts of the work.—*Am. Journ. of Pharm.,* Philadelphia, July, 1874.

The volume will be found useful, not only to students, but to many others who may desire to refresh their memories with the smallest possible expenditure of time. - *N. Y. Med. Journ.,* Sept. 1874.

The student will find this the most convenient and useful book of the kind on which he can lay his hand.—*Pacific Med. and Surg. Journ.,* Aug. 1874.

By the same Author.

HANDBOOK OF ANATOMY AND PHYSIOLOGY. Second Edition, revised. In one royal 12mo. volume, with 220 wood-cuts; cloth, $1 75. *(Just Issued.)*

Jones (C. Handfield), M.D.,
Physician to St. Mary's Hospital. &c.

CLINICAL OBSERVATIONS ON FUNCTIONAL NERVOUS DISORDERS. Second American Edition. In one handsome octavo volume of 348 pages; cloth, $3 25.

Kirkes (William Senhouse), M.D.

A MANUAL OF PHYSIOLOGY Edited by W. MORRANT BAKER, M.D., F.R.C.S. A new American from the eighth and improved London edition. With about two hundred and fifty illustrations. In one large and handsome royal 12mo. volume: cloth, $3 25 ; leather, $3 75. *(Lately Issued.)*

On the whole, there is very little in the book which either the student or practitioner will not find of practical value and consistent with our present knowledge of this rapidly changing science; and we have no hesitation in expressing our opinion that this eighth edition is one of the best handbooks on physiology which we have in our language.—*N. Y. Med. Record.* April 15, 1873.

This volume might well be used to replace many of the physiological text-books in use in this country. It represents more accurately than the works of Dalton or Flint, the present state of our knowledge of most physiological questions, while it is much

less bulky and far more readable than the larger text-books of Carpenter or Marshall. The book is admirably adapted to be placed in the hands of students.—*Boston Med. and Surg Journ.,* Apr. 10, '73.

In its enlarged form it is, in our opinion, still the best book on physiology, most useful to the student.—*Philadelphia Med Times,* Aug. 30, 1873.

This is undoubtedly the best work for students of physiology extant.—*Cincin. Med. News,* Sept. '73.

It more nearly represents the present condition of physiology than any other text-book on the subject.—*Detroit Review of Med. and Pharm.,* Nov. 1873.

KNAPP'S TECHNOLOGY ; or Chemistry Applied to the Arts, and to Manufactures. With American additions, by Prof. WALTER R. JOHNSON. In two

very handsome octavo volumes, with five hundred wood engravings; cloth, $6.

Leishman (William), M.D.,

Regius Professor of Midwifery in the University of Glasgow, etc.

A SYSTEM OF MIDWIFERY, INCLUDING THE DISEASES OF

PREGNANCY AND THE PUERPERAL STATE. Second American, from the Second and revised English Edition, with additions by J. S. PARRY, M.D., Obstetrician to the Phila. Hospital. In one large and very handsome octavo volume of nearly 800 pages, with about 200 illustrations: cloth, $5; leather, $6. *(Just Ready.)*

From the Preface of the American Editor.—In preparing for the press the Second American Edition of Dr. Leishman's System of Midwifery, the Editor has added such notes only as he believed would make the book more useful to the profession in this country. The additions are distinguished from the text by being inclosed in brackets [—P.], and will be found chiefly in the chapters on the Use of the Forceps, Lactation, and the Puerperal Diseases. A chapter on Diphtheria of Puerperal Wounds has been added, and a few new illustrations have been introduced, representing the principal modifications of obstetrical instruments generally employed in this country. The Editor trusts that these additions will increase the usefulness of a work of which the value is attested by the simultaneous exhaustion of both the English and American Editions.

But the most valuable additions to the volume are those made by the American editor. One of the best tests of a man's ability is for him to take a standard work in our profession, like this of Dr. Leishman, and materially improve it. Many a one, with more ambition than wisdom, has attempted it with other books and failed. But Dr. Parry has succeeded most admirably. We know no obstetrical work that has anything better on the use of the forceps than that which Dr. Parry has given in this, and no work that has the rational and intelligent views upon lactation with which he has enriched this. Having used "Leishman" for two years, as a text-book for students we can cordially commend it, and are quite satisfied to continue such use now.—*Am. Practitioner,* Mar. '76.

This new edition decidedly confirms the opinion which we expressed of the first edition of the work, in the May, 1874, number of this Journal, that this is "the best modern work on the subject in the English language." The excellent practical notes contributed by Dr. Parry refer principally to the use of the forceps, lactation, and the puerperal diseases, and are intended to increase the usefulness of the work in this country. An entirely new chapter on diphtheria of puerperal wounds has been added (Dr. P has had unusual experience in this form of puerperal fever), and also a number of illustrations of the principal obstetrical instruments in use in America. We have no hesitation in saying that the work, in

its present shape, is a great improvement on its predecessor, and in recommending it as the one obstetrical text book which we should advise every English speaking practitioner and student to buy.—*Am. Journ. of Obstetrics,* Feb. 1876.

Perhaps the most useful one the student can procure. Some important additions have been made by the editor, in order to adapt the work to the profession in this country, and some new illustrations have been introduced, to represent the obstetrical instruments generally employed in American practice. In its present form, it is an exceedingly valuable book for both the student and practitioner.—*New York Med. Journ.,* Jan. 1876.

In about two years after the issue of this excellent treatise a second edition has been called for. We regard the treatise as thoroughly sound and practical, and one which may with confidence be consulted in any emergency.—*The London Lancet,* Dec. 11, 1875.

The appearance of a second edition of this System is the fulfilment of the prophecy which we made in a former review, that the book was destined to " become a favorite." The additions by Dr. Parry are usually not abundant, but certain places which are pointed out as the weak part of Dr. Leishman's handicraft have been greatly strengthened by abundant and very judicious addenda.—*Phila. Med. Times,* Dec. 25, 1875.

Lincoln (D. F.), M.D.,

Physician to the Department of Nervous Diseases, Boston Dispensary.

ELECTRO-THERAPEUTICS; A Concise Manual of Medical Electricity.

In one very neat royal 12mo. volume; cloth, with illustrations, $1 50. *(Just Issued.)*

The work is convenient in size, its descriptions of methods and appliances are sufficiently complete for the general practitioner, and the chapters on Electrophysiology and diagnosis are well written and readable. For those who wish a handy-book of directions for the employment of galvanism in medicine, this will serve as a very good and reliable guide.—*New Remedies,* Oct. 1874.

Eminently practical in character. It will amply repay any one for a careful perusal.—*Leavenworth Med. Herald,* Oct. 1874.

This little book is, considering its size, one of the very best of the English treatises on its subject that has come to our notice, possessing, among others, the rare merit of dealing avowedly and actually with principles, mainly, rather than with practical details, thereby supplying a real want, instead of helping merely to flood the literary market. Dr. Lincoln's style is usually remarkably clear, and the whole book is readable and interesting.—*Boston Medical and Surgical Journal,* July 23, 1874.

Lee (Henry),

Prof. of Surgery at the Royal College of Surgeons of England, &c.

LECTURES ON SYPHILIS AND ON SOME FORMS OF LOCAL

DISEASE, AFFECTING PRINCIPALLY THE ORGANS OF GENERATION. In one handsome octavo volume of 246 pages: cloth, $2 25. *(Now Ready.)*

The long-established reputation of this eminent surgeon as an author on venereal diseases, and the easy style of his writings make anything from his pen on the subjects indicated by the title of this book, engerly sought after and read. The present work consists principally of a collection and revision of the author's numerous papers and lectures on venereal diseases, which have been published in various medical journals, through which channels his views have already become familiar to the medical world. It will be remembered that he is a dualist, and is an earnest advocate of the mercurial plan of treatment of syphilis—the treatment being carried out preferably by means of calomel vapor baths Indeed, were demonstrative facts asked to establish the value of mercury in syphilis, they would not be called for a second time after perusal of the fourth chapter (*Treatment of Syphilis*). The other portion of the work is alike interesting, instructive, and

authoritative. We are compelled to abbreviate our notice; but we cannot lay our pen aside without commending this book to physicians who propose to practise on venereal diseases—whether or not they already have the more systematic works of Van Buren and Keyes or of Bumstead, of our own country.—*Va. Med. Monthly,* Nov. 1875.

Mr. Henry Lee's Hunterian Lectures attracted much attention when they first appeared in the English journals, and will be widely read, now that they are published entire in book form. No man in England has a higher or wider reputation as a syphilographer than the author, and his views are the matured fruit of years of study and very extensive observation. John Hunter could have had no abler nor more conscientious reviewer of his doctrines as tested by the experience of medical men during more than three-quarters of a century.—*The Clinic,* Nov. 6, 1875.

Lea (Henry C.).

SUPERSTITION AND FORCE: ESSAYS ON THE WAGER OF

LAW, THE WAGER OF BATTLE, THE ORDEAL, AND TORTURE. Second Edition, Enlarged. In one handsome volume, royal 12mo., of nearly 500 pages: cloth, $2 75. (*Lately Published.*)

We know of no single work which contains, in so small a compass, so much illustrative of the strangest operations of the human mind. Foot-notes give the authority for each statement, showing vast research and wonderful industry. We advise our *confrères* to read this book and ponder its teachings.—*Chicago Med. Journal*, Aug. 1870.

As a work of curious inquiry on certain outlying points of obsolete law, "Superstition and Force" is one of the most remarkable books we have met with —*London Athenæum*, Nov. 3, 1866.

He has thrown a great deal of light upon what must

be regarded as one of the most instructive as well as interesting phases of human society and progress. . . The fulness and breadth with which he has carried out his comparative survey of this repulsive field of history [Torture], are such as to preclude our doing justice to the work within our present limits. But here, as throughout the volume, there will be found a wealth of illustration and a critical grasp of the philosophical import of facts which will render Mr. Lea's labors of sterling value to the historical student.—*London Saturday Review*, Oct. 8, 1870.

As a book of ready reference on the subject, it is of the highest value.—*Westminster Review*, Oct. 1867.

By the same Author. (*Lately Published.*)

STUDIES IN CHURCH HISTORY—THE RISE OF THE TEM-

PORAL POWER—BENEFIT OF CLERGY—EXCOMMUNICATION. In one large royal 12mo. volume of 516 pp. : cloth, $2 75.

The story was never told more calmly or with greater learning or wiser thought. We doubt, indeed, if any other study of this field can be compared with this for clearness, accuracy, and power.—*Chicago Examiner*, Dec. 1870.

Mr. Lea's latest work, "Studies in Church History," fully sustains the promise of the first. It deals with three subjects—the Temporal Power, Benefit of Clergy, and Excommunication, the record of which has a peculiar importance for the English student, and is a chapter on Ancient Law likely to be regarded as final. We can hardly pass from our mention of such works as these—with which that on "Sacerdotal Celibacy" should be included—without noting the

literary phenomenon that the head of one of the first American houses is also the writer of some of its most original books.—*London Athenæum*, Jan. 7, 1871.

Mr Lea has done great honor to himself and this country by the admirable works he has written on ecclesiological and cognate subjects. We have already had occasion to commend his "Superstition and Force" and his "History of Sacerdotal Celibacy." The present volume is fully as admirable in its method of dealing with topics and in the thoroughness—a quality so frequently lacking in American authors—with which they are investigated.—*N. Y. Journal of Psychol. Medicine*, July, 1870.

By the same Author. (*Lately Published.*)

AN HISTORICAL SKETCH OF SACERDOTAL CELIBACY IN

THE CHRISTIAN CHURCH. In one handsome octavo volume of 600 pages: extra cloth, $3 75.

In freshness and exactness of detail, in conscientious citation of authorities, in the impartiality with which all possible sources of information have been searched, in learning and scholarly finish, it is absolutely unapproached by any similar treatise which has issued from the American press. Indeed, the number of foreign historical works which have equalled it in these particulars might be readily

counted on the fingers.—*Quarterly Journ. of Psychological Medicine*, Oct. 1867.

Thus his chapter on the Anglican church is perhaps the most accurate and most satisfactory account of our own Reformation, as to the question of celibacy or marriage, that could be found.—*Quarterly Review*, London, Oct. 1867.

Laurence (John Z.), F.R.C.S.,

Editor of the Ophthalmic Review, &c.

A HANDY-BOOK OF OPHTHALMIC SURGERY, for the use of Practitioners. Second edition, revised and enlarged. With numerous illustrations. In one very handsome octavo volume, cloth, $3 00.

Lawson (George), F.R.C.S. Engl.,

Assistant Surgeon to the Royal London Ophthalmic Hospital. Moorfields, &c.

INJURIES OF THE EYE, ORBIT, AND EYELIDS: their Immediate and Remote Effects. With about one hundred illustrations. In one very handsome octavo volume, cloth, $3 50.

It is an admirable practical book in the highest and best sense of the phrase.—*London Medical Times and Gazette*, May 18, 1867.

LA ROCHE ON YELLOW FEVER, considered in its Historical, Pathological, Etiological, and Therapeutical Relations. In two large and handsome octavo volumes of nearly 1500 pages, cloth, $7 00.

LA ROCHE ON PNEUMONIA. 1 vol. 8vo., cloth, of 500 pages. Price $3 00.

LAYCOCK'S LECTURES ON THE PRINCIPLES AND METHODS OF MEDICAL OBSERVATION AND RESEARCH. For the use of advanced students and junior practitioners. In one very neat royal 12mo. volume, cloth, $1 00.

LEHMANN'S PHYSIOLOGICAL CHEMISTRY.

Translated from the second edition by GEORGE E. DAY, M.D., F.R.S., &c ; edited by R. E. ROGERS, M.D. Complete in two large and handsome octavo volumes, containing 1200 pages, with nearly two hundred illustrations: cloth, $6

LEHMANN'S MANUAL OF CHEMICAL PHYSIOLOGY. Translated from the German, with Notes and Additions, by J. CHESTON MORRIS, M.D. With illustrations on wood. In one very handsome octavo volume of 336 pages ; cloth, $2 25.

LYONS'S TREATISE ON FEVER. In one octavo volume of 362 pages ; cloth, $2 15.

Ludlow (J. L.), M.D.

A MANUAL OF EXAMINATIONS upon Anatomy, Physiology, Surgery, Practice of Medicine, Obstetrics, Materia Medica, Chemistry, Pharmacy, and Therapeutics. To which is added a Medical Formulary. Third edition, thoroughly revised and greatly extended and enlarged. With 370 illustrations. In one handsome royal 12mo. volume of 816 large pages : cloth, $3 25; leather, $3 75.

Maclise (Joseph).

SURGICAL ANATOMY. By JOSEPH MACLISE, Surgeon. In one volume, very large imperial quarto ; with 68 large and splendid plates, drawn in the best style and beautifully colored. containing 190 figures, many of them the size of life ; together with copious explanatory letter-press. Strongly and handsomely bound in cloth. Price $14 00.

Marshall (John), F.R.S.,

Professor of Surgery in University College, London, &c.

OUTLINES OF PHYSIOLOGY, HUMAN AND COMPARATIVE. With Additions by FRANCIS GURNEY SMITH, M.D., Professor of the Institutes of Medicine in the University of Pennsylvania, &c. With numerous illustrations. In one large and handsome octavo volume, of 1026 pages, cloth, $6 50; leather, raised bands, $7 50.

MEIGS ON THE NATURE, SIGNS, AND TREATMENT OF CHILDBED FEVER. 1 vol. 8vo., pp. 365, cloth, $2 00.

MILLER'S PRINCIPLES OF SURGERY Fourth American, from the third and revised Edinburgh edition. In one vol. of 700 pages, with 240 cuts : cloth, $3 75.

MILLER'S PRACTICE OF SURGERY. Fourth American, from the last Edinburgh edition. In one vol. 8vo., of nearly 700 pages, cloth, with 364 cuts: $3 75.

MONTGOMERY'S EXPOSITION OF THE SIGNS AND SYMPTOMS OF PREGNANCY. With two exquisite colored plates, and numerous wood-cuts. In 1 vol. 8vo., of nearly 600 pp., cloth, $3 75.

Neill (John), M.D., and Smith (Francis G.), M.D.,

Prof of the Institutes of Med. in the Univ. of Penna.

AN ANALYTICAL COMPENDIUM OF THE VARIOUS BRANCHES OF MEDICAL SCIENCE; for the Use and Examination of Students. A new edition, revised and improved. In one very large and handsomely printed royal 12mo. volume, of about one thousand pages, with 374 wood cuts, cloth, $4 ; strongly bound in leather, with raised bands, $4 75.

The Compend of Drs. Neill and Smith is incomparably the most valuable work of its class ever published in this country. Attempts have been made in various quarters to squeeze Anatomy, Physiology, Surgery, the Practice of Medicine, Obstetrics, Materia Medica, and Chemistry into a single manual; but the operation has signally failed in the hands of all up to the advent of "Neill and Smith's" volume, which is quite a miracle of success. The outlines of the whole are admirably drawn and illustrated, and the authors are eminently entitled to the grateful consideration of the student of every class.—*N. O. Med. and Surg. Journal.*

There are but few students or practitioners of medicine unacquainted with the former editions of this unassuming, though highly instructive work. The whole science of medicine appears to have been sifted, as the gold bearing sands of El Dorado, and the precious facts treasured up in this little volume. A complete portable library so condensed that the student may make it his constant pocket companion.—*Western Lancet.*

Neligan (J. Moore), M.D., M.R.I.A.

ATLAS OF CUTANEOUS DISEASES. In one beautiful quarto volume, with exquisitely colored plates, &c., presenting about one hundred varieties of disease. Cloth, $5 50.

Odling (William),

Lecturer on Chemistry at St. Bartholomew's Hospital, &c.

A COURSE OF PRACTICAL CHEMISTRY, arranged for the Use of Medical Students. With Illustrations. From the Fourth and Revised London Edition. In one neat royal 12mo. volume, cloth, $2.

Playfair (W. S.), M.D., F.R.C.P.,

Professor of Obstetric Medicine in King's College, etc. etc.

A TREATISE ON THE SCIENCE AND PRACTICE OF MIDWIFERY. In one handsome octavo volume, with several hundred illustrations. (*In Press.*)

Pirrie (William), F.R.S.E.,

Professor of Surgery in the University of Aberdeen.

THE PRINCIPLES AND PRACTICE OF SURGERY. Edited by JOHN NEILL, M.D., Professor of Surgery in the Penna. Medical College, Surgeon to the Pennsylvania Hospital, &c. In one very handsome octavo volume of 780 pages, with 316 illustrations, cloth, $3 75.

Parry (John S.), M.D., ·

Late Obstetrician to the Phila. Hospital, Vice-Prest. of the Obstet Society of Philadelphia.

EXTRA-UTERINE PREGNANCY: ITS CLINICAL HISTORY, DIAGNOSIS, PROGNOSIS, AND TREATMENT.

In one handsome octavo volume of 274 pages: cloth, $2 50. (*Just Ready.*)

It is with genuine satisfaction, therefore, that we read the work before us, which is far in advance of any monograph upon the subject in the English language, and exceeding very much, in the number of cases upon which it is based. we believe. any work of the kind ever published. The author has given great care and study to the work, and has handled his statistics with judgment; so that, whatever was to be gained from them, he has gained and added to our knowledge on the subject. We owe the author much for giving us a clear, readable look upon this topic. He has, so far as it is at present possible, removed the obscurity attending certain points of the subject. He has brought order out of something very like chaos.—*Philadelphia Med. Times*, Feb. 19, 1876.

In this work Dr. Parry has added a most valuable contribution to obstetric literature, and one which meets a want long felt by those of the profession who have ever been called upon to deal with this class of cases.—*Boston Med. and Surg. Journal*, March 9, 1876.

This work, being as near as possible a collection of the experiences of many persons, will afford a most useful guide, both in diagnosis and treatment, for this most interesting and fatal malady. We think it should be in the hands of all physicians practising midwifery.—*Cincinnati Clinic*, Feb. 5, 1876.

This work is based upon an analysis of five hundred cases of misplaced pregnancy, and the author has succeeded in giving a most interesting and valuable work as the result of this labor.—*Med. and Surg. Reporter*, Jan. 29, 1876.

We scarcely know which most to admire in this work, the labor and industry exhibited in the collection from the medical literature of the world, of 500 cases of extra-uterine pregnancy, or the ingenuity and skill with which the cases are appropriated to the illustration of various points in the diagnostic and clinical relations of the subject. The work is a most important addition to American medical literature.—*Pacific Med. and Surg. Journal*, Feb. 1876.

Parrish (Edward),

Late Professor of Materia Medica in the Philadelphia College of Pharmacy.

A TREATISE ON PHARMACY.

Designed as a Text-Book for the Student, and as a Guide for the Physician and Pharmaceutist. With many Formulæ and Prescriptions. Fourth Edition, thoroughly revised, by THOMAS S. WIEGAND. In one handsome octavo volume of 977 pages, with 280 illustrations: cloth, $5 50; leather, $6 50. (*Just Issued.*)

Of Dr. Parrish's great work on pharmacy it only remains to be said that the editor has accomplished his work so well as to maintain, in this fourth edition, the high standard of excellence which it had attained in previous editions, under the editorship of its accomplished author. This has not been accomplished without much labor, and many additions and improvements, involving changes in the arrangement of the several parts of the work, and the addition of much new matter. With the modifications thus effected, it constitutes, as now presented, a compendium of the science and art indispensable to the pharmacist, and of the utmost value to every practitioner of medicine desirous of familiarizing himself with the pharmaceutical preparation of the articles which he prescribes for his patients.—*Chicago Med. Journ.*, July, 1874.

The work is eminently practical, and has the rare merit of being readable and interesting, while it preserves a strictly scientific character. The whole work reflects the greatest credit on author, editor, and publisher. It will convey some idea of the liberality which has been bestowed upon its production when we mention that there are no less than 280 carefully executed illustrations. In conclusion, we heartily recommend the work, not only to pharmacists, but also to the multitude of medical practitioners who are obliged to compound their own medicines. It will ever hold an honored place on our own bookshelves.—*Dublin Med Press and Circular*, Aug. 12, 1874.

With these few remarks we heartily commend the work, and have no doubt that it will maintain its old reputation as a text-book for the student, and a work of reference for the more experienced physician and pharmacist.—*Chicago Med. Examiner*, June 15, 1874.

Perhaps one, if not the most important book upon pharmacy, which has appeared in the English language, has emanated from the transatlantic press. "Parrish's Pharmacy" is a well-known work on this side of the water, and the fact shows us that a really useful work never becomes merely local in its fame. Thanks to the judicious editing of Mr. Wiegand, the posthumous edition of "Parrish" has been saved to the public with all the mature experience of its author, and perhaps none the worse for a dash of new blood.—*London Pharm Journ.*, Oct. 17, 1874.

Pavy (F. W.), M.D., F.R.S.,

Senior Asst. Physician to, and Lecturer on Physiology at, Guy's Hospital, etc.

A TREATISE ON FOOD AND DIETETICS, PHYSIOLOGICALLY AND THERAPEUTICALLY CONSIDERED.

In one handsome octavo volume of nearly 600 pages: cloth, $4 75. (*Just Ready.*)

The present book is a result of his work in this direction, and is well calculated to do credit to his perseverance in collecting facts, and his judgment in arranging them in an entertaining, as well as a practical form. It is but rarely that we have had offered us so much practical information in so agreeable a manner as is done by Dr Pavy in the present instance.—*New Remedies*, July, 1874.

No modern treatise on this subject having existed in the English language, Dr. Pavy's work supplies a want which has been very seriously felt, and in a manner which shows that the author is an extensive reader and has judiciously arranged the numerous facts and theories, together with the most striking experiments and the deductions drawn therefrom. It seems to us that he has truly conferred a great benefit upon all interested in the subject-matter of his work, and that nobody will study its pages without having derived valuable instruction therefrom, and without considering it not only useful, but next to indispensable.—*Amer. Journ. of Pharmacy*, Aug. 1874.

By the same Author.

A TREATISE ON THE FUNCTION OF DIGESTION; ITS DISORDERS AND TREATMENT.

From the Second London Edition. In one handsome volume, small octavo; cloth, $2 00

Roberts (William), M.D.,
Lecturer on Medicine in the Manchester School of Medicine, etc.

A PRACTICAL TREATISE ON URINARY AND RENAL DIS-
EASES, including Urinary Deposits. Illustrated by numerous cases and engravings. Second American, from the Second Revised and Enlarged London Edition. In one large and handsome octavo volume of 616 pages, with a colored plate: cloth, $4 50. (*Lately Published.*)

The plan, it will thus be seen, is very complete, and the manner in which it has been carried out is in the highest degree satisfactory. The characters of the different deposits are very well described, and the microscopic appearances they present are illustrated by numerous well-executed engravings. It only remains to us to strongly recommend to our readers Dr Roberts's work, as containing an admirable *résumé* of the present state of knowledge of urinary diseases, and as a safe and reliable guide to the clinical observer —*Edin. Med. Jour.*

The most complete and practical treatise upon renal diseases we have examined. It is peculiarly adapted to the wants of the majority of American practitioners from its clearness and simple announcement of the facts in relation to diagnosis and treatment of urinary disorders, and contains in condensed form the investigations of Bence Jones, Bird, Beale, Hassall, Prout, and a host of other well known writers upon this subject. The characters of urine, physiological and pathological, as indicated to the naked eye as well as by microscopical and chemical investigations, are concisely represented both by description and by well-executed engravings.—*Cincinnati Journ. of Med.*

Ramsbotham (Francis H.), M.D.

THE PRINCIPLES AND PRACTICE OF OBSTETRIC MEDICINE
and Surgery, in reference to the Process of Parturition. A new and enlarged edition, thoroughly revised by the author. With additions by W. V. KEATING, M.D., Professor of Obstetrics, etc., in the Jefferson Medical College, Philadelphia. In one large and handsome imperial octavo volume of 650 pages, strongly bound in leather, with raised bands; with sixty four beautiful plates, and numerous wood-cuts in the text, containing in all nearly 200 large and beautiful figures: leather, $7 00.

RIGBY'S SYSTEM OF MIDWIFERY. With Notes and Additional Illustrations. Second American edition. One volume octavo, cloth, 422 pages. $2 50.
SHARPEY AND QUAIN'S HUMAN ANATOMY. Revised, with Notes and Additions, by JOSEPH LEIDY, M.D., Professor of Anatomy in the University of Pennsylvania. Complete in two large octavo volumes, of about 1300 pages, with 511 illustrations: cloth, $6 00.

Smith (J. Lewis), M.D.,
Physician to Infants' Hospital, Ward's Island, New York, etc.

A PRACTICAL TREATISE ON THE DISEASES OF INFANCY AND
CHILDHOOD. Third Edition, enlarged and thoroughly revised. With illustrations on wood. In one handsome 8vo. volume of 726 pages: cloth, $5; leather, $6. (*Just Ready.*)

The eminent success which this work has achieved has encouraged the author, in preparing this third edition, to render it even more worthy than heretofore of the favor of the profession. It has been thoroughly revised, and very considerable additions have been made throughout. To accommodate these the volume has been printed in a smaller type, so as to prevent any notable increase in its size, and it is presented in the hope that it may attain the position of the American text-book on this important department of medical science.

This work took a stand as an authority from its first appearance, and every one interested in studying the diseases of which it treats is desirous of knowing what improvements are apparent in the successive editions. The principal additions to which we refer and which will be the distinguishing features of the third edition, are chapters on diphtheria, cerebro-spinal meningitis, and rötheln. The former disease is considered much more in detail than formerly, and a great amount of very practical information is added, and altogether it is one of the most comprehensive and one of the best written chapters of the subject we have thus far read. His description of cerebro-spinal meningitis, founded also for the most part on personal experience, is admirably clear and exhaustive.—*The Med. Record*, Feb. 19, 1876.

In presenting this deservedly popular treatise for the third time to the profession, Dr. Smith has given it a careful preparation, which will make it of decided superiority to either of the former editions. The position of the author, as physician and consultant to several large children's hospitals in New York city, has furnished him with constant occasions to put his treatment to the test, and his work has at once that practical and thoughtful tone which is a marked characteristic of the best productions of the American medical press.—*Med. and Surg. Reporter*, Feb. 1876.

There is now no work on the diseases of infancy and childhood better adapted to the uses of the profession in this country than this one of Dr. Smith's as regards either its completeness, reliability, practical nature, or style of composition.—*New Remedies*, March, 1876.

The former editions of this book have given it the highest rank among works of its class, and the present edition will confirm and add to its reputation. Having been brought up to the present mark in the rapid advance of medical science, it is the best work in our language, on its range of topics, for the American practitioner.—*Pacific Med. and Surg. Journ.*, Feb. 1876.

Dr. Smith's Diseases of Children is certainly the most valuable work on the subjects treated that the practitioner can provide himself with. It is fully abreast with every advance: it should be in the hands of practitioners generally, while, because of the conciseness and clearness of style of the writing of the author, every professor of diseases of children, if he has not already done so, should adopt this as his text-book.—*Va. Med. Monthly*, Feb. 1876.

We can cordially recommend the work to students and practitioners as one of the very best with which we are acquainted.—*Cincin. Med. News*, Feb 1876.

The third edition of this really valuable work is now before us, with a hundred pages of additional matter, an altered size of page, new illustrations, and new type. Of the diseases treated of for the first time, we notice rötheln and cerebro-spinal fever, which lately prevailed in epidemic form in some parts of the country. The article upon diphtheria, containing the latest developments in the pathology and treatment of that dread disease, which so lately ravaged our country, is peculiarly interesting to every practitioner. We gladly welcome this standard work, and cheerfully recommend it to our readers as the best on this subject in the English language.—*Nashville Journ. of Med. and Surg.*, March, 1876.

Stillé (Alfred), M.D.,
Professor of Theory and Practice of Medicine in the University of Penna.

THERAPEUTICS AND MATERIA MEDICA; a Systematic Treatise on the Action and Uses of Medicinal Agents, including their Description and History. Fourth Edition, Revised and Enlarged. In two large and handsome 8vo. vols. of about 2000 pages: cloth, $10 00; leather, $12 00. *(Just Issued.)*

The care bestowed by the author on the revision of this edition has kept the work out of the market for nearly two years, and has increased its size about two hundred and fifty pages. Notwithstanding this enlargement, the price has been kept at the former very moderate rate.

The prominent feature of Dr. Stillé's great work is sound, good sense. It is learned, but its learning is of interior value compared with the discriminating judgment which is shown by its author in the discussion o his subjects, and which renders it a trustworthy guide in the sick-room. This treatise, if it has not already taken the place of Pereira's learned volumes on materia medica, must ultimately supersede that elaborate work, as having all its learning and being at the same time more practical and more fully up with the therapeutics of the day. It constitutes a sort of encyclopedia on the subject, and is issued in a style as to paper and binding, suitable for a book likely to be so constantly referred to.— *Am. Practitioner*, Jan. 1875.

We can hardly admit that it has a rival in the multitude of its citations and the fulness of its research into clinical histories, and we must assign it a place in the physician's library; not, indeed, as fully representing the present state of knowledge in pharmacodynamics, but as by far the most complete treatise upon the clinical and practical side of the question.—*Boston Med. and Surgical Journ.*, Nov. 5, 1874.

For all who desire a complete work on therapeutics and materia medica for reference, in cases involving medico-legal questions, as well as for information concerning remedial agents, Dr. Stillé's is "*par excellence*" the work. The work being out of print, by the exhaustion of former editions, the author has laid the profession under renewed obligations, by the careful revision, important additions, and timely re-issuing a work not exactly supplemented by any other in the English language, if in any language. The mechanical execution handsomely sustains the well-known skill and good taste of the publisher.—*St. Louis Med. and Surg. Journ.*, Dec. 1874.

We need not dwell on the merits of the third edition of this magnificently conceived work. It is the work on Materia Medica, in which Therapeutics are primarily considered—the mere natural history of drugs being briefly disposed of. To medical practitioners this is a very valuable conception. It is wonderful how much of the riches of the literature of Materia Medica has been condensed into this book. The references alone would make it worth possessing. But it is not a mere compilation. The writer exercises a good judgment of his own on the great doctrines and points of Therapeutics. For purposes of practice, Stillé's book is almost unique as a repertory of information, empirical and scientific, on the actions and uses of medicines.—*London Lancet*, Oct. 31, 1868.

Swayne (Joseph Griffiths), M.D.,
Physician-Accoucheur to the British General Hospital, &c.

OBSTETRIC APHORISMS FOR THE USE OF STUDENTS COMMENCING MIDWIFERY PRACTICE. Second American, from the Fifth and Revised London Edition, with Additions by E. R. HUTCHINS, M.D. With Illustrations. In one neat 12mo. volume. Cloth, $1 25. *(Lately Issued.)*

Stokes (William), M.D., D.C.L., F.R.S.
LECTURES ON FEVER. *(See p. 7.)*

SMITH'S PRACTICAL TREATISE ON THE WASTING DISEASES OF INFANCY AND CHILDHOOD. In one 8vo. volume, cloth, $2 50.

STURGES' INTRODUCTION TO CLINICAL MEDICINE. In one volume 12mo., cloth, $1 25.

SKEY'S OPERATIVE SURGERY. In 1 vol. 8vo., cloth, of over 600 pages; with about 100 woodcuts. $3 25.

SARGENT ON BANDAGING AND OTHER OPERATIONS OF MINOR SURGERY. In one 12mo. volume of 383 pp., with 184 illustrations, cloth, $1 75.

SLADE ON DIPHTHERIA. In one 12mo. volume, cloth, $1 25.

SMITH ON CONSUMPTION; ITS EARLY AND REMEDIABLE STAGES. 1 vol. 8vo., pp. 254. $2 25.

Smith (Henry H.), M.D., and Horner (William E.), M.D.,
Prof. of Surgery in the Univ. of Penna., &c.   *Late Prof. of Anatomy in the Univ. of Pa., &c.*

AN ANATOMICAL ATLAS, illustrative of the Structure of the Human Body. In one volume, large imperial octavo, cloth, with about six hundred and fifty beautiful figures. $4 50.

Tuke (Daniel Hack), M.D.,
Joint author of " The Manual of Psychological Medicine," &c.

ILLUSTRATIONS OF THE INFLUENCE OF THE MIND UPON THE BODY IN HEALTH AND DISEASE. Designed to illustrate the Action of the Imagination. In one handsome octavo volume of 416 pages, cloth, $3 25. *(Just Issued.)*

The object of the author in this work has been to show not only the effect of the mind in causing and intensifying disease, but also its curative influence, and the use which may be made of the imagination and the emotions as therapeutic agents. Scattered facts bearing upon this subject have long been familiar to the profession, but no attempt has hitherto been made to collect and systematize them so as to render them available to the practitioner, by establishing the several phenomena upon a scientific basis. In the endeavor thus to convert to the use of legitimate medicine the means which have been employed so successfully in many systems of quackery, the author has produced a work of the highest freshness and interest as well as of permanent value.

Thomas (T. Gaillard), M.D.,

Professor of Obstetrics, etc., in the College of Physicians and Surgeons, N. Y., etc.

A PRACTICAL TREATISE ON THE DISEASES OF WOMEN.
Fourth Edition, enlarged and thoroughly Revised. In one large and handsome octavo volume of 800 pages, with 191 illustrations. Cloth, $5 00; leather, $6 00. (*Just Issued.*)

The author has taken advantage of the opportunity afforded by the call for another edition of this work to render it worthy a continuance of the very remarkable favor with which it has been received. Every portion has been subjected to a conscientious revision, and no labor has been spared to make it a complete treatise on the most advanced condition of its important subject.

This volume of Prof. Thomas in its revised form is classical without being pedantic, full in the details of anatomy and pathology, without ponderous translations of pages of German literature, describes distinctly the details and difficulties of each operation, without wearying and useless minutiæ, and is in all respects a work worthy of confidence, justifying the high regard in which its distinguished author is held by the profession.—*Am. Supplement, Obstet. Journ.*, Oct. 1874.

Reluctantly we are obliged to close this unsatisfactory notice of so excellent a work, and in conclusion would remark that, as a teacher of gynæcology, both didactic and clinical, Prof. Thomas has certainly taken the lead far ahead of his *confrères*, and as an author he certainly has met with distinguished and merited success.—*Am. Journ. of Obstetrics*, Nov. 1874.

The latest edition of this well-known text-book retains the essential characters which rendered the earliest so deservedly popular. It is still pre-eminently a practical manual intended to convey to students in a clear and forcible manner a sufficiently complete outline of gynæcology. In a word, we should say that any one who intended to make a special study of gynæcology could hardly do better than to begin with a minute perusal of this book, and that any one who intended to keep gynæcology subordinate to general practice, should hardly fail to have it on hand for future reference.—*N. Y. Med. Journ.*, Jan. 1875.

Thomas's Diseases of Women is one of the few books regarded by American physicians with feelings of national pride. Few works in the English language equal it, none surpass it, as a text-book for students or a reference book for practitioners. No medical book ever published in this country has a wider European reputation.—*Cincinnati Clinic*, Nov. 7, 1874.

A standard and almost classical work on the subject by an eminent American obstetrician. It well deserves its popularity.—*British Med. Journ.*, Oct. 31, 1874.

Thompson (Sir Henry),

Surgeon and Professor of Clinical Surgery to University College Hospital.

LECTURES ON DISEASES OF THE URINARY ORGANS. With
illustrations on wood. Second American, from the Third English Edition. In one neat octavo volume: cloth, $2 25. (*Now Ready.*)

By a change in the typographic arrangement, the very considerable additions of the author have been accommodated with but little increase of size, and the work has been kept at its former very moderate price.

The author is well known as one of the best and most esteemed authorities on diseases of the urinary organs. Those who read this book cannot fail to admire him also as a teacher and a writer, for in one hundred and ninety-five well leaded pages he gives us a perfectly clear and readable treatise upon the diseases peculiar to this portion of the system, sufficiently comprehensive in its extent to serve the purposes of most physicians, and show them the way to gain a practical knowledge of the subject.—*New Remedies*, Jan. 1875.

By the same Author.

ON THE PATHOLOGY AND TREATMENT OF STRICTURE OF
THE URETHRA AND URINARY FISTULÆ. With plates and wood-cuts. From the third and revised English Edition. In one very handsome octavo volume: cloth, $3 50. (*Lately Published.*)

This classical work has so long been recognized as a standard authority on its perplexing subjects that it should be rendered accessible to the American profession. Having enjoyed the advantage of a recent revision at the hands of the author, it will be found to present his latest views, and to be on a level with the most recent advance of surgical science.

With a work accepted as *the* authority upon the subjects of which it treats, an extended notice would be a work of supererogation. The simple announcement of another edition of a work so well and favorably known by the profession as this before us, must create a demand for it from those who would keep themselves well up in this department of surgery.—*St. Louis Med. Archives*, Feb. 1870.

The subjects are treated with the precision of a teacher and the authority of a master, of one who learned his art, and never subordinates practical experience to theory. One of the chief merits of the book is its brevity; what the author has to say is said well and concisely, the volume of less than two hundred pages containing more than in many instances would be diluted with five or six hundred of words.—*Chicago Med. Journ.*, April, 1875.

By the same Author. (*Just Issued.*)

THE DISEASES OF THE PROSTATE, THEIR PATHOLOGY AND
TREATMENT. Fourth Edition, Revised. In one very handsome octavo volume of 355 pages, with thirteen plates, plain and colored, and illustrations on wood. Cloth, $3 75.

This work is recognized in England as the leading authority on its subject, and in presenting it to the American profession, it is hoped that it will be found a trustworthy and satisfactory guide in the treatment of an obscure and important class of affections.

TODD'S CLINICAL LECTURES ON CERTAIN ACUTE DISEASES. In one neat octavo volume of 30; pages: cloth, $2 50.

Taylor (Alfred S.), M.D.,
Lecturer on Med. Jurisp. and Chemistry in Guy's Hospital.

POISONS IN RELATION TO MEDICAL JURISPRUDENCE AND MEDICINE. Third American, from the Third Revised English Edition. In one large octavo volume of 788 pages, and 104 illustrations : cloth, $5 50; leather, $6 50. (*Now Ready.*)

From the Preface to the Third Edition.

But few words are required to introduce this volume. It is based on the two previous editions ; but the complete revision, rendered necessary by time, has converted it into a new work. As a rule, I have omitted a description of those poisonous substances which have not hitherto given rise to investigations before our legal tribunals, and which are otherwise of little interest to the profession. In short, as the reader will perceive, the subject of poisons has been treated only in relation to Medical Jurisprudence and Medicine, and as fully as the space at my disposal would permit.

The present is based upon the two previous editions; "but the complete revision rendered necessary by time has converted it into a new work." This statement from the preface contains all that it is desired to know in reference to the new edition. The works of this author are already in the library of every physician who is liable to be called upon for medico-legal testimony (and what one is not?), so that all that is required to be known about the present book is that the author has kept it abreast with the times. What makes it now, as always, especially valuable to the practitioner is its conciseness and practical character, only those poisonous substances being described which give rise to legal investigations.— *The Clinic,* Nov. 6, 1875.

. Prof. Taylor's work on Poisons has been so long before the profession, and is so universally recognized as a classic, that we do not think it worth while to do more than announce the appearance of a new edition, and to state that an examination of it has shown that its learned author has honestly and successfully endeavored to bring his book fully up to the most recent progress in toxicology.- *Phila. Med. Times,* Oct. 2, .875.

Dr. Taylor has brought to bear on the compilation of this volume stores of learning, experience, and practical acquaintance with his subject, probably far beyond what any other living authority on toxicology could have amassed or utilized. He has fully sustained his reputation by the consummate skill and legal acumen he has displayed in the arrangement of the subject-matter, and the result is a work on Poisons which will be indispensable to every student or practitioner in law and medicine.— *The Dublin Journ. of Med. Sci.,* Oct. 1875.

By the same Author. (*Just Issued.*)

THE PRINCIPLES AND PRACTICE OF MEDICAL JURISPRUDENCE. Second Edition, Revised, with numerous Illustrations. In two large octavo volumes : cloth, $10 ; leather, $12.

This great work is now recognized in England as the fullest and most authoritative treatise on every department of its important subject. In laying it, in its improved form, before the American profession, the publisher trusts that it will assume the same position in this country.

By the same Author. (*Lately Published.*)

MEDICAL JURISPRUDENCE. Seventh American Edition. Edited by JOHN J. REESE, M.D., Prof. of Med. Jurisp. in the Univ. of Penna. In one large octavo volume of nearly 900 pages. Cloth, $5 00; leather, $6 00.

To the members of the legal and medical profession it is unnecessary to say anything commendatory of Taylor's Medical Jurisprudence. We might as well undertake to speak of the merit of Chitty's Pleadings.—*Chicago Legal News,* Oct. 16, 1873.

Little can be added to what has already been said of this standard work of Dr. Taylor's. As a manual it is doubtless the most comprehensive extant, meeting fully the demands of the student of medicine and law.—*Western Lancet,* Nov. 1873.

It is beyond question the most attractive as well as most reliable manual of medical jurisprudence published in the English language.—*Amer. Journal of Syphilography,* Oct. 1873.

It is altogether superfluous for us to offer anything in behalf of a work on medical jurisprudence by an author who is almost universally esteemed to be the best authority on this specialty in our language. On this point, however, we will say that we consider Dr. Taylor to be the safest medico-legal authority to follow, in general, with which we are acquainted in any language.—*Va. Clin. Record,* Nov. 1873.

This last edition of the Manual is probably the best of all, as it contains more material and is worked up to the latest views of the author as expressed in the last edition of the Principles. Dr. Reese, the editor of the Manual, has done everything to make his work acceptable to his medical countrymen.—*N. Y. Med. Record,* Jan. 15, 1874.

Tanner (Thomas H.), M.D.,
Physician to the Skin Department in University College Hospital, &c.

ON THE SIGNS AND DISEASES OF PREGNANCY. First American from the second and enlarged English edition. With four colored plates and illustrations on wood. In one handsome octavo volume of about 500 pages, cloth, $4 25.

By the same Author.

A MANUAL OF CLINICAL MEDICINE AND PHYSICAL DIAGNOSIS. Third American from the second London edition. In one neat volume small 12mo., of about 375 pages, cloth, $1 50.

*** By reference to the "Prospectus of Journal" on page 3, it will be seen that this work is offered as a premium for procuring new subscribers to the "AMERICAN JOURNAL OF THE MEDICAL SCIENCES."

Watson (Thomas), M.D., etc.

LECTURES ON THE PRINCIPLES AND PRACTICE OF PHYSIC.

Delivered at King's College, London. A new American, from the Fifth revised and enlarged English edition Edited, with additions, and several hundred illustrations, by HENRY HARTSHORNE, M.D., Professor of Hygiene in the University of Pennsylvania. In two large and handsome 8vo. vols. Cloth, $9 00; leather, $11 00. (*Lately Published.*)

It is a subject for congratulation and for thankfulness that Sir Thomas Watson, during a period of comparative leisure, after a long, laborious, and most honorable professional career, while retaining full possession of his high mental faculties, should have employed the opportunity to submit his Lectures to a more thorough revision than was possible during the earlier and busier period of his life. Carefully passing in review some of the most intricate and important pathological and practical questions, the results of his clear insight and his calm judgment are now recorded for the benefit of mankind, in language which, for precision, vigor, and classical elegance, has rarely been equalled, and never surpassed. The revision has evidently been most carefully done, and the results appear in almost every page.—*Brit. Med. Journ.,* Oct. 14, 1871.

The lectures are so well known and so justly appreciated, that it is scarcely necessary to do more than call attention to the special advantages of the last over previous editions. The author's rare combination of great scientific attainments combined with wonderful forensic eloquence has exerted extraordinary influence over the last two generations of physicians. His clinical descriptions of most diseases have never been equalled; and on this score at least his work will live long in the future. The work will be sought by all who appreciate a great book.—*Am. Journ. of Syphilography,* July, 1872.

Wells (J. Soelberg),

Professor of Ophthalmology in King's College Hospital, &c.

A TREATISE ON DISEASES OF THE EYE. Second American,

from the Third and Revised London Edition, with additions; illustrated with numerous engravings on wood, and six colored plates. Together with selections from the Test-types of Jaeger and Snellen. In one large and very handsome octavo volume of nearly 800 pages: cloth, $5 00; leather, $6 00. (*Lately Published.*)

The continued demand for this work, both in England and this country, is sufficient evidence that the author has succeeded in his effort to supply within a reasonable compass a full practical digest of ophthalmology in its most modern aspects, while the call for repeated editions has enabled him in his revisions to maintain its position abreast of the most recent investigations and improvements. In again reprinting it, every effort has been made to adapt it thoroughly to the wants of the American practitioner. Such additions as seemed desirable have been introduced by the editor, Dr. I. Minis Hays, and the number of illustrations has been largely increased. The importance of test-types as an aid to diagnosis is so universally acknowledged at the present day that it seemed essential to the completeness of the work that they should be added, and as the author recommends the use of those both of Jaeger and of Snellen for different purposes, selections have been made from each, so that the practitioner may have at command all the assistance necessary. Although enlarged by one hundred pages, it has been retained at the former very moderate price, rendering it one of the cheapest volumes before the profession.

Of all the numerous treatises on the eye which exist, this possesses qualities which must specially recommend it to the general practitioner who wishes to know something of the cases he certainly will be called on to give an opinion about, if not to treat, or as a text-book for the student. The style is clear, simple, and straightforward; the manner in which the different subjects are treated is eminently practical, and the discussion of varying views as to details, which, valuable as it might be to the specialist, would only embarrass the physician, who has neither time nor opportunity to study the subject at length, is as much as possible avoided.— *Boston Med. and Surg. Journ.,* April 30, 1874.

West (Charles), M.D.,

Physician to the Hospital for Sick Children, &c

LECTURES ON THE DISEASES OF INFANCY AND CHILDHOOD.

Fifth American from the sixth revised and enlarged English edition. In one large and handsome octavo volume of 678 pages. Cloth, $4 50; leather, $5 50. (*Just Issued.*)

The continued demand for this work on both sides of the Atlantic, and its translation into German, French, Italian, Danish, Dutch, and Russian, show that it fills satisfactorily a want extensively felt by the profession. There is probably no man living who can speak with the authority derived from a more extended experience than Dr. West, and his work now presents the results of nearly 2000 recorded cases, and 600 post-mortem examinations selected from among nearly 40,000 cases which have passed under his care. In the preparation of the present edition he has omitted much that appeared of minor importance, in order to find room for the introduction of additional matter, and the volume, while thoroughly revised, is therefore not increased materially in size.

By the same Author.

LECTURES ON THE DISEASES OF WOMEN. Third American,

from the third London edition. In one neat octavo volume of about 550 pages, cloth, $3 75; leather, $4 75.

We have to say of it, briefly and decidedly, that it is the best work on the subject in any language and that it stamps Dr. West as the *facile princeps* of British obstetric authors.—*Edin. Med. Journal.*

By the same Author.

ON SOME DISORDERS OF THE NERVOUS SYSTEM IN CHILDHOOD; being the Lumleian Lectures delivered at the Royal College of Physicians of London, in March, 1871. In one volume, small 12mo., cloth, $1 00.

Winckel (F.),

Professor and Director of the Gynæcological Clinic in the University of Rostock.

THE PATHOLOGY AND TREATMENT OF CHILDBED. A Treatise for Physicians and Students. From the Second German Edition, with additions by the author. Translated by JAMES READ CHADWICK, M.D., Clinical Lecturer on Diseases of Women in Harvard University. In one handsome octavo volume. (*In Press.*)

Williams (C. J. B.), M.D.,

Senior Consulting Physician to the Hospital for Consumption, Brompton, and

Williams (Charles T.), M.D.,

Physician to the Hospital for Consumption.

PULMONARY CONSUMPTION; Its Nature, Varieties, and Treatment. With an Analysis of One Thousand Cases to exemplify its duration. In one neat octavo volume of about 350 pages: cloth, $2 50. (*Lately Published.*)

He can still speak from a more enormous experience, and a closer study of the morbid processes involved in tuberculosis, than most living men. He owed it to himself, and to the importance of the subject, to embody his views in a separate work, and we are glad that he has accomplished this duty.

After all, the grand teaching which Dr. Williams has for the profession is to be found in his therapeutical chapters, and in the history of individual cases extended, by dint of care, over ten, twenty, thirty, and even forty years.—*London Lancet*, Oct. 21, 1871.

Wilson (Erasmus), F.R.S.

ON DISEASES OF THE SKIN. With Illustrations on wood. Seventh American, from the sixth and enlarged English edition. In one large octavo volume of over 800 pages, $5 00.

A SERIES OF PLATES ILLUSTRATING "WILSON ON DISEASES OF THE SKIN:" consisting of twenty beautifully executed plates, of which thirteen are exquisitely colored, presenting the Normal Anatomy and Pathology of the Skin, and embracing accurate representations of about one hundred varieties of disease, most of them the size of nature. Price in extra cloth, $5 50.

Also, the Text and Plates, bound in one handsome volume. Cloth, $10 00.

By the same Author.

A SYSTEM OF ANATOMY, General and Special. Edited by W. H. GOBRECHT, M.D., Professor of General and Surgical Anatomy in the Medical College of Ohio. Illustrated with three hundred and ninety-seven engravings on wood. In one large and handsome octavo volume of over 600 large pages: cloth, $4 00; leather, $5 00.

By the same Author.

THE STUDENT'S BOOK OF CUTANEOUS MEDICINE and Diseases OF THE SKIN. In one very handsome royal 12mo. volume. $3 50.

Wöhler and Fittig.

OUTLINES OF ORGANIC CHEMISTRY. Translated with Additions from the Eighth German Edition. By IRA REMSEN, M.D., Ph.D., Professor of Chemistry and Physics in Williams College, Mass. In one handsome volume, royal 12mo., of 550 pages: cloth, $3 00.

Winslow (Forbes), M.D., D.C.L., etc.

ON OBSCURE DISEASES OF THE BRAIN AND DISORDERS OF THE MIND; their incipient Symptoms, Pathology, Diagnosis, Treatment, and Prophylaxis. Second American, from the third and revised English edition. In one handsome octavo volume of nearly 600 pages: cloth, $4 25.

WALSHE ON THE DISEASES OF THE HEART AND GREAT VESSELS. Third American edition. In 1 vol. 8vo., 420 pages: cloth. $3 00. WHAT TO OBSERVE AT THE BEDSIDE AND AFTER DEATH IN MEDICAL CASES. Published under the authority of the London Society for Medical Observation. From the second London edition. 1 vol. royal 12mo., cloth. $1 00.

Zeissl (H.), M.D.

A COMPLETE TREATISE ON VENEREAL DISEASES. Translated from the Second Enlarged German Edition, by FREDERIC R. STURGIS, M.D. In one octavo volume, with illustrations. (*Preparing.*)